Amino Acid
Metabolism

Amino Acid Metabolism

David A. Bender

Courtauld Institute of Biochemistry,
The Middlesex Hospital Medical School,
London

A Wiley–Interscience Publication

JOHN WILEY & SONS

London · New York · Sydney · Toronto

Library of Congress Cataloging in Publication Data:

Bender, David A.
Amino acid metabolism.
Bibliography: p.
Includes index.
1. Amino acid metabolism. I. Title.
[DNLM: 1. Amino acids—Metabolism. QU60 B458a]
QP561.B46   574.1′33   74-20863

ISBN 0 471 06498 X

Printed in Great Britain by William Clowes & Sons Ltd.,
London, Beccles and Colchester

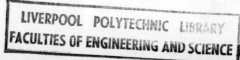

PREFACE

I am probably biased, because it is my field of research, but I consider that the metabolism of amino acids is one of the more fascinating areas of biochemistry. There are several excellent multi-author reference books on amino acid metabolism, and reviews frequently appear in various secondary journals, but these are all directed at the specialist research worker and are generally very much more detailed than a student would want, or need, to read. At the same time, the many modern textbooks of biochemistry deal with amino acids only very briefly, so that the topic is poorly covered in many undergraduate courses. I have written this book in the hope of filling the gap, and providing a book which will be useful to undergraduate and post-graduate students.

Because this is a book on a specialized aspect of biochemistry, it does not contain very much general biochemistry. With the exception of Chapter 1, where I have covered the incorporation of inorganic nitrogen into amino acids, I have kept fairly strictly to amino acid metabolism, and have not dealt with general intermediary metabolism, protein synthesis or biochemical genetics at all, except where specific aspects have required some explanation. Some background knowledge is therefore required for this book to be useful.

I have written the book to be of use mainly in the final year of a British BSc course in biochemistry, or during a post-graduate course in biochemistry; an appropriate level of background information would also be that of a medical student taking a one year intercalated BSc following second MB or part II of a basic medical sciences course. I also hope that it will be of some use to specialist research workers in other fields.

Comparative studies of biochemistry aid our understanding of evolution and the differentiation of species, but in general the major interest of biochemistry is its application to medicine and agriculture. Studies of bacterial biochemistry are mainly of interest, apart from specific studies directed towards finding more efficient methods of curing bacterial infections, in so far as they are useful as models of human systems. Studies of bacterial biochemistry, and especially *Escherichia coli*, have been especially useful in elucidating the biochemistry of protein synthesis and biochemical genetics: with a generation time of the order of 20 minutes, bacteria are obviously more suitable for genetic research than animals. The other widely studied organism is the rat; the reasons for this are fairly obvious. The animal is small enough to be housed and handled easily and relatively economically, yet large enough for even relatively unskilled workers to be able to dissect out most tissues. We piously hope that the biochemistry of the rat is sufficiently close to that of man for it to serve as a useful model; such comparative studies as have been performed reassure us that it is possible to extrapolate from animal experiments to the human situation in many cases.

I have attempted in this book not only to give an insight into the fascinating field of amino acid biochemistry, but also to indicate where that information is of relevance to the solution of medical and other human problems. I hope that I have shown that the study of basic biochemistry is not merely self-indulgence, but also justifiable in the terms of the most rigorous criteria of relevance and economic necessity.

D. A. BENDER

April 1974

CONTENTS

THE LANGUAGE OF BIOCHEMISTRY

Throughout this book, I have assumed that the reader has a basic knowledge of chemistry and biochemistry, as well as an understanding of the principles of cell fractionation and the culture of micro-organisms. One term used in connection with bacterial culture requires definition for the non-specialist; a **minimal medium** is a culture medium which contains glucose or a similar compound as the sole source of carbon, and ammonium ions as the nitrogen source. An organism which can grow on minimal medium is therefore capable of synthesizing all its cellular constituents from these simple compounds. An organism which has a defect in a biosynthetic pathway will require to be cultured on a medium which contains the product of the defective pathway, and will not grow on minimal medium. Organisms which require a source of carbon other than carbon dioxide are termed **heterotrophic**; by contrast, **autotrophic** organisms are capable of reduction of carbon dioxide to carbohydrate, and therefore do not require any complex carbon compound in the culture medium. This fixation of carbon dioxide can be either photosynthetic (**photo-autotrophs**), or linked to an inorganic chemical reaction, such as the oxidation of ammonia to nitrogen or sulphide to sulphate; such organisms are termed **chemo-autotrophs**.

Perhaps the most jargon-ridden area of biochemistry is the subject of **enzyme regulation**. There are two mechanisms by which the activity of an enzyme can be altered to meet changes in the environment: the activity of existing enzyme protein can be altered by activation or inhibition, or the amount of enzyme protein present can be altered. This latter is a long-term response to changed requirements, while alteration of the activity of existing enzyme protein is a rapid response.

When an enzyme is **induced** by a substrate or precursor (i.e., there is new synthesis of enzyme protein in response to a stimulus), there is a moderate time-lag between the application of the stimulus and the detection of new protein. In bacteria this may be of the order of minutes, while in mammals it may be several hours before there is any detectable change in enzyme activity. An enzyme which is not normally produced at all, but which can be induced in response to a suitable stimulus, is termed an **inducible enzyme**; by contrast, an enzyme which is normally produced is termed a **constitutive enzyme**.

The amount of an enzyme which is synthesized can also be modified by **repression**: inhibition of protein synthesis by a specific repressor substance, frequently the end-product of the pathway. The rate at which enzyme activity changes after repression depends on the rate at which existing enzyme protein is being degraded, and in general repression yields a response very much more slowly than does induction. Many enzymes which are normally repressed when there is an adequate supply of the end-product of the pathway are **derepressed** when that product is required in greater amount. Thus, derepression can be visualized as induction by the absence of the end-product of the pathway.

In some cases, all the enzymes of a pathway can be shown to be induced or repressed together in response to a stimulus; this is **coordinate induction** or **repression**, and indicates that the genes coding for these enzymes are located in the same region of the genome of the organism, so that a single regulator gene can control the activity of all the structural genes.

The activity of an enzyme can be controlled according to conditions on a short-term basis by **inhibition** or **activation**. *In vitro*, product analogues are frequently used as **competitive** enzyme inhibitors; they compete with the substrate for the catalytic site of the enzyme, and thus reduce the apparent affinity of the enzyme for its substrate (i.e., they increase K_m), but have no effect on the maximum possible activity of the enzyme in the presence of saturating amounts of substrate (V_{max}). **Non-competitive** inhibitors generally interact with the enzyme–substrate complex, rather than with the free enzyme, and thus do not affect the K_m of the enzyme, but reduce the V_{max}. A great many drugs are non-competitive inhibitors of enzymes. A third class of *in vitro* enzyme inhibition, which is seen less frequently than competitive or non-competitive inhibition is termed **uncompetitive**. An uncompetitive enzyme inhibitor reduces the V_{max} of the enzyme, but also enhances the enzyme–substrate reaction, so that the K_m is reduced (i.e., the enzyme has an enhanced affinity for its substrate).

In vivo, such patterns of enzyme inhibition are probably of little importance in the regulation of enzyme activity. It has become obvious over the last few years that many key enzymes in pathways (normally the first reaction unique to a given reaction sequence is the key regulatory step) have multiple affinity sites. Such sites can bind either precursors, which activate the enzyme, or end-products, which inhibit the enzyme. Such interactions are **allosteric**, in that they involve some change in the conformation of the catalytic site of the enzyme.

Abbreviations and nomenclature

In general, abbreviations have been used in the text as allowed by the *Biochemical Journal*, as in the following list. Other abbreviations are defined in the text where they are used. The standard three-letter code has been used for the amino acids in diagrams; this code is shown in Appendix I.

References have been cited in the text by the author and date of publication, as in the *Biochemical Journal*. They are listed in the bibliography by alphabetical order of the first author, then date order.

Enzymes have been named in the text and in diagrams only by trivial names. The Enzyme Commission classification numbers of enzymes cited in the text are listed in Appendix III. The standard Unit of enzyme activity has been used:

1 unit = 1 μmol of substrate converted per min, under specified conditions, at 30°C.

The following abbreviations have been used undefined in the text:

DNA	deoxyribonucleic acid
RNA	ribonucleic acid
mRNA	messenger-RNA
tRNA	transfer-RNA
ATP	adenosine triphosphate
ADP	adenosine diphosphate
AMP	adenosine monophosphate
UTP	uridine triphosphate
GTP	guanidine triphosphate
CTP	cytidine triphosphate
TTP	thymidine triphosphate
dAMP	deoxyadenosine monophosphate
P_i	inorganic phosphate
PP_i	inorganic pyrophosphate
$-P$ or ⓅP	organic phosphate esters
NAD	nicotinamide adenine dinucleotide
NADP	nicotinamide adenine dinucleotide phosphate
NAD(P)	NAD or NADP (oxidation state undefined)
NAD(P)$^+$	oxidized form
NAD(P)H	reduced form
FAD	flavin adenine dinucleotide
FMN	flavin mononucleotide

CHAPTER 1

THE ECOLOGY OF NITROGEN

Antoine Lavoisier gave the name 'azote' to the gas nitrogen, meaning 'without life', because of its lack of chemical reactivity. The N≡N bond is highly resistant to chemical attack, with a bond energy of 0·94 MJ (225 kcal) per mol. This stable bond must be broken before any use can be made of gaseous nitrogen, which makes up 78 % of the atmosphere, for formation of the amino acids and nucleic acids essential to all living systems. Chemically, this bond can be broken for example by burning magnesium metal in air, or by catalytic reduction with hydrogen, using an iron or other metal catalyst at a temperature of about 300 °C and a pressure of 100–200 atm—the Haber–Bosch chemical fixation of nitrogen.

The overall fixation of nitrogen into soluble ammonium salts, nitrates and nitrites by all means, has been estimated at about 10^{12}–10^{13} kg per year. About $2·2 \times 10^{10}$ kg are accounted for by chemical reduction. A further 5×10^{10}–50×10^{10} kg per year can be accounted for by the production in the atmosphere of oxides of nitrogen, which are washed into the soil as nitrites and nitrates. This is mainly by the action of lightning, but the contribution made by high compression internal combustion engines cannot be ignored. It has been estimated that as much as 3×10^9 kg of nitrogen may be fixed annually by automobiles in the United States, while the American fertilizer industry fixes about 8×10^9 kg per year. The rest, 9×10^{10} kg per year, is bacterial. At the same time, chemoautotrophic bacteria use ammonia as a substrate for respiration, returning nitrogen gas to the atmosphere, and thus maintaining the *status quo*. This cycle, the classic nitrogen cycle, is shown in Figure 1.1.

The only organisms capable of fixing nitrogen from the atmosphere into forms that can be used by other organisms are the relatively primitive prokaryotic bacteria, and some of the blue-green algae, although slight nitrogen-fixing ability has been demonstrated in many other bacterial and fungal species. Most studies of the biochemistry of nitrogen fixation have been carried out using the free-living nitrogen-fixing organisms, because their system is less complex than that of the photosynthetic organisms or the plant–micro-organism symbiont pairs. However, the latter two groups of organisms make a considerably greater contribution to nitrogen ecology than do the free-living organisms.

These organisms form ammonia and ammonium salts which, together with organically and inorganically formed nitrates and nitrites, can be used by other bacteria and green plants for synthesis of all the nitrogenous constituents of the cell. Animals are not in general capable of using inorganic nitrogen compounds, although some urea can be used even by man, but must satisfy their requirements for nitrogen by eating bacterial, plant and other animal proteins. The other nitrogenous compounds produced by plants and bacteria are not generally

1

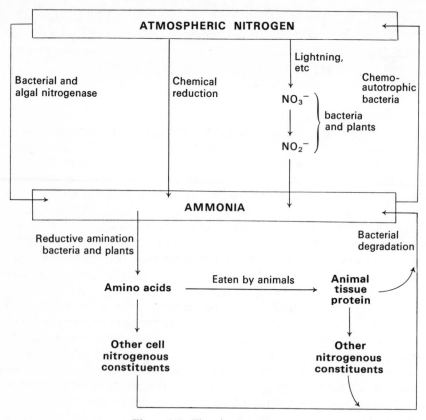

Figure 1.1. The nitrogen cycle

used by animals, but are excreted, either unchanged or after moderate oxidation. Ruminants, which have a large enteric population of commensal bacteria, can indirectly use non-amino acid nitrogen sources, a factor of great economic importance; it has been estimated that in 1969–70 in the United States the 680,000 tons of chemically-synthesized urea fed to cattle released, for consumption by monogastric livestock and man, about 3×10^6 tons of protein-rich oil-seed cake.

By bacterial mating and bacteriophage transduction it has been possible to transfer the genetic information for nitrogen fixation from wild-type *Klebsiella pneumoniae* into *Escherichia coli* strains which normally lack it (Dixon and Postgate, 1972). The aim of much current plant genetic work is to achieve a transfer of the genetic information for nitrogen fixation to other organisms which cannot normally reduce nitrogen. Alfalfa, a legume which has nitrogen-fixing, *Rhizobium*-containing root nodules, can contribute as much as 300–600 kg of fixed nitrogen per hectare per year (1 hectare = 2·47 acres). A mutation allowing similar nodule formation in wheat or other non-leguminous crops, would be of enormous economic and agricultural advantage.

MICROBIAL NITROGEN FIXATION

Systems capable of incorporating gaseous nitrogen into amino acids have been detected in a variety of organisms, occupying a wide variety of ecological niches, as can be seen from the partial list in Table 1.1. Both strict (obligate) anaerobes (e.g., *Clostridium pasteurianum*) and obligate aerobes (e.g., *Azotobacter vinelandii*) as well as facultative anaerobes such as *Klebsiella pneumoniae* among the heterotrophic bacteria, and a number of autotrophic (photosynthetic) bacteria, including *Rhodospirillum rubrum* and *Chromatium* species can be classed together as free-living nitrogen-fixing organisms.

A number of plant-bacteroid symbiont pairs are also known to be capable of reducing nitrogen to ammonia; the best known is the association of leguminous plants with bacteroids of the genus *Rhizobium*, but there are also associations of other organisms, which have been assigned the genus *Frankia*, with non-legumes, including the alder (*Alnus* spp.), a common pioneer of virgin land. A number of blue-green algae also form symbiotic associations with plants, either as leaf nodules or associated with the roots of water plants. Some plants support a mycelial growth of fungi around the roots which fix nitrogen at least to a slight extent. The leaf nodule symbionts are very much more casually associated with their hosts than the root nodule symbionts, in that they are capable of independent, free-living existence, while *Rhizobium* and *Frankia* are not.

Table 1.1. Some organisms capable of fixing nitrogen

Free-living organisms	
Obligate aerobic heterotrophs	*Azotobacter* and *Mycobacterium* spp.
Facultative anaerobic heterotrophs	*Klebsiella pneumoniae*
	Bacillus polymyxa
Obligate anaerobic heterotrophs	*Clostridium pasteurianum* and *butyricum*
	Desulphovibrio spp.
Facultative anaerobic photo-autotrophs	*Rhodospirillum rubrum*
	Rhodopseudomonas palustris
Obligate anaerobic photo-autotrophs	*Chromatium* spp.
	Clorobium spp.
Aerobic photo-autotrophs	Blue–green algae—representatives of 16 genera, including: *Anabena*, *Nostoc* and *Plectonema*
Symbiotic associations	
Blue–green algae with:	Fungi (the lichens)
	Liverworts
	Azolla (the water fern)
Bacterial symbionts with higher plants:	
	Klebsiella in leaf nodules
	Azotobacter associated with roots and leaves
	Rhizobium in legume root nodules
	Frankia in non-legume root nodules
Bacterial symbionts or commensals in the gut of animals	

The nitrogen-fixing system has three essential components: an enzyme capable of reducing nitrogen to ammonia, nitrogenase; a source of reductant for this reaction; and an electron carrier to couple the reductant with the enzyme. ATP is also required; in *Azotobacter* as many as 15 mol of ATP may be consumed per mol of nitrogen reduced to ammonia.

The electron carrier for nitrogen reduction is frequently ferredoxin, the ferroprotein found in all photosynthetic organisms, with a redox potential sufficiently negative to allow the reduction of NAD^+ to NADH. It is probable that in photosynthetic organisms the source of reducing power for nitrogen reduction is the same photoreduction as is used in the reduction of carbon dioxide. Winter and Arnon (1970) have shown that cell-free preparations from *Chromatium* will slowly reduce nitrogen in the dark if they are provided with hydrogen as a

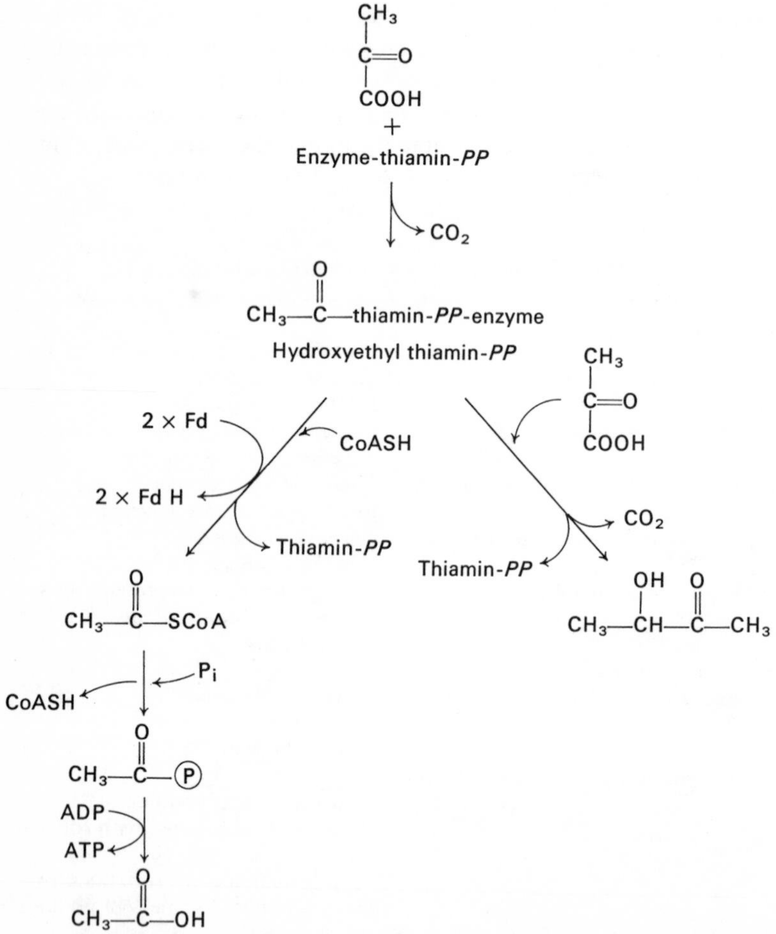

Figure 1.2. The oxidation of pyruvate in *Clostridium pasteurianum*

reducing agent. Reduced ferredoxin from a variety of sources can also be used as a reducing agent in cell-free preparations in the dark. When the photoreduction system is present in the extract, a number of weak reducing agents can be used by illuminated preparations.

In non-photosynthetic (heterotrophic) nitrogen-fixing organisms, the reductant is frequently pyruvate, the oxidation of which is linked to the reduction of ferredoxin, rather than through lipoate to NAD as in other organisms. *C. pasteurianum* has two pathways of pyruvate utilization, as shown in Figure 1.2. The oxidative pathway involves the reduction of ferredoxin, and the production of acetyl phosphate which is used in a substrate level phosphorylation reaction to form ATP. *K. pneumoniae* and other organisms can also use the oxidation of formate as a reductant for nitrogen fixation.

Ferredoxins from plants and bacteria contain non-haem iron atoms (i.e., they are iron–sulphur proteins). Some bacteria grown in iron-deficient media form flavodoxin, a flavin-mononucleotide containing protein functionally similar to ferredoxin, but not containing a metal ion. Under similar conditions, the blue-green algae form phytoflavin, and *Azotobacter* forms azotoflavin. Azotoflavin and flavodoxin have been shown to carry electrons *in vitro* between illuminated chloroplasts and nitrogenase, but to date no biological activity has been demonstrated for phytoflavin.

Ferredoxins from different sources have very different molecular weights and redox potentials. Bacterial ferredoxins carry two electrons per molecule, while the protein from plants is generally a single electron carrier. It has, however, been possible to reconstitute active nitrogen-fixing systems using plant ferredoxin as the electron carrier. The chemical properties of the ferredoxins have been reviewed by Buchanan and Arnon (1970).

Nitrogenase

All nitrogenase systems examined to date have been shown to consist of two components: a small ferro-protein, and a larger protein containing both iron and molybdenum. The larger protein from *K. pneumoniae* contains one molybdenum and 17 iron atoms (bound to acid labile sulphide) per molecule. Both

Table 1.2. The reactions of nitrogenase

$$N_2 \rightarrow NH_3$$
$$NH_2OH \rightarrow NH_3 + H_2O$$
$$CH{\equiv}CH \rightarrow CH_2{=}CH_2 \text{ (and other alkynes } \rightarrow \text{ alkenes)}$$
$$CH_2{=}CH{=}CH_2 \rightarrow CH_3{-}C{\equiv}CH \rightarrow CH_3{-}CH{=}CH_2$$
$$CN^- \rightarrow CH_4 + NH_3 \text{ (also some } CH_3NH_2 \text{ formed)}$$
$$R{-}CN \rightarrow RCH_3 + NH_3$$
$$R{-}NC \rightarrow RNH_2 + CH_4 \text{ (also some } C_2H_6 \text{ and } C_3H_8 \text{ formed)}$$

$N_3^- \rightarrow N_2 + NH_3$ $\Big\rbrace$ (some of the N_2 formed is further reduced to
$N_2O \rightarrow N_2 + H_2O$ $\Big\rfloor$ NH_3)
$$H^+ \rightarrow H_2$$

proteins have been purified from a number of sources since the original demonstration of nitrogen fixation in a cell-free preparation from *C. pasteurianum* by Carnahan and coworkers (1960).

Both proteins are required for the fixation of nitrogen, or for any of the other reactions catalysed by nitrogenase (see Table 1.2). Attempts to reconstitute active nitrogenase from isolated components, or to assign functions to the separate proteins, have been largely frustrated by the extreme sensitivity of isolated nitrogenase to irreversible denaturation by oxygen.

It has been demonstrated that for the reduction of nitrogen to ammonia, or acetylene to ethylene, the optimum composition is 2 mol of ferro-protein to 1 mol of ferro–molybdeno-protein, while for the reduction of cyanide to methane and ammonia, or of methyl isocyanide to methane and methylamine, the optimum ratio is 1:1. Whether this indicates that there are more cyanide reducing sites on the molecule than there are nitrogen reducing sites, or whether there are other molecular configurations that can reduce cyanide but not nitrogen, is unclear. It has been suggested that the substrate binds to the molybdenum atoms of the larger subunit, which also reacts with ferredoxin, and the two ferro-protein units function mainly as ATPases. It has been shown by Mössbauer spectroscopy of ^{57}Fe-labelled nitrogenase that the iron is involved in the formation of the active enzyme–substrate complex, but there is no evidence of a direct iron–substrate bond.

Nitrogenase is found mainly in rather primitive organisms, and is believed to have played a part in early evolution. The discovery of the cyanide reduction reaction has led to the suggestion that the original reaction of this enzyme was not the reduction of nitrogen to ammonia, which would have been a rather superfluous reaction at the stage of evolution when there is believed to have been a great deal of atmospheric ammonia, but rather a method of rendering harmless the cyanide thought to have been abundant in the primeval atmosphere and seas.

No such convenient teleological explanation can be put forward for the reduction of acetylene to ethylene, which is also catalysed by nitrogenase. However, this reaction has been greatly used in studies of nitrogenase. Ethylene can be measured readily by gas–liquid chromatography, and no other system catalysing its formation from acetylene has yet been discovered. Furthermore, use of the acetylene reduction reaction allows a three-fold increase in the sensitivity of the assay for nitrogenase, since it is a two-electron reduction, while the reduction of nitrogen to ammonia is a six-electron process. It is mainly on the evidence of reduction of acetylene that the presence of small numbers of nitrogen-fixing bacteria in human intestinal flora has been established.

In the reduction of alkyl isocyanides to methane and alkylamines, there is some formation of ethane and propane, suggesting that the reaction may proceed by way of formation of a methylene radical at the catalytic site of the enzyme. Such a radical would be capable of polymerization to higher hydrocarbons. Although nitrogenase will catalyse the reduction of a number of alkynes to alkenes, the only alkene which is a substrate for reduction is allene,

$CH_2\!=\!CH\!=\!CH_2$. There is some evidence that the reduction of this compound requires an initial isomerization to methyl acetylene ($CH_3\!-\!C\!\equiv\!CH$), so that the reduction is mechanistically the same as the reduction of acetylene and other alkynes.

All nitrogenase systems studied evolve hydrogen gas by reduction of protons; however, such a reaction is not characteristic of nitrogenase since many enzyme systems are known which will evolve gaseous hydrogen. The reaction is ATP utilizing, and as well as occurring in the absence of other reducible substrates, it can be shown to occur as a parallel reaction together with substrate reduction. To some extent, the presence of substrate inhibits this hydrogen evolution. Some strains of *Rhizobium* have an active hydrogenase, which recovers the hydrogen evolved by nitrogenase and so conserves the reducing power which would otherwise be lost.

Nitrogenase is irreversibly inhibited by oxygen, and systems are present in most nitrogen fixing organisms (except those which are obligate anaerobes), which control the activity of the enzyme in response to changes in PO_2. This has been studied in *A. vinelandii*, an obligate aerobe, where there is a switching off of nitrogenase activity in response to increasing PO_2. This appears to be mediated by a conformational change in the enzyme, to an inactive form which is protected from oxygen in some way.

Cultures of *Azotobacter* grown under high oxygen tension contain more cytochrome a_2 than do those grown under lower oxygen tension. It has been proposed that this represents an oxygen scavenging system to reduce the intracellular PO_2 to as low a value as possible. Cytochrome a_2 is one of two terminal cytochrome oxidases which have been identified in *Azotobacter*; the other consists of cytochromes a_1 and o. As can be seen from Figure 1.3, the electron

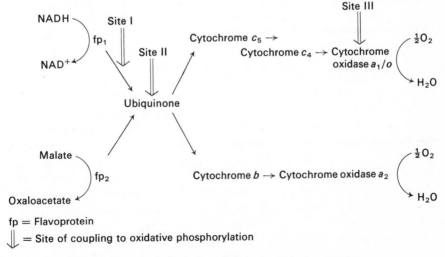

fp = Flavoprotein

⇓ = Site of coupling to oxidative phosphorylation

Figure 1.3. The respiratory chain of *Azotobacter vinelandii*

transport chain of *Azotobacter* is envisaged as consisting of two parallel cytochrome chains to the oxygen side of ubiquinone. One terminates in cytochrome oxidase a_1/o, and incorporates phosphorylation site III, while the other terminates in cytochrome oxidase a_2, and is not coupled to phosphorylation of ADP to ATP. Growth under conditions of high oxygen tension leads to the synthesis of cytochrome a_2, and therefore encourages use of the electron transport pathway with a P:O ratio of 2 rather than 3 for the oxidation of NADH. Hence for the same ATP yield, more substrate and more oxygen will have to be consumed. This pathway therefore represents a mechanism for effectively uncoupling respiration from electron transport to a limited extent, and so maintaining the PO_2 below the level at which nitrogenase would suffer damage. Growth of *Azotobacter* on media which are limited by phosphate renders the cells more sensitive to inhibition by oxygen. This has been interpreted as representing respiratory control of the kind seen in mammalian mitochondria when ADP (or occasionally phosphate) is present in limiting amounts. In the absence of phosphate, the rate of respiration cannot be increased sufficiently to remove all the oxygen entering the cell, and there is increased inhibition of nitrogenase.

For the blue-green algae which fix nitrogen, the problem of oxygen inhibition is more complex, since they release oxygen during photosynthesis. In the filamentous alga *Anabena* this has been overcome by the development of specialized heterocysts along the algal filament. In these cysts there appears to be no photosynthesis, although the light reaction of photosynthesis is the ultimate source of reducing power for ammonia formation. Nitrogen fixation is limited to these heterocysts, where there is a highly reducing environment, and it has been shown that heterocyst formation is related to the availability of ammonium salts in the culture medium.

The unicellular blue-green alga, *Plectonema*, which can be either free-living or symbiotic in leaf cavities of the water fern *Azolla*, fixes nitrogen only under conditions of low oxygen tension, and only when the level of illumination is so low that photolysis of water cannot occur. There is evidence that the nitrogenase of *Plectonema* can undergo a conformational switch of the type proposed above for the enzyme from *Azotobacter*. The symbiotic pair of *Plectonema* in the leaf cavities of *Azolla* can live entirely without an exogenous source of fixed nitrogen, and makes a considerable contribution to the fertility of rice paddies.

Legume root nodules, containing symbiotic *Rhizobium* are aerobic, but again the nitrogenase, which is contained entirely in the bacteroids, must be protected from oxygen, while ensuring adequate penetration of oxygen to the actively metabolizing tissues of the root. Bergerson and coworkers (1973) have shown that leghaemoglobin, a haemoglobin-like protein in the root nodules, both stimulates the nitrogenase activity of the bacteroids and increases oxygen uptake by intact nodules. In intact nodules, nitrogenase is inhibited by carbon monoxide, while in isolated bacteroids it is not; carbon monoxide pretreated leghaemoglobin will not enhance the activity of isolated bacteroids, while the native protein will. Bergerson and coworkers therefore propose that the function of leghaemoglobin in the intact nodule is to maintain a sufficiently low oxygen tension around the bacteroids to allow nitrogen reduction, while ensuring transport of an adequate amount of oxygen into the remainder of the tissue for normal respiration to continue. The kinetics of association of leghaemoglobin with oxygen would support this hypothesis.

Little is known about the requirements of bacteria of the genus Frankia, which nodulate the roots of some non-leguminous plants. They appear to be free-living in the soil until they form a symbiotic association, but have not yet been isolated in culture.

Very little is known about the regulation in vivo of nitrogen fixation; it is known that bacterial nitrogenase is repressed by growth on ammonia-rich media, but pre-formed nitrogenase appears not to be inhibited under such conditions. E. coli hybrids which form nitrogenase after bacterial mating with nitrogen-fixing organisms can be shown to be sensitive to ammonia repression of nitrogenase synthesis, which suggests that the regulator gene is located very close to the structural gene for nitrogenase.

THE ASSIMILATION OF NITRATE AND NITRITE

Nitrates applied to the soil as fertilizer, or washed into soil together with nitrites formed by atmospheric oxidation of nitrogen, are reduced to ammonia before they are used by plants for amino acid synthesis. Nitrate reductase uses nitrate as an electron acceptor, forming nitrite which is then reduced to ammonia by nitrite reductase. Both enzymes are widely distributed in plants and bacteria.

High nitrate levels in drinking water and food can give rise to methaemoglobinaemia in young children. Intestinal bacteria reduce nitrate to nitrite, which combines more or less irreversibly with haemoglobin, especially with foetal haemoglobin (HbF), which persists in infant blood for some time.

The six-electron reduction of nitrite to ammonia occurs without any detectable intermediate in algae and the green tissue of higher plants; the enzyme is found in the chloroplasts and uses ferredoxin as an electron carrier. Nitrite reduction appears to be coupled with photosynthesis, occurring together with photophosphorylation and oxygen evolution. Iron, but not molybdenum, is found in chloroplast nitrite reductase.

In the alga Chlorella, the regulatory step of nitrate assimilation appears to be nitrate reductase; the enzyme is stimulated by exposure to light, showing an 80–100% increase in activity within 1 h of illumination, and a similar fall within 1 h of restoration of darkness, responses probably too rapid to be accounted for by de novo enzyme synthesis.

As well as this requirement for light for maximal nitrate reductase activity, there also appears, in some plants, to be a requirement for light for synthesis of the two reductases. Etiolated rice seedlings require about 3 h after exposure to light before there is any detectable activity of nitrate or nitrite reductase activity. However, seedlings which have been raised in the light and then kept in the dark for up to 36 h do not show any such lag in the activation of the reductases after exposure to light.

Like nitrite reductase, nitrate reductase appears to use ferredoxin as an electron donor, coupled through NAD or NADP to the enzyme, which is a molybdeno-flavo-protein. In the mould *Neurospora crassa*, nitrate reductase can be shown to consist of two subunits, a particulate molybdenum-containing protein, which is constitutive, and a nitrate-inducible protein, which solubilizes the metallo-protein, and also acts as an NADPH-cytochrome *c* reductase. A functional nitrate reductase complex can be reconstituted from the fungal inducible protein together with xanthine oxidase, xanthine dehydrogenase or aldehyde oxidase prepared from animal tissues.

While photosynthetic organisms generally reduce nitrate and nitrite at the expense of photosynthetically-generated reductant to allow the incorporation of inorganic nitrogen into tissue components, the fungi and heterotrophic bacteria use nitrate and nitrite as terminal electron acceptors under conditions of low oxygen availability. The production of usable nitrogenous compounds is coincidental. Van't Riet and coworkers (1972) have suggested that in *K. aerogenes* the same nitrate reductase can function either aerobically for nitrate assimilation, when the nitrite produced is further reduced to ammonia, or anaerobically as a terminal electron acceptor, when the nitrite may be allowed to accumulate. Different electron transport chains are involved in the provision of

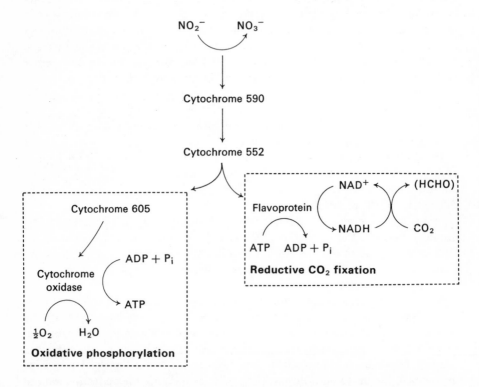

Figure 1.4. The utilization of nitrite in *Nitrobacter* species

reductant for these two processes; in anaerobic respiration cytochrome *b* is required, as in normal oxygen-terminated respiration, while in anaerobic assimilation of nitrate the cytochrome is not used, but the process is energy requiring. In the presence of oxygen there is competition between oxygen and nitrate for electrons generated by substrate oxidation.

Some chemo-autotrophic bacteria use nitrite or ammonia as electron donors for respiration. In *Nitrobacter*, the oxidation of nitrite to nitrate is linked to cytochrome reduction, as shown in Figure 1.4. Cytochrome 552, reduced by nitrite, can be re-oxidized either by reduction of oxygen to water, coupled to the phosphorylation of 1 mol of ADP to ATP per pair of electrons transported, or by reduction of flavin and NAD, associated with the assimilation of carbon dioxide. The reduction of NAD^+ by nitrite is thermodynamically unfavourable, and requires ATP to force the reaction, as in mammalian mitochondria when NAD^+ is reduced by succinate.

The nitrite ion is relatively toxic, and it is interesting to note that the enzymes involved in nitrite utilization in *Nitrobacter* are membrane-bound, and that the cell is protected by concentric rings of membrane. Thus, the toxic nitrite does not reach the cytoplasm, but is presumably converted to the less dangerous nitrate during passage through the series of membrane envelopes.

Nitrosomonas uses the oxidation of ammonia directly to nitrogen gas as an electron source, the classic denitrifying reaction.

THE ASSIMILATION OF AMMONIA

Reductive amination

The major pathway by which ammonia is incorporated into amino acids is the reductive amination of α-oxo-glutarate to glutamate, catalysed by glutamate dehydrogenase, as shown in Figure 1.5. As discussed in Chapter 2, there are a great many aminotransferase reactions, and aminotransferases are found in all organisms. Many use the α-oxo-glutarate-glutamate pair as amino donor–acceptor, so that ammonia incorporated into glutamate can readily be transferred to form the α-amino group of any amino acid for which the organism has an aminotransferase, and can form the α-oxo-acid.

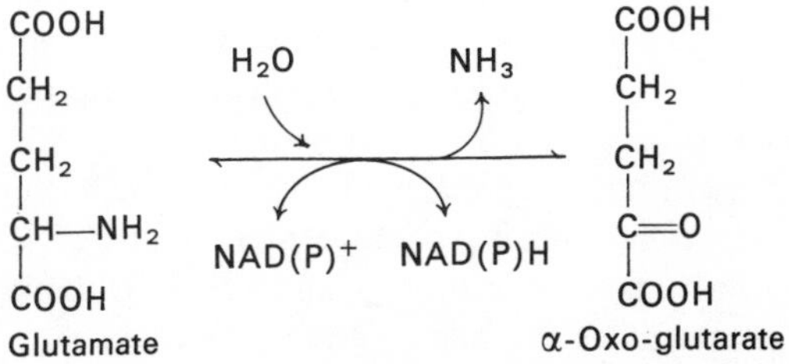

Figure 1.5. The reaction of glutamate dehydrogenase

In general, glutamate dehydrogenase from plant and animal sources can use either NAD or NADP as the proton carrier; the relative activity with the two cofactors differs not only with species, but also with the tissue of origin of the enzyme. Most appear to show a preference for NAD. In bacteria and yeasts the enzyme will use only one of the two pyridine nucleotides, depending upon the species of origin.

In *Neurospora crassa* there are two separate glutamate dehydrogenases, one which functions primarily in the direction of reductive amination (glutamate synthesis), and uses NADP, while the other functions primarily in the direction of oxidative deamination, and is NAD-dependent. The two enzymes show co-ordinate induction and repression, depending on the culture conditions.

All glutamate dehydrogenases examined to date show slight alanine dehydrogenase activity, which persists throughout purification. This appears to represent a genuine secondary activity of the enzyme rather than contamination with bacterial alanine dehydrogenase, which has a somewhat broader specificity.

Beef liver glutamate dehydrogenase normally exists as a readily-dissociated polymer, with eight NAD binding sites which show no cooperativity. The enzyme is allosterically activated by ADP and AMP, and inhibited by GTP, apparently by alteration of the coenzyme affinity. These allosteric effects would be compatible with a primary role of the enzyme in mammalian liver in glutamate catabolism, to yield the citrate cycle intermediate α-oxo-glutarate. Thus, catabolism of glutamate is enhanced when there is a relative deficit of ATP (an excess of ADP and AMP), and reduced when there is an excess of GTP produced by substrate level phosphorylation in the citrate cycle. However, as will be shown below, reductive amination of α-oxo-glutarate to glutamate is an important reaction in mammalian tissues, especially liver and brain.

In *E. coli*, glutamate dehydrogenase appears to function almost solely for the assimilation of ammonia. Vender and coworkers (1965) showed that in a mutant capable of using glutamate as the sole source of nitrogen and carbon, there was a repression of glutamate dehydrogenase when the organism was grown on a glutamate-containing medium. They proposed that the main route of glutamate catabolism was by transamination to α-oxo-glutarate, with oxaloacetate acting as the amino acceptor, forming aspartate. Growth on glutamate stimulated the production of aspartase which catalyses the direct removal of ammonia from aspartate to yield fumarate, a reaction analogous to the direct addition and removal of water catalysed by fumarase; no coenzyme requirement has been shown. Thus, in *E. coli* the pathway for the deamination of glutamate can be represented as shown in Figure 1.6. The same pathway can also operate in other bacteria and plants, but not in animals, where aspartase has not been reported.

The aspartase reaction can also operate in reverse, for the assimilation of ammonia, at least in bacterial mutants which have no glutamate dehydrogenase but can still use ammonia as the sole source of nitrogen. Ammonia can also be incorporated into amino acids in a variety of bacteria by a number of more or less specific reductive aminations, which, at least formally, are the reverse of the mammalian and bacterial oxidative deaminations discussed below, although

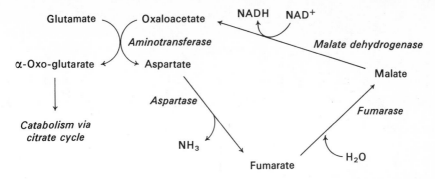

Figure 1.6. A proposed catabolism of glutamate in *E. coli*

they are probably mechanistically different. Thus, in *Bacillus subtilis*, pyruvate is reductively aminated to alanine as a major pathway of ammonia incorporation, the alanine dehydrogenase reaction.

The formation of amino acid amides

Ammonia is highly toxic to animals. Baldwin (1966) has cited an experiment by Sumner in which purified urease was injected into the bloodstream of rabbits. They died in convulsions before there was any change in the pH of the blood from released ammonia. He showed that this was not an effect of the injected enzyme *per se* by injecting it into chickens, which have little or no blood urea; they were unaffected.

The mechanism of ammonia toxicity is not clear, but it is assumed that the effect is mainly on the central nervous system, since ammonia intoxication is always accompanied by vomiting, dizziness and finally convulsions. The brain has a very active glutamate dehydrogenase, and it has been suggested that reductive amination of α-oxo-glutarate to glutamate depletes the brain mitochondrial pool of α-oxo-glutarate. Chalupa (1972) has shown that high levels of ammonia also inhibit the oxidative decarboxylation of pyruvate and α-oxo-glutarate, two reactions which are important in the energy-yielding metabolism of the brain and other tissues.

The ammonia concentration of normal human peripheral blood is less than 1 mg/litre, while the concentration in the hepatic portal vein is ten times as high. Thus, a single pass through the liver removes the greater part of the ammonia absorbed from the intestine as a result of bacterial action. In experimental animals, it has been shown that as much as 70% hepatectomy has no effect on the capacity of the liver to remove excess ammonia from the portal blood at a single pass. Shunting the portal blood into the peripheral circulation leads to neurological signs like those seen during the infusion of ammonium salts into the peripheral circulation (Visek, 1972).

As well as formation of glutamate from α-oxo-glutarate, ammonia is detoxicated by formation of glutamine, the γ-amide of glutamate. This is an energy-requiring reaction catalysed by glutamine synthetase, as shown in Figure 1.7.

14

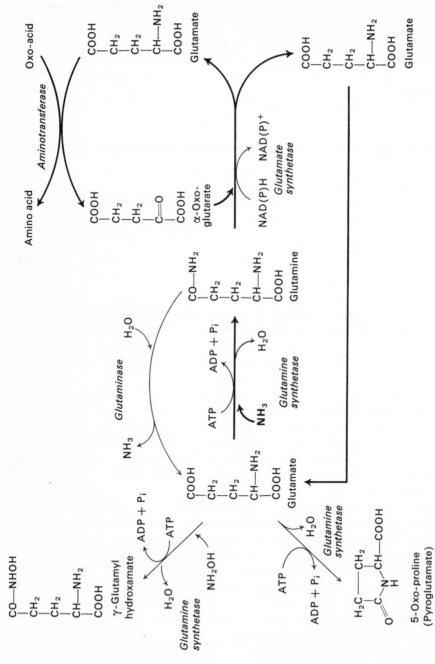

Figure 1.7. The reactions of glutamine synthetase and the role of glutamate synthetase in ammonia incorporation

Berl (1962) showed that when [^{15}N]ammonium salts were infused into cats, the most highly labelled compound was the amide nitrogen of glutamine, with rather less labelling in the α-amino group of glutamine, and almost no labelling in the α-amino group of glutamate. This has been interpreted as showing the presence of two separate pools of glutamate in the brain. Glutamine synthetase obviously does not deplete the brain glutamate pool, neither does it draw glutamate from the blood, since either of these would have an unlabelled amino group. There appears to be a separate pool of newly synthesized glutamate (incorporating the label from the $^{15}NH_4^+$) which is the substrate for glutamine synthetase. This pool does not appear to mix significantly with that pool of brain glutamate which is mainly concerned with neurotransmitter function (either *per se*, or in GABA synthesis, see page 91). In the liver, the label after infusion of $^{15}NH_4^+$ is evenly distributed in glutamate, glutamine, aspartate, asparagine and urea.

As well as this role as a non-toxic carrier of ammonia in animals, glutamine has an important role *per se*, both as a constituent of proteins (unlike hydroxyproline and hydroxylysine, see page 99, glutamine and asparagine are incorporated into proteins as amides, and are not formed *in situ*), and as a nitrogen donor in many reactions, including the synthesis of urea, histidine, tryptophan, purines, pyrimidines and amino sugars.

A role for glutamine in the overall incorporation of ammonia into amino acids has been postulated following the isolation of glutamate synthetase from a number of micro-organisms, both nitrogen-fixing organisms and others. Glutamate synthetase catalyses a reductive reaction, using NADH or NADPH, between glutamine and α-oxo-glutarate to yield two molecules of glutamate. The enzyme appears to be an iron–sulphur flavo-protein, containing both FMN and FAD; the reaction is shown in Figure 1.7.

The other amino acid amide is asparagine. In some bacteria (e.g., *Lactobacillus arabinosa* and *Streptococcus bovis*) asparagine is formed from aspartate and ammonia in a reaction essentially similar to that of glutamine synthetase, except that ATP is hydrolysed to AMP and pyrophosphate, rather than to ADP and phosphate. This suggests that the enzyme-bound intermediate may be β-adenosyl-aspartate, rather than the phosphate derivative of glutamate. Like glutamine synthetase, this asparagine synthetase is repressed by growth on ammonia-rich media.

In most animals, asparagine is synthesized by amide transfer from glutamine. Ammonia is not active as a donor except at unphysiologically high levels. The asparagine synthetase isolated from Novikoff hepatoma cells normally uses glutamine as the amide donor, but can use hydroxylamine to form β-aspartyl hydroxamate. Like the bacterial systems, this enzyme hydrolyses ATP to AMP and pyrophosphate, and again the intermediate activated form has been postulated to be β-adenosyl aspartate (Patterson and Orr, 1968). A similar glutamine-dependent asparagine synthetase has been demonstrated in plant tissues. However, other plants have an ammonia-dependent asparagine synthetase, like that in some bacteria, and asparagine can also be formed in some plants by hydrolysis of β-cyano-alanine, a product of cyanide incorporation (see below).

The finding that some mammalian tumours have very high levels of asparagine synthetase (like the Novikoff hepatoma referred to above), has led to the suggestion that asparagine may be essential for tumour growth, although no precise function for this amide in tumour metabolism has been determined. Presumably, as well as its role in protein synthesis, asparagine may function in an amino-transfer capacity, as does glutamine in normal mammalian tissue. Since the normal circulating levels of asparagine in man are very low, it was considered feasible to starve the tumours of asparagine by treatment with asparaginase, a treatment which has met with success in some cases. In general, those tumours which regress under asparaginase therapy are those which do not have a very active asparagine synthetase, but depend on the host for most of their asparagine. As would be expected, those tumours which have an active endogenous asparagine synthetase are less dependent on the host for this amino acid, and are therefore less susceptible to therapy with asparaginase.

THE ASSIMILATION OF CYANIDE

As was noted above, organisms which have nitrogenase are able to detoxicate cyanide by reduction to methylamine; other organisms have to use alternative pathways to remove this potentially dangerous cytochrome inhibitor. There is some evidence that in man cyanide is complexed with coenzyme B_{12}, and after reduction the methyl-coenzyme B_{12} enters the pool of 'one-carbon' compounds (see page 72), while the ammonia produced by this cyanide reduction is metabolized as described above.

Bacteria, fungi and higher plants have a variety of pathways for the assimilation of cyanide into cell constituents. Thus, in some fungi the carbon atom of cyanide becomes the carbon atom of the carboxyl group of alanine, while the nitrogen enters the cell ammonia pool after a reaction between the cyanide, ammonia and acetaldehyde. A number of higher plants incorporate cyanide into β-cyano-alanine, by displacement of the sulphydryl group of cysteine as sulphide. The enzyme responsible, β-cyano-alanine synthetase, has been purified and characterized (Hendrickson and Conn, 1969); it is a mitochondrial enzyme which reacts only with cysteine and to a very limited extent with O-acetyl serine. No cofactor requirement has been demonstrated. The β-cyano-alanine can be metabolized to asparagine or, after hydrolysis, to aspartate and ammonia.

THE PRODUCTION OF AMMONIA FROM AMINO ACIDS

One obvious route for the removal of excess α-amino nitrogen is via the synthesis of glutamate from α-oxo-glutarate by amino transfer followed by oxidative deamination, catalysed by glutamate dehydrogenase. However, most available evidence suggests that in mammals, glutamate dehydrogenase acts mainly in the reductive direction to assimilate ammonia rather than forming it by oxidative deamination, despite the apparent evidence of the regulatory factors in mammalian liver referred to above. There is considerable evidence that a major pathway for oxidative deamination involves the flavo-protein glycine oxidase, which forms glyoxylate and ammonia from glycine. Glyoxylate is an excellent substrate for amino-transfer; indeed, glycine aminotransferase does not appear to act *in vivo* at all readily in the direction of glycine deamination, but almost entirely in the direction of glycine formation from glyoxylate. Hence, it is probable that a considerable proportion of mammalian ammonia production from amino acids is by trans-deamination involving glycine aminotransferase and oxidase.

More generally applicable are the D- and L-amino acid oxidases, i.e., mitochondrial flavo-protein oxidases which are coupled directly to the electron transport chain at the level of ubiquinone, and which remove ammonia from amino acids to form the corresponding α-oxo-acids. While both D- and L-amino acid oxidases are widely distributed, it is interesting to note that in mammalian tissues the activity of L-amino acid oxidase is very low, while, especially in the kidney there is a great deal of the apparently useless D-amino acid oxidase. Because this enzyme can be purified readily, it has been greatly studied as a model of flavo-protein oxidases; it was using this enzyme that it was first observed that although flavins can accept two electrons per molecule, in most enzymes they are single electron carriers cycling between the fully oxidized form and the free radical. It is difficult to see any physiological function for this enzyme, since it is almost wholly inactive towards glycine and L-amino acids—the naturally occurring forms. It probably serves mainly as a detoxication mechanism, removing the traces of D-amino acids which are absorbed from some foods, and especially from digestion of bacterial proteins. Because they are not readily utilized, many D-amino acids are extremely toxic, and inhibit some of the enzymes which use the L-isomers. Most insects contain large amounts of D-serine, and it is possible that D-amino acid oxidase was evolved initially in insectivorous species to allow utilization of this amino acid. It has been demonstrated that germ-free rats have extremely low levels of renal D-amino acid oxidase compared with normal animals, thus supporting the view that the primary function of this enzyme is the detoxication of D-amino acids produced by intestinal bacteria, and absorbed on digestion of their proteins after death. It is also interesting that at least in sheep the enzyme activity alters with the season, being maximal in spring-time, presumably associated with altered composition of spring pasture.

Ammonia is also released in the non-oxidative deamination of serine and threonine, yielding respectively pyruvate and α-oxo-butyrate, and in the oxidation of amines to aldehydes catalysed by amine oxidases.

The amino acid amides, glutamine and asparagine, are deaminated by specific hydrolases, glutaminase and asparaginase, to form dicarboxylic amino acids. In mammals, the action of glutaminase in the kidneys is important in the regulation of urinary pH, and the activity of the enzyme is regulated by a variety of factors which affect the initial pH of the urine (diet, metabolic acidosis or alkalosis, etc.). In bacteria, the activity of glutaminase is closely regulated to avoid wastage of the metabolic energy used in the synthesis of glutamine—factors which enhance the activity of the synthetase reduce glutaminase activity, and *vice versa*.

In rat kidney, Katanuma and coworkers (1966) have demonstrated the presence of two separate glutaminase isoenzymes, a phosphate-independent form which is activated by carbonate and maleate, with a low K_m (4×10^{-3} M), and a phosphate-dependent isoenzyme with a higher K_m (4×10^{-2} M), induced by a high protein intake. Both the isoenzymes are located in the mitochondria of the kidney cortex, and both respond to the intra-mitochondrial pH. The phosphate-independent kidney glutaminase is found mainly in the proximal straight tubules, while the phosphate-dependent isoenzyme is found in the distal straight and convoluted tubules. It is this latter enzyme which responds to metabolic acidosis (20-fold increase in ammonium chloride-induced acidosis) and alkalosis (40% decrease in sodium bicarbonate-induced alkalosis).

In rat liver, glutaminase activity is mediated not only by amide hydrolysis, as described above, but also by a 'glutaminase II' system. This system has been separated into two enzyme activities, one of which removes the α-amino group from glutamine to form α-oxo-glutaramic acid in an amino transfer reaction, while the second enzyme, ω-amidase, hydrolyses the amide group of α-oxo-glutaramic acid to form α-oxo-glutarate and ammonia (Cooper and Meister, 1972).

A number of amide transfer reactions are known, in which the amide group of a protein-incorporated glutaminyl or asparaginyl residue is displaced by an amine, liberating ammonia. Such reactions are thought to be responsible for the incorporation into proteins of the polyamines, and for the long-term effects of the hallucinogen mescaline, which can be shown to be bound covalently to proteins in the central nervous system. The transamidase appears to be a soluble enzyme, with a broad specificity for the acceptor protein; *in vitro* casein, fibrinogen and human α-globulin have all been used. When insulin was used as the acceptor, it was shown that the mammalian amidotransferase acted only on glutaminyl residues in the protein, and not on asparaginyl residues (Mycek *et al.*, 1959). It has also been demonstrated that thalidomide, the sedative which was later found to have a severe teratogenic effect in man and some experimental animals, can be incorporated into proteins in the same way, which may explain its effect on the foetus.

Pisano and coworkers (1969) have shown that the stable cross-links formed in fibrin clots under the influence of clotting factor XIII, a later stage than the formation of the initially non-covalently-linked fibrin clot, are formed by transamidation to glutaminyl residues, the ammonia being displaced by the ε-amino groups of lysyl residues in the chain. Similar ε-(γ-glutamyl)-lysyl cross-links have been identified in native wool keratin, where there are also links from lysyl to aspartyl residues.

THE EXCRETION OF NITROGENOUS WASTE

For a small organism, the excretion of nitrogenous waste presents no problem. Ammonia is a freely diffusible material, and the organism is sufficiently small for the ammonia produced by catabolism of nitrogenous materials to cross a relatively large surface area readily. For larger aquatic animals, there is still no problem. As much as 60% of the nitrogenous excretion of fishes is ammonia with little urea production (apart from the elasmobranchs, see below), and about 30% is trimethylamine oxide which may represent an oxidation product of trimethylamine taken in with the food rather than a general nitrogenous end-product.

The tadpole excretes most of its nitrogenous waste as ammonia, but upon metamorphosis its terminal nitrogen metabolism changes, and the adult frog excretes mainly urea. The *Xenopus* toad, an amphibian which has made a secondary return to a wholly aquatic environment, excretes 70–80% of its nitrogenous waste as ammonia (the remainder is urea), but if it is removed from water it can form more urea, and store it in the body for several days until it is returned to water. In the same way, osmotic stress (the provision of brackish or salt rather than fresh water) also leads to urea synthesis in *Xenopus*, both as a means of avoiding ammonia intoxication and of increasing the osmolarity of the blood. The spade-foot toad (*Scaphiopus hammondii*) aestivates, and as the osmolarity of the soil water rises, so does the blood urea, thus maintaining a constant osmotic gradient to encourage the movement into the animal of such water as is available. The lung-fish, which is probably related to the ancestral amphibians, also accumulates urea during aestivation, when considerable dehydration occurs, although in some species of lung-fish urea is not the normal end-product of ammonia metabolism. After a prolonged period of aestivation as much as 1% of the body weight of the fish may consist of urea.

In terrestrial vertebrates which produce cleidoic eggs, the main end-product of nitrogen metabolism is uric acid, probably as a result of the limited water supply in the egg. Most insects and other terrestrial invertebrates also produce uric acid as a water conservation mechanism: it is sparingly soluble in water, and can be deposited in the eggs or excreted by the adult as dry crystals. Some invertebrates metabolize uric acid further to allantoin or allantoic acid, and the arachnids excrete most of their nitrogenous waste as guanine. Some of the land snails, although they produce mainly uric acid, also excrete large amounts of guanine and xanthine. It is therefore preferable to use the term *purinotelic* to describe those animals which excrete their nitrogenous waste as uric acid, by analogy with the terms *ammonotelic* and *ureotelic* for animals which excrete mainly ammonia and urea respectively. Some insects put their nitrogenous waste to specific use: waste accumulating during pupation is used for synthesis of the leucopterine pigments of butterfly wings and the xanthopterine of wasps.

Viviparous terrestrial vertebrates generally produce urea as an end-product of nitrogen catabolism. The general evolutionary and environmental succession of nitrogen excretion is most clearly seen in the turtles and tortoises. Aquatic members of this family are ammonotelic, the amphibian members are ureotelic, and of the dry-land living members, some produce urea, some urea and uric acid, and at least one produces uric acid only.

The earthworm is the only terrestrial invertebrate to produce urea as the main nitrogenous end-product, and then only under specialized conditions such as starvation. Under normal conditions the worm excretes mainly ammonia, and it appears that the stimulus for urea production in starvation is ammonia intoxication. In general, invertebrates are considerably more tolerant of ammonia than are vertebrates, and a number of terrestrial invertebrates excrete fairly large amounts of ammonia gas, a situation very different from the excretion of ammonium ions in an aquatic environment.

The salt content of fish blood is intermediate between that of fresh and sea water, so that whatever their environment, fishes have problems of osmoregulation. Marine teleosts (bony fishes) with a blood osmotic pressure less than that of the surrounding sea water, continually drink large amounts of water and excrete small amounts of hypotonic urine while excreting salts actively through the gills. Freshwater teleosts have the opposite problem: water continually enters the body, and they drink very little, excrete copious amounts of very dilute urine, and actively absorb salts through the gills. The elasmobranchs (cartilaginous fishes) have tackled the problem differently. Marine elasmobranchs form urea as an end-product of nitrogen metabolism and maintain a high blood urea level (as much as 20 g/l) by active resorption from the glomerular filtrate. They thus maintain their blood isotonic with sea water. They have, however, only a limited capacity to synthesize urea since they have little carbamyl phosphate synthetase and are still primarily ammonotelic. Freshwater elasmobranchs retain some of the uraemia of their marine ancestors (about 6 g/l) and therefore have a high blood osmotic pressure compared with the surrounding water. Like the freshwater teleosts, they produce a very dilute urine to rid themselves of the water that continually enters the body. Ammonotelism in freshwater fishes may also serve to allow conservation of sodium; there is some evidence that there is a linked transport of NH_4^+ and Na^+ across the gills. Bicarbonate and chloride may be similarly linked.

Figure 1.8 shows the pathway for the synthesis of uric acid from the purines adenine and guanine, and its subsequent conversion to allantoin and allantoic acid. In those animals where uric acid is the main product of amino acid catabolism, the nitrogen is incorporated into the purines by the same route followed in all organisms for the synthesis of purines for nucleic acid synthesis.

In ureotelic animals, uric acid is produced only as a product of purines taken in in the diet, or from nucleic acid breakdown. Apart from man and the higher apes, which lack uric acid oxidase, the main product of purine catabolism is allantoin. In fishes and amphibians, allantoin is further degraded, through allantoic acid, to urea and glyoxylate.

In man, the disease of gout is characterized by swelling of the joints, and intense pain, due to the accumulation in cartilage of crystals of uric acid produced vastly in excess of the capacity of the kidneys to excrete it. Although there is some evidence that renal clearance of uric acid may be impaired in gout, and in glycogen storage diseases the elevated blood lactate certainly causes gout by inhibition of uric acid excretion, in general it is thought that the defect is the failure to regulate purine synthesis. Purines are synthesized greatly in excess of demand, and are catabolized to uric acid; this accumulates, and finally crystal-

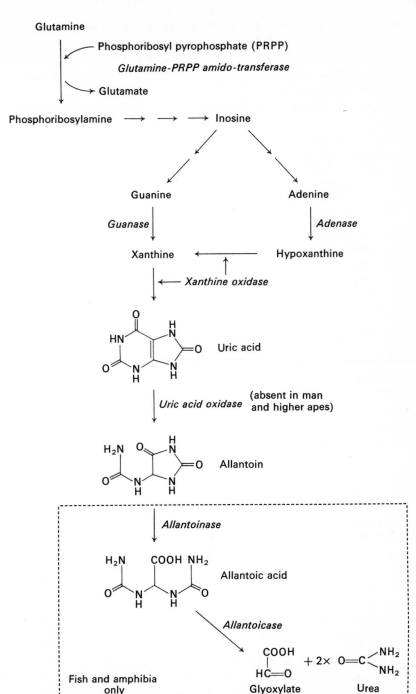

Figure 1.8. The purinotelic excretion pathway

lizes in the cartilage of joints and elsewhere. Gout is extremely rare in young women, who have very much lower plasma uric acid levels than men or post-menopausal women. Nicholls and coworkers (1973) have shown that oestrogen therapy of male patients (other than for gout) lowers plasma uric acid and increases its renal clearance.

Katunuma and coworkers (1970) have studied the differences in regulation of glutamine metabolism in birds and mammals. In mammals, glutamine is important in the detoxication of ammonia produced by amino acid deamination, but for the synthesis of urea it must be hydrolysed to ammonia and glutamate, while in birds, glutamine is used directly for the synthesis of phosphoribosylamine, the first step of purine synthesis. Katunuma *et al.* showed that in birds the hepatic glutaminase activity is only about one tenth of that found in mammals, and this activity is strongly inhibited by its product, glutamate. Mammalian glutaminase is induced by feeding a high protein diet, when there will be a need for more glutaminase as an early step in the synthesis of urea, while in birds, as would be expected, the dietary protein intake does not affect glutaminase activity. Conversely, while in mammals the activity of glutamine–phosphoribosyl pyrophosphate amidotransferase is strongly inhibited by IMP, AMP and GMP, in birds, where the production of purine phosphates is not the sole function of this enzyme, this is not so, and avian PRPP amidotransferase and glutamine synthetase are both induced by feeding a high protein diet; the mammalian enzymes are not. Mammals on a high protein diet have a raised blood urea level, while in birds it is the blood uric acid which is raised. These findings are summarized in Table 1.3.

Table 1.3. The responses of birds and mammals to a high protein diet

| | Normal activity | | Response to high protein diet | |
	Rabbit	Chicken	Rabbit	Chicken
Glutamine synthetase	Low	High	Unchanged	Raised
Glutaminase	High	Low	Raised	Unchanged
Glutamine-PRPP amidotransferase	Low	High	Unchanged	Raised
Urea cycle enzymes	High	Absent	Raised	—
Serum uric acid	—	—	Unchanged	Raised
Serum urea	—	—	Raised	Unchanged

The synthesis of urea

The urea synthesis pathway was first elucidated by Krebs and Henseleit in 1932; it was the first cyclic metabolic pathway to be described. In Figure 1.9, heavy type has been used to show those parts of the intermediates which are added at various stages, to emphasize the simplicity of the pathway. Krebs (1973) in a brief essay describing the discovery of the urea cycle, has commented on the 'admirable evolutionary economy' shown in the development of pathways

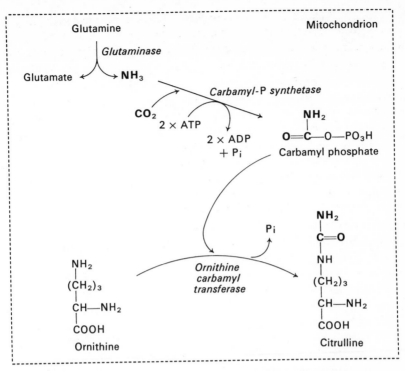

Figure 1.9. The synthesis of urea

for the elimination of nitrogenous waste. The urea synthesis cycle in ureotelic animals is essentially the same as the pathway used by all animals for the synthesis of ornithine and arginine; in the same way, the pathway used by purinotelic animals for the synthesis of excretory uric acid is the same as that used by all animals for purine synthesis.

The first step in the synthesis of urea is the formation of carbamyl phosphate; the same precursor is also required for pyrimidine synthesis and it is interesting to see how the production of the same precursor for two distinct pathways, with very different types of end-product, has been separated in ureotelic animals and a number of other organisms. In *E. coli* there is a single carbamyl phosphate synthetase, using glutamine as the amino donor, which is used for the synthesis of both arginine and the pyrimidines. In yeasts and moulds there are two distinct enzymes, one associated with arginine biosynthesis, and the other with the pyrimidine pathway. Both use glutamine as the nitrogen donor.

In higher animals there are two separate enzymes, one associated with the biosynthesis of pyrimidines, and using glutamine, and the other associated with arginine (and where appropriate also urea) synthesis, and using ammonia as the nitrogen source. In the vertebrate liver, these two pools of carbamyl phosphate are also physically separated with the ammonia-dependent synthetase and the next enzyme of the arginine pathway, ornithine carbamyl transferase, located inside the mitochondrion, while the carbamyl phosphate associated with pyrimidine synthesis, using glutamine, and the second enzyme of the pathway, aspartate carbamyl transferase, are in the cytosol. A similar physical separation probably occurs in other organisms which have separate pools of carbamyl phosphate for the two pathways.

Ammonia-dependent carbamyl phosphate synthetase of mammalian liver requires *N*-acetyl glutamate as an allosteric activator, and the mechanism is believed to proceed by way of the formation of an initial enzyme–carboxyphosphate complex, which then reacts with ammonia to form enzyme-bound carbamate and release phosphate. The enzyme–carbamate complex then reacts with a further molecule of ATP to form carbamyl phosphate and release the enzyme for further reaction.

Carbamyl phosphate then reacts, again intramitochondrially, with ornithine, in a reaction catalysed by ornithine carbamyl transferase, to form citrulline. Citrulline then leaves the mitochondrion, and reacts with aspartate to form argininosuccinic acid. This reaction is catalysed by argininosuccinate synthetase and is believed to proceed by way of the intermediate formation of an enzyme-bound AMP-citrulline derivative. Formation of this intermediate is reversible, and the equilibrium is maintained in the direction of argininosuccinate synthesis by the action of pyrophosphatase on the inorganic pyrophosphate released. The AMP-citrulline complex then reacts with aspartate to form argininosuccinate and release AMP. The remaining two reactions of the cycle are simple hydrolyses, the first, catalysed by argininosuccinase, cleaving argininosuccinate to form arginine and fumarate, and the other, catalysed by arginase, cleaving arginine to release urea, and reform ornithine.

Since the original description of the urea cycle there have been many suggestions that some alternative pathway for the synthesis of urea must exist, since in argininosuccinic aciduria, although there is an accumulation of argininosuccinate in the blood and urine, indicating a deficit of argininosuccinase which can be demonstrated by biopsy, the total production of urea is normal. However, despite intense investigation, no alternative pathway has been demonstrated. Although argininosuccinase activity is low on assay of biopsy samples from patients, this is mainly because the enzyme has an abnormally high K_m, so that there would not be any significant hydrolysis of argininosuccinate until there is a considerable accumulation of the substrate. Once the enzyme is saturated with substrate, the reaction can proceed at a normal rate, and as long as the overall concentration of argininosuccinate is high, the throughput of the cycle is normal.

The known inborn errors of the urea cycle are listed in Table 1.4; all of them must be assumed to be of the same type as argininosuccinic aciduria, with abnormalities of the K_m of the enzyme, since any defect of the cycle involving the total absence of an activity would, in the absence of an alternative mechanism for urea synthesis, prove lethal soon after birth because of ammonia intoxication.

Table 1.4. Metabolic defects of the urea synthesis cycle

Syndrome	Enzyme absent
Ammonaemia*	Carbamyl phosphate synthetase
Ornithinaemia / Ornithinuria	Ornithine carbamyl transferase
Citrullinaemia	Argininosuccinate synthetase
Argininosuccinic aciduria	Argininosuccinase
Argininaemia	Arginase

* Note that in all defects of the urea synthesis cycle there will also be some degree of ammonaemia, leading to ammonia intoxication.

Colombo and coworkers (1964) showed an interesting defect of urea synthesis in a patient with defective lysine catabolism. The patient showed congenital lysine intolerance with periodic ammonia intoxication. They concluded that the symptoms arose as a result of inhibition of arginase by lysine, which, although not a substrate for the enzyme, is a potent competitive inhibitor. This inhibition led to an accumulation of all the intermediates of the cycle, and eventually to an accumulation of ammonia which precipitated the attack.

Regoeczi and coworkers (1965) showed that the half-life of administered [^{15}N]urea was considerably greater than that of [^{14}C]urea. They attributed this to catabolism of urea to carbon dioxide and ammonia; while the ammonia was then reassimilated into amino acids, and ultimately reformed into urea, the carbon dioxide was not used. Work with sterile tissue preparations and germ-free animals has shown that mammals have no endogenous urease and that this recirculation of urea nitrogen is via the gastro-intestinal tract. Bacterial urease hydrolyses urea to carbon dioxide and ammonia; the ammonia is then absorbed and removed from the portal blood by the liver. Sterilization of the human gut with antibiotics leads to a faecal urea level which is about the same as that of blood, while normally there is no urea in faeces. Although the colon is impermeable to urea, the latter readily diffuses across the stomach and the wall of the small intestine. Saliva, gastric juice and bile all contain considerable amounts of urea. As much as 25 % of the urea synthesized in the body is broken down in this entero–hepatic circulation, and must be resynthesized for excretion.

Other nitrogenous compounds in human urine

Table 1.5 lists the normal levels of a number of nitrogenous compounds in human urine. Apart from conversion to urea, as much as 3 g/day of amino acids may be excreted, approximately one third each as free amino acids, small peptides and conjugates (mainly of glycine and glutamate). There are also traces of small proteins; the presence of large amounts of protein, or of proteins as large as haemoglobin, is indicative of renal damage or dysfunction. The amino acid conjugates are detoxication products of exogenous materials, or catabolites of endogenous materials such as the steroids.

Table 1.5. Levels of nitrogenous compounds in human urine

Urea	10–35 g/day (depends on protein intake)
NH_4^+	340–1200 mg/day (depends on acid–base status)
Amino acids	1300–3200 mg/day: 1/3 as free amino acids
	1/3 as peptides
	1/3 as conjugates
Protein	up to 60 mg/day
Uric acid	250–750 mg/day
(traces of xanthine, hypoxanthine, guanine and adenine)	
Amino sugars	10–40 mg/day
Creatinine	males 1·8 g/day
	females 1·2 g/day
Creatine	0–50 mg/day
Vitamins	Degradation products and amounts surplus to requirements

Aminoaciduria occurs in many cases of inborn errors of amino acid metabolism. A partial list of such metabolic errors is given in Appendix II, and a number are noted at various points in the text, with discussion of the metabolism of the amino acids concerned. A primary renal defect may be responsible for the aminoaciduria; for example, in Hartnup disease there is a defect of amino-acid transport in both kidney and intestine, so that neutral amino acids, and especially tryptophan, are not adequately absorbed from the diet, and are not resorbed from the glomerular filtrate, resulting in signs of tryptophan deficiency. In this case, the aminoaciduria will consist of members of a specific group of amino acids sharing a common transport mechanism (see page 106). It is also possible that aminoaciduria will occur as a result of a more general renal defect, in which case not only amino acids but other abnormal compounds, possibly including proteins and glycopeptides, will appear in the urine. The commoner aminoacidurias, however, are due to much elevated blood levels of amino acids, because of a metabolic block. The capacity of the kidney to resorb these amino acids from the glomerular filtrate will then be overwhelmed. Again, several amino acids sharing the same transport mechanism may be found in the urine together.

Creatinine concentration in urine is reasonably constant: it arises spontaneously by cyclization of creatine phosphate in muscle, and the amount formed depends more on the amount of creatine present in the body (i.e., the muscle mass) than on any other factor. The biochemistry of creatine and creatinine is discussed on page 86.

PROTEIN TURNOVER

Early in this century it was noticed that even with diets which contained no source of nitrogen, nitrogenous waste was still excreted in the urine of man and experimental animals, an observation which led to the concept of separate pools of endogenous and exogenous nitrogenous materials. It was not until the work of Schoenheimer in 1942 that this was resolved, although it had been postulated in 1935 that all mammalian proteins are continually broken down and replaced, and Magendie in 1829 had stated intuitively that 'all parts of the body of man experience an intestine movement which has the double effect of expelling molecules that can or ought no longer to compose the organs, and replacing them with new molecules'.

Schoenheimer used ^{15}N-labelled amino acids, and reasoned that if the endogenous and exogenous pools of nitrogen were separate then all of the administered ^{15}N should appear in the urine almost immediately. This did not occur; less than one third of the label from administered [^{15}N]leucine, and less than half of that from [^{15}N]glycine appeared in the urine within 24 h. He therefore formulated the hypothesis that a considerable proportion of dietary protein is sequestered in the tissues, presumably as tissue proteins, and that there must be some delicate regulatory mechanism which allows this to occur without increasing the total amount of tissue protein. The tissue proteins, and indeed all tissue components, are in a state of dynamic equilibrium, with new protein being synthesized and old protein being degraded continually. This process appears to be wholly random in that there is no apparent selection of older molecules for degradation, and after proteolysis the constituent amino acids are mixed randomly with newly ingested or synthesized amino acids for new protein or metabolite synthesis.

If radioactive or other labelled amino acids are given to experimental animals, the specific activity is, predictably, higher in those tissues with the fastest rate of turnover, i.e. in those tissues whose constituent proteins have the shortest metabolic half-lives. Therefore the specific activity of an amino acid will be highest in the intestinal tract, liver, pancreas and serum proteins, lower in skeletal muscle, and lower still in the skin. Almost none will normally be detected in bone and connective tissue, which have a very low rate of turnover. The protein turnover of the pancreas, which secretes many of the digestive enzymes, is extremely high: as much as 25% of the total protein content of the organ is secreted every day in the exocrine secretions alone. Administration of radioactive amino acids leads to a very rapid (within 40–60 min) accumulation of radioactivity in the exocrine cells of the pancreas, initially in the cytosol and microsomes, then rapidly in the zymogen granules.

Not only do different proteins show characteristic turnover rates, but whole cells can be shown to divide more frequently than the observed increase in organ weight would suggest, so there must be a turnover of whole cells at a rate very different from that of any of the component proteins. Individual cell organelles also show turnover, again at rates different from either that of their constituent proteins or their parent cells. In the rat liver, 70% of the total protein is replaced in 4–5 days, while the life span of individual liver cells is estimated at between 160 and 400 days. Therefore protein turnover must be due to intracellular exchange, not to whole cell turnover. The half-lives of some proteins are shown in Table 1.6.

Table 1.6. Half-lives of some mammalian liver enzymes and other proteins

Protein	Half-life
Liver ornithine decarboxylase	11 min
Liver δ-amino-laevulinic acid synthetase	70 min
Liver tyrosine aminotransferase	1·5 h
Liver tryptophan pyrrolase	2 h
Liver alanine aminotransferase	0·7–1·0 d
Liver glucokinase	1·25 d
Liver peroxosomal catalase	1·4 d
Serum albumin	3·5 d
Liver cytochrome c reductase	3–4 d
Liver arginase	4–5 d
Liver cytochrome b_5	5–6 d
Liver lactate dehydrogenase (type H_4)	16 d
Adult collagen	300 d
Infant collagen	1–2 d and 150 d

Figure 1.10 shows the specific activity of ^{15}N in various proteins after pulse administration of ^{15}N-labelled amino acids. In all cases the decay of labelling follows first-order kinetics; the degradation of proteins is random, and does not depend on the age of the protein molecule. Proteins with a short half-life will be more rapidly labelled, and will show a higher maximum specific activity than those with longer half-lives. The specific activity curve for haemoglobin and other erythrocyte proteins shows an extensive plateau because there is no protein turnover in mature mammalian erythrocytes. The turnover time of all erythrocyte proteins will be the same as that of the whole cells.

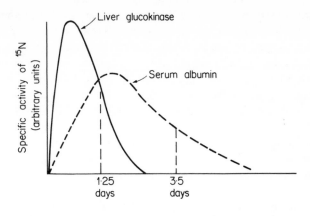

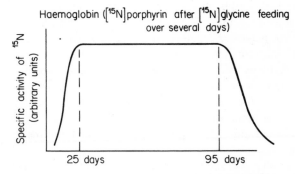

Figure 1.10. The accumulation and loss of ^{15}N-label in proteins

In exponentially-growing bacterial cultures it is not possible to demonstrate any protein turnover, but in non-growing cultures, 4–6% of the total protein may be broken down and resynthesized each hour. It is possible that the effect in exponentially growing cultures may be due to immediate re-utilization of the amino acids released after proteolysis, rather than to a cessation of turnover. It can be shown in rapidly growing cultures of *E. coli* that [^{14}C]glycine is speedily incorporated almost entirely into protein. Later the label can be shown to be present to a great extent in the nucleic-acid fraction, presumably reflecting protein catabolism and re-utilization of the amino acids. It is also possible to demonstrate some exchange of radioactive material between different bacterial cells in rapidly growing cultures. In human cell cultures, the rate of protein turnover appears to be constant, regardless of the rate of growth of the culture.

For an adult mammal in dynamic equilibrium, the excretion of nitrogenous waste will be exactly the same as the dietary intake of nitrogenous material. This is nitrogen equilibrium or balance. For accurate measurement of the state of *nitrogen balance* of man or experimental animals, the losses of nitrogen not only in the urine and faeces, but also in sweat and shed skin cells must be measured.

Some nitrogen is lost from the body even on a nitrogen-free diet and this is referred to as the obligatory nitrogen loss. The most recent estimate of the obligatory nitrogen losses for adult man (World Health Organization Report number 522, 1973), is 54 mg/kg body weight per day. This figure is the summation of 37 mg in urine, 12 mg in faeces, 3 mg in shed skin cells, and 2 mg in minor losses. It is important to quantify these figures for obligatory nitrogen loss in order to estimate the minimum dietary nitrogen intake required for its replacement.

Some nitrogen-fixing organisms have been identified in human intestinal cultures, suggesting that some fixation of nitrogen may occur in the human gut. However, the number of organisms present is extremely small, and there is no evidence that they make any contribution to nitrogen equilibrium. This is therefore a factor of importance only in studies on ruminants.

An individual who is losing more nitrogen from the body than he is consuming (i.e., is overall degrading tissue protein without replacing it), is said to be in negative nitrogen balance. The converse, the net retention of nitrogen in the body, is termed positive nitrogen balance. Positive balance is, of course, expected and desirable in children, but is seen in adults only when tissues are being replaced. For example, there is a considerable loss of tissue protein in fever, surgical trauma, broken bones, starvation, and even prolonged bed rest, and patients recovering from these conditions are in positive nitrogen balance. It is interesting to note that a terminal cancer patient may appear to be in nitrogen equilibrium, while in fact the tumour is in positive balance, at the expense of the rest of the body.

Figure 1.11 shows in diagrammatic form the turnover of protein through the intestinal tract of a normal adult man, in nitrogen equilibrium. The total amount of protein passing through the intestine may average about 90 g of dietary protein, plus active secretion into the gut lumen of serum albumin, digestive enzymes, and mucopolysaccharides which serve both as a lubricant for the gut contents and to protect the mucosa against attack by the digestive enzymes. Almost all of this protein (totalling about 150 g) is digested and the resultant amino acids absorbed. The equivalent of 80 g of protein is excreted in the urine, and 10 g is lost in the faeces as undigested food (about 5% of dietary protein), residues of the digestive juices, shed mucosal cells, and bacteria.

Total daily protein synthesis in an adult man has been estimated at about 300 g per day without any change in the total size of the protein pool, i.e., to replace degraded proteins and desquamated epithelial cells. The liver synthesizes about 12 g per day of serum albumin; the same amount is degraded daily, half by proteolysis in the liver, and half by secretion into the gut. This continual turnover of proteins serves to maintain a pool of readily-available amino acids for protein synthesis despite the fact that storage of free amino acids in the body is very small. Thus, the body retains a buffer supply to even up the availability in spite of infrequent meals. This is most important in the case of the essential amino acids, but is also important as a source of raw material for synthesis of the non-essential amino acids. However, such storage of amino acids as does occur is of limited use; it has been shown that if an animal is fed with all

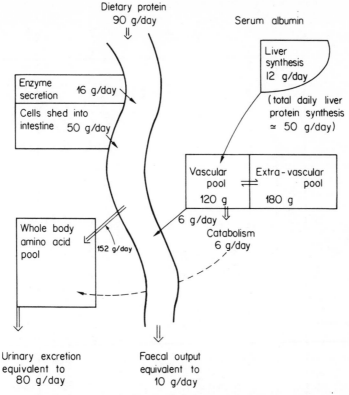

Figure 1.11. Protein turnover through the gastro-intestinal
tract—a normal man in nitrogen balance

the amino acids except tryptophan at one meal, and then is given tryptophan
about 6 hours later, it is unable to use this tryptophan, goes into negative nitrogen
balance and eventually dies. An incomplete amino acid mixture cannot be stored
for any length of time.

In the same way as amino acids are stored in a relatively labile protein pool,
so fixed nitrogen is maintained in an available form for some considerable time.
Although surplus amino acids are deaminated rapidly, and the ammonia converted to urea, this urea is not excreted immediately, but is to a certain extent
broken down in the entero-hepatic circulation described above, thus allowing
re-utilization of the ammonia.

Digestion

The major mammalian digestive proteases, and some other proteolytic
enzymes, are listed in Table 1.7, together with the source of the enzyme, and its
specificity for the hydrolysed peptide bond. All the mammalian proteases are
secreted as inactive zymogens which are subsequently activated by limited
proteolysis. This causes a rearrangement to yield an active configuration at

Table 1.7. The specificity of some proteolytic enzymes

Enzyme	Source	Specificity
Mammalian digestive enzymes		
Pepsin	Gastric juice	Endopeptidase—adjacent to aromatic, leucyl or methionyl residue
Trypsin	Pancreatic juice	Endopeptidase—lysyl or arginyl esters
Chymotrypsin	Pancreatic juice	Endopeptidase—aromatic esters
Elastase	Pancreatic juice	Endopeptidase—neutral aliphatic esters
Carboxypeptidase A	Pancreatic juice	Exopeptidase—C-terminal aromatic or branched-chain amino acid
Carboxypeptidase B	Pancreatic juice	Exopeptidase—C-terminal arginine or lysine
Aminopeptidases	Succus entericus	Exopeptidases—various N-terminal amino acids
Dipeptidases	Mucosal cells	Various dipeptides
Other proteases		
Papain	Paw-paw fruit	Endopeptidase—amides of arginine or lysine
Ficin	Latex of *Ficus* spp.	Endopeptidase—amides of arginine, lysine, glutamine, histidine, glycine and tyrosine
Bromelain	Pineapple fruit	Endopeptidase—esters of arginine, glutamate, phenylalanine, tyrosine, leucine and lysine
Subtilisin	*B. subtilis*	Endopeptidase—any bond adjacent to neutral or acidic residue
Collagenase	Various bacteria	Endopeptidase—glycyl-proline or glycyl-hydroxyproline

the catalytic site. Pepsin is secreted as pepsinogen, which is activated either by pre-existing pepsin, or by the action of gastric hydrochloric acid. Gastric acid also aids the digestion of proteins by denaturation, rendering them more susceptible to proteolytic attack. Most native proteins are relatively resistant to proteolysis, so that the digestive enzymes are poor substrates for each other or themselves. Trypsinogen in the pancreatic juice is activated to trypsin by the action of a specific protease, enteropeptidase, secreted by the intestinal cells. In turn trypsin activates procarboxypeptidases A and B, chymotrypsinogen, and probably also pro-elastase. This activation by limited proteolysis, followed by resistance to further proteolytic attack, indicates that the digestive proteases have a rigid tertiary structure, and do not reveal any bonds susceptible to hydrolysis.

The endopeptidases will only hydrolyse internal peptide bonds in a protein molecule, and will not remove terminal amino acids from a peptide. Carboxy- and aminopeptidases are exopeptidases, and will only remove carboxyl and amino terminal amino acids respectively. They do not act on dipeptides, which are absorbed by the intestinal brush border cells and degraded to free amino acids intracellularly by specific dipeptidases. As well as this cellular uptake of dipeptides, there is some evidence that small peptides, 2–6 amino acyl residues long, can be absorbed directly into the blood stream, even in adults. Such a mechanism may be of importance in such conditions as Hartnup disease where there is an impairment of the absorption of free amino acids, and small peptides can be utilized as a source of the amino acids for which the transport mechanism is defective. Cook (1973) has shown that glycyl dipeptides are absorbed more rapidly across jejunal mucosa than is free glycine. Glycyl dipeptidase in the mucosal cells hydrolyses these peptides to free amino acids which then enter the blood stream. Kinetic studies of the absorption of glycine and glycyl glycine across the human jejunum indicate that the two transport mechanisms are separate.

In young children, there is evidence that there may be considerable absorption of whole proteins, especially during the first few days of life, when preformed immunoglobulins can be transmitted to the infant in the mother's milk. At this stage of life there is no gastric acid secretion, and intestinal proteolysis is largely inhibited by specific protease inhibitors present in colostrum. The mouse milk factor, implicated in transmission of susceptibility to mouse mammary tumours, may also be transmitted in this way. It has been suggested, although without good evidence, that a similar absorption of whole proteins may occur in adults who have specific allergic reactions to certain dietary proteins.

Blood clotting

Limited proteolysis leading to the activation of an inactive precursor is also shown in the sequence of events involved in blood clotting. The factors involved are shown in Figure 1.12. The mechanism of the activation of factor XII by injury is unclear, but each of the activated factors is a specific protease which removes an inhibitory peptide sequence from the next inactive precursor to

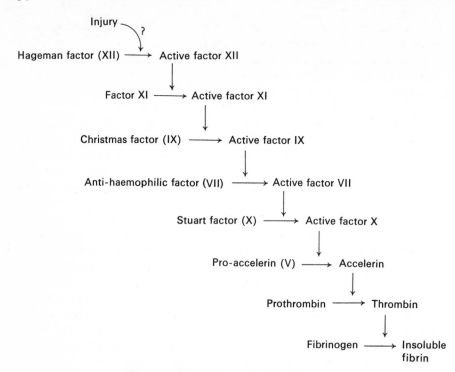

Figure 1.12. The blood clotting factors

give the active factor. The final step, the conversion of fibrinogen into the insoluble fibrin clot, is also a proteolysis. Removal of a protective peptide sequence allows the fibrin molecules to form a hydrogen-bonded polymer. Later this is stabilized by formation of ε-(γ-glutamyl)–lysyl cross-links, as described above. In the process, the clot shrinks, exuding serum: the process of syneresis. Both thrombin, the enzyme response for clotting, and plasmin, the enzyme responsible for fibrin degradation and clot liquefaction, have the same specificity as trypsin.

Further reading

Munro, H. N. and Allison, J. B. (1964). *Mammalian Protein Metabolism*, Vol. I. Academic Press, London and New York.

Postgate, J. (1972). *Biological Nitrogen Fixation*. Merrow, Watford (England).

Spickett, R. G. W. (1971). Proteolytic enzymes, *Chem. and Ind.*, 83–94.

Stewart, W. D. P. (1972). Nitrogen fixation by photosynthetic micro-organisms. *Ann. Rev. Microbiol.*, **27**, 283–316.

Streicher, S. L. and Valentine, R. C. (1973). Comparative aspects of nitrogen fixation. *Ann. Rev. Biochem.*, **42**, 279–302.

Tavill, A. S. (1972). The synthesis and degradation of liver produced proteins. *Gut*, **13**, 225–241.

Yagi, K. (1971). Reaction mechanisms of D-amino acid oxidase. *Adv. Enzymol.*, **34**, 1–40.

References cited in the text are listed in the bibliography

CHAPTER 2

THE ROLE OF VITAMIN B₆ IN AMINO ACID METABOLISM

The importance of vitamin B_6 in the metabolism of amino acids is demonstrated by the lactic acid bacteria: when grown in the absence of the vitamin, all amino acids must be supplied for growth, but in the presence of the vitamin, none of the added amino acids is essential as all can be synthesized.

The chemical forms of vitamin B_6 are shown in Figure 2.1. There is some confusion in the earlier literature arising from the fact that the term pyridoxine was initially used to describe the alcohol form of the vitamin, and then was recommended as the generic descriptor for all the vitamers in the early IUPAC–IUB recommended nomenclature. The revised nomenclature [for example, *Eur. J. Biochem.*, (1973) **40**, 325–7] recommends the use of the term vitamin B_6 as a generic descriptor for compounds with the activity *in vivo* of the vitamin, and 'pyridoxine', 'pyridoxal' and 'pyridoxamine' for the alcohol, aldehyde and amine respectively. The alcohol is also occasionally called 'pyridoxol' but this is no longer a recommended trivial name.

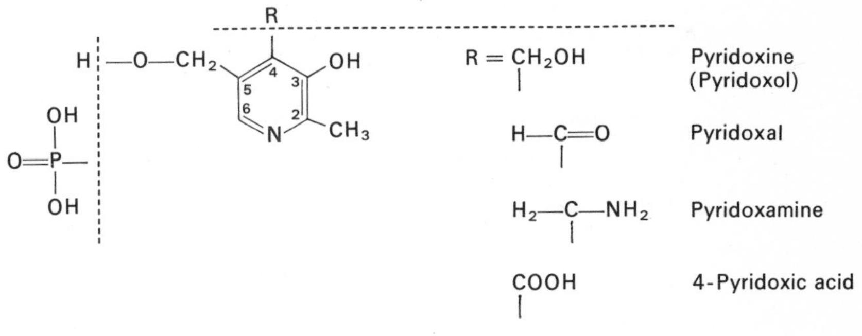

Figure 2.1. The chemical forms of vitamin B_6

The biologically active vitamer is pyridoxal phosphate. As will be discussed in more detail in this chapter, it is the cofactor for enzymes catalysing a number of reactions of amino acids: racemization, which is mainly important in bacteria, decarboxylation to form primary amines, and transfer of the amino group from an amino acid to an oxo-acid. This last reaction is central to biosynthesis and catabolism of most amino acids.

35

THE METABOLISM OF VITAMIN B$_6$

The pathway of vitamin B$_6$ biosynthesis in bacteria has not yet been elucidated in any detail. Hill and coworkers (1972) have shown that in *E. coli* the molecule is formed from three triose units: the 2'-methyl and adjacent carbon 2 are derived from pyruvate via acetaldehyde; carbons 3, 4 and 4' from one triose, and carbons 5', 5 and 6 from another. They have thus ruled out both the possibility that the methyl group is derived from methionine or formate, and the earlier hypothesis that the branched-chain amino acids were precursors of vitamin B$_6$. The origin of the heterocyclic nitrogen has not yet been determined.

The interconversions of the B$_6$ vitamers are shown in Figure 2.2 and the same pattern of metabolism is shown in both bacteria and mammals. A single enzyme, pyridoxal phosphokinase, acts on all three non-phosphorylated vitamers although in different species, and even in different tissues of the same species, it has different relative affinities for the three substrates. Bacterial kinases are activated by magnesium ions, but in mammals this function is performed by zinc ions. Both pyridoxine-*P* and pyridoxal-*P* can be dephosphorylated by a phosphorylase. Pyridoxine oxidase acts on both pyridoxine and its phosphate to yield the pyridoxal derivative. The enzyme is a flavoprotein with the rather unusual prosthetic group, riboflavin-5'-phosphate. FAD will only reactivate the apoenzyme at concentrations 10^3-times greater than the natural cofactor. Pyridoxine oxidase is strongly inhibited by pyridoxal-*P*, the end product of the pathway.

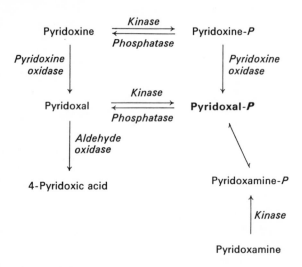

Figure 2.2. The metabolism of vitamin B$_6$

Because the vitamers are so readily interconverted *in vivo*, it is difficult to measure their individual levels in biological materials. In general, it is probably most useful to measure the total vitamin B$_6$ present although this might obscure any defect in, for example, phosphorylation of the non-phosphorylated vitamers, and might suggest the presence of more vitamin than is actually available to the enzyme in a usable form. There are also some occasions when it is desirable to measure the different vitamers separately, for example nitrate reductase in some green plants is inhibited by pyridoxamine-P, but not by pyridoxal-P. The ratio of pyridoxamine-P to pyridoxal-P will reflect the nitrogen nutritional status of the plant (i.e., the availability of reduced nitrogen compounds), and hence to what extent further nitrate reduction is required. In such cases, the vitamers are generally assayed by reactivation of apoenzymes which specifically require one form; chemical assay procedures and chromatographic separations are generally not sufficiently sensitive or precise for most biological purposes, although they can be used when large amounts of tissue are available, for example in some of the vitamin B_6 metabolic studies described below.

Studies by Johansson and coworkers (1968) and Colombini and McCoy (1970) on the metabolism of radioactive pyridoxine have shown that it was metabolized in liver and brain within 60 min of administration. Equal amounts of the label are found in pyridoxine-P and pyridoxal, both of which can act as precursors of pyridoxal-P. While liver, kidney and brain are rich sources of pyridoxine phosphokinase, muscle is a poor source, and in skeletal muscle the first product from radioactive pyridoxine is almost entirely pyridoxal, with phosphorylation occurring very much more slowly. It has been suggested that much vitamin B_6 may be stored in muscle in the relatively inert form of pyridoxal. Pyridoxamine-P is formed very much more slowly, and apparently only from pyridoxal-P by aminotransfer. Although administered pyridoxamine is a substrate for phosphorylation, free pyridoxamine does not appear to be formed normally.

Once formed, pyridoxal-P and pyridoxamine-P are lost only slowly: between 4 and 7 days after the administration of radioactive pyridoxine to mice, the specific activity of these two vitamers is almost constant. The excretion product of vitamin B_6 in animals is 4-pyridoxic acid, an inactive metabolite formed by the action of aldehyde oxidase on pyridoxal but not on pyridoxal-P. There is no evidence that the 4-pyridoxic acid-5-phosphate, which has been identified in tissue preparations, arises as a result of enzymic action; it is almost certainly formed by photo-oxidation of pyridoxal-P in the course of tissue preparation. Hence the rate of pyridoxal-P catabolism is not regulated so much by the activity of aldehyde oxidase as by the relative activities of the kinase and phosphatase.

McCoy and coworkers (1972) have reviewed some aspects of vitamin B_6 metabolism in rabbit brain. Factors which lead to an increase in the biogenic (neurotransmitter) amine concentrations in the brain also lead to inhibition of pyridoxal phosphokinase. This enzyme is also inhibited *in vitro* by high concentrations of the amines and their precursors, especially DOPA. It is possible that when large doses of DOPA are used in the therapy of Parkinson's disease there may be a disturbance of vitamin B_6 metabolism. A fall in the brain biogenic amine levels (for example, following reserpine administration) causes an increase in the activity of the kinase. Cannabinol administration leads to an inhibition of pyridoxine oxidase so that there is an increase in the proportion of the brain vitamin B_6 in the form of pyridoxine-P, and a fall in pyridoxal-P. Raised brain pyridoxal-P following pyridoxine administration also leads to inhibition of the kinase, while reduction in brain pyridoxal-P (for example following administration of 2-deoxy-pyridoxine, an analogue without coenzyme activity) leads to an increase in kinase activity. Hence the activity of pyridoxal phosphokinase appears to be a major regulatory factor in the metabolism of vitamin B_6 in the brain.

ENZYMIC REACTIONS INVOLVING VITAMIN B_6

Only pyridoxal-P and pyridoxamine-P show coenzyme activity in the majority of systems. Aminotransferases can use either, while all other vitamin B_6-dependent enzymes require pyridoxal-P for reconstitution of an active holoenzyme. With the exception of glycogen phosphorylase, in which pyridoxal-P does not appear to have a coenzyme role (see below), all enzymes requiring pyridoxal-P are concerned with amino acid metabolism. The range of B_6-catalysed reactions is shown in Table 2.1; some of these reactions are discussed in greater detail in this chapter, and others are discussed together with the metabolism of the amino acids involved, in later chapters.

The initial reaction of an amino acid with pyridoxal-P is the formation of an intermediate complex, a Schiff base, by condensation between the α-amino group of the substrate and the 4'-aldehyde group of pyridoxal-P, as shown in Figure 2.3.

The reaction undergone by the Schiff base depends on which of the bonds about the α-carbon of the amino acid moiety is broken prior to hydrolysis of the complex. Cleavage of the α-carbon–carbonyl bond releases carbon dioxide, and the hydrolysis product is the primary amine corresponding to the amino acid. Cleavage of the α-carbon–hydrogen bond will result in a complex symmetrical about the α-carbon, and rehydrogenation followed by cleavage yields a racemic product, so that the overall reaction is racemization of the amino acid substrate. If hydrolysis of the symmetrical product of α-hydrogen removal proceeds with cleavage of the α-carbon–nitrogen bond rather than the α-amino–pyridoxal-4'-carbon bond (as in the case of racemization), then the products will be the α-oxo-acid corresponding to the substrate amino acid and pyridoxamine-P. Reaction of pyridoxamine-P with another oxo-acid, in the reverse of the sequence shown in Figure 2.3, results in the formation of the amino acid corresponding to the second oxo-acid, and reformation of pyridoxal-P. The overall reaction of aminotransfer (transamination) is shown in Figure 2.4.

The α-oxo-acid product of transamination is the same as that formed by amino acid oxidase (see page 17). Thus, although amino acid oxidases are generally irreversible, the oxo-acid can be reaminated provided that a suitable donor amino acid is available. The exception here is lysine, which does not have a stable oxo-acid: α-oxo-ε-amino caproic acid cyclizes spontaneously to pipecolic acid. Threonine is only poorly transaminated, but its amino group can be shown to be in slow equilibrium with the general nitrogen pool, unlike that of lysine. Thus, if any ^{15}N-labelled amino acid is given to an experimental animal, the

Table 2.1. Vitamin B_6 catalysed enzymic reactions

Type	Bond broken	Reaction
Reactions at α-carbon		
Racemization (EC 5.1.1.X)	α-C—H	D-Amino acid ⇌ L-amino acid
Aminotransfer (EC 2.6.1.X)	α-C—NH$_2$	Amino acid ⇌ oxo-acid + PMP
α-Decarboxylation (EC 4.1.1.X)	α-C—COOH	Amino acid → primary amine + CO$_2$
		Histaminase
Oxidative deamination	α-C—NH$_2$	Histamine → urocanic acid
	α-C—H	*Threonine aldolase*
Loss of side-chain	α-C—β-C	Threonine → glycine + acetaldehyde
		Serine hydroxy-methyl transferase
		Serine → glycine + methylene-THF
Reactions at β-carbon		
Elimination of β-substituent	β-C—X	*Tryptophanase*
	α-C—H	Tryptophan → indole + pyruvate + ammonia
		Serine deaminase
		Serine → pyruvate + ammonia + water
		Aspartate β-decarboxylase
		Aspartate → alanine + carbon dioxide
Replacement at β-carbon	β-C—X	*Tryptophan synthetase*
	α-C—H	Indole + serine → tryptophan
Reactions at γ-carbon		
Elimination of the γ-substituent	γ-C—X	*Homocysteine desulphydrylase*
	α-C—H	Homocysteine → α-oxo-butyrate + ammonia + hydrogen sulphide
Replacement at γ-carbon	γ-C—X	*Cystathionine-γ-synthetase*
	α-C—H	Succinyl homoserine + cysteine → cystathionine

40

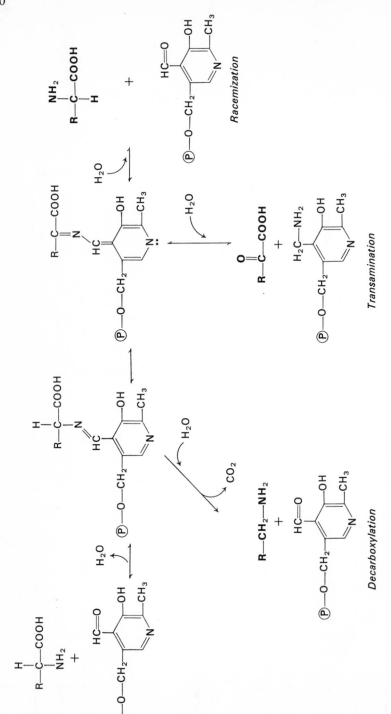

Figure 2.3. The reactions of pyridoxal phosphate with amino acids: racemization, α-decarboxylation and transamination

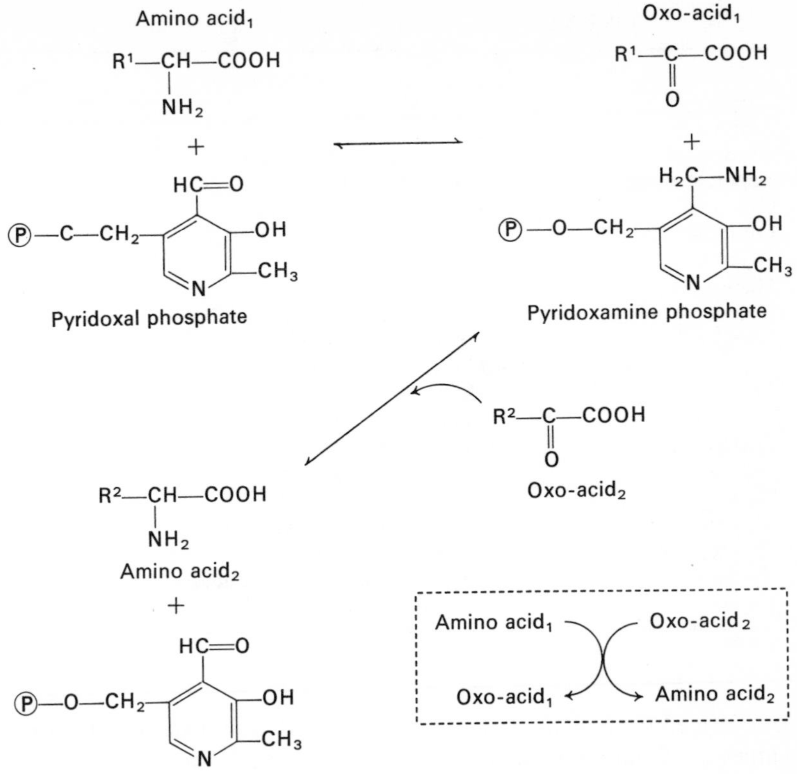

Amino acid₁

R¹—CH—COOH
|
NH₂

Oxo-acid₁

R¹—C—COOH
‖
O

+

$$\text{Amino acid}_1 + \text{Pyridoxal phosphate} \rightleftharpoons \text{Oxo-acid}_1 + \text{Pyridoxamine phosphate}$$

HC=O

(P)—C—CH₂—[ring]—OH, —CH₃, N

Pyridoxal phosphate

H₂C—NH₂

(P)—O—CH₂—[ring]—OH, —CH₃, N

Pyridoxamine phosphate

R²—C—COOH
‖
O

Oxo-acid₂

R²—CH—COOH
|
NH₂

Amino acid₂

+

HC=O

(P)—O—CH₂—[ring]—OH, —CH₃, N

Amino acid₁ ⟶ Oxo-acid₂

Oxo-acid₁ ⟶ Amino acid₂

Figure 2.4. The aminotransferase reaction

label will be recovered in the α-amino groups of all the amino acids except lysine, although the label in the α-amino group of threonine will be very much less than that in the others.

As can be seen from Table 2.2, many of the oxo-acids produced by transamination of the amino acids are common metabolic intermediates and therefore, as well as providing a pathway for degradation of surplus amino acids which is integrated with other metabolic sequences, transamination allows synthesis of many of the amino acids from intermediates of carbohydrate metabolism. Other amino acids are referred to as *essential* or indispensable; they are dietary essentials for man and most mammals (although there are differences in detail in the list of essential amino acids for some species). These amino acids have oxo-acids which cannot be synthesized by the animal concerned from any source other than the amino acid itself. For man, leucine, isoleucine, valine, threonine, lysine, methionine, phenylalanine and tryptophan are essential. In children, histidine and arginine are also essential, since, although they can be synthesized, the requirement for growth is greater than the synthetic capacity. Thus, an essential amino acid is one which cannot be synthesized, or not in sufficient quantity, by the animal or organism concerned. Tyrosine, formed from phenylalanine, and

Table 2.2. Transamination products of amino acids

Amino acid	Oxo-acid
Alanine	Pyruvic acid
Arginine	α-Oxo-γ-guanido-acetic acid
Aspartic acid	Oxaloacetic acid
Cysteine	β-Mercapto-pyruvic acid
Glutamic acid	α-Oxo-glutaric acid
Glycine	Glyoxylic acid
Histidine	Imidazole-pyruvic acid
Isoleucine	α-Oxo-β-methyl-valeric acid
Leucine	α-Oxo-isocaproic acid
(Lysine	(α-Oxo-ε-amino-caproic acid) → pipecolic acid)
Methionine	S-Methyl-β-thiol-α-oxo-propionic acid
Ornithine	Glutamic-γ-semi-aldehydre
Phenylalanine	Phenyl-pyruvic acid
Proline	γ-Hydroxy-glutamic acid
Serine	Hydroxy-pyruvic acid
Threonine	α-Oxo-β-hydroxy-butyric acid
Tryptophan	Indole-pyruvic acid
Tyrosine	p-Hydroxyphenyl-pyruvic acid
Valine	α-Oxo-isovaleric acid

cysteine, formed from methionine, are not essential amino acids, but since they are synthesized from essential amino acids their synthesis places a strain on the available precursor. Plants, bacteria and other micro-organisms can generally synthesize all the amino acids. However, an amino acid can be a growth factor for a bacterial mutant which has a block in the biosynthetic pathway. In this case, either the amino acid or a precursor formed after the defective stage must be provided for growth. Such mutants have been greatly used in the mapping of metabolic pathways and in bacterial genetic studies.

According to their products of catabolism, the amino acids can also be classified as glucogenic (those which give rise to intermediates of glucose synthesis), and ketogenic (those which give rise to acetyl-SCoA, and hence ketone bodies). Some, such as phenylalanine, give rise to both glucogenic and ketogenic fragments.

It has been suggested that to combat the uraemia which accompanies chronic renal failure (accounting for some 7000 deaths annually in the United Kingdom) it may be advantageous to feed the oxo-acids of the essential amino acids, so as to utilize some of the nitrogen which would otherwise have to be converted to urea. However, Walser and coworkers (1973) have shown that although the essential oxo-acids can be used by perfused rat liver to form the essential amino acids, this has no effect on the rate or amount of urea synthesized. On perfusion with an oxo-acid-rich medium, there is a fall in the perfusate glutamine, and a rise in α-oxo-glutarate. It is therefore unlikely that oxo-acid administration would be of any benefit to uraemic patients.

Table 2.3. Glutamate and aspartate aminotransferase levels in human tissue

	Enzyme activity (U/g fresh tissue)					Serum (U/1)
	Heart	Liver	Muscle	Kidney	Pancreas	
Glutamate	156	142	99	91	28	10
Aspartate	7	44	4·8	19	2	10

1 enzyme unit, U = 1 μmol of substrate converted/min under optimal conditions.

Table 2.3 shows the activities of glutamate–oxaloacetate (GOT) and glutamate–pyruvate (GPT) aminotransferases in a number of human tissues. Any increase in the serum level of either of these enzymes above about twice the normal level of 10 U/litre of each activity, indicates damage to a tissue rich in the enzyme. A high serum level of both GPT and GOT indicates liver damage, tissue necrosis allowing the enzymes to escape into the blood. A rise in GOT without so great a change in GPT indicates damage to heart, skeletal muscle or pancreas. Heart and skeletal muscle can be distinguished by the characteristic lactate dehydrogenase and creatine phosphokinase isoenzymes released in tissue damage. In acute hepatitis, serum GPT can rise to 600 U/litre, and GOT to 400 U/litre. Figure 2.5 shows the level of serum GOT after a single, moderately severe, myocardial infarct. Within 48 h of the incident, the enzyme has reached its maximum value, and then declines towards normal values. The activity at maximum reflects the severity of the infarct, and the extent of tissue necrosis. When there are repeated ischaemic episodes, the tissue level of the enzyme remains high, indicating poor prognosis.

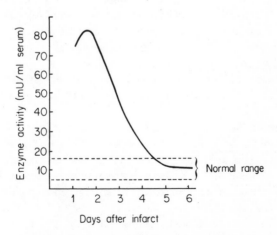

Figure 2.5. Serum glutamate–oxaloacetate aminotransferase activity after myocardial infarct

THE MECHANISM OF B_6-CATALYSED REACTIONS

It can be shown that under physiological conditions of temperature and pressure, pyridoxal will react non-enzymically with α-amino acids to form: (a) α-oxo-acids, (b) primary amines by decarboxylation and (c) the racemic mixture from an initially stereo-specific substrate, i.e. the same reactions listed above as the general reactions of pyridoxal-P enzymes with amino acids. These non-enzymic reactions have been studied as models for enzyme-catalysed pyridoxal-P dependent reactions. In a review of the structural requirements for non-enzymic and coenzymic activity of vitamin B_6 analogues, Snell (1972) noted that although the 2'-methyl and 5'-phosphorylated hydroxymethyl groups are essential for coenzyme activity, substitution at these positions has no effect on the activity of analogues in non-enzymic systems. However, the heterocyclic nitrogen, the 4'-formyl group and the phenolic hydroxyl group are all essential to both enzymic and non-enzymic reactions.

The model reactions are generally catalysed by metal ions, especially Cu^{2+}, Fe^{3+} and Al^{3+}. The initial step in the reaction is the formation of a Schiff base aldimine by condensation between the α-amino group of the amino acid and the 4'-carbonyl group of the pyridoxal, as shown in Figure 2.6. In the model systems, this intermediate is stabilized by the metal ion; it is assumed that a similar stabilization is provided by suitable charged groups in the catalytic site of the enzyme. The Schiff base chelates of copper formed at 37 °C are stable at neutral pH, and can be isolated chromatographically for spectral characterization. At pH 5·0 and below, the Schiff base tends to break down to a mixture of amino and oxo-acids, and pyridoxal and pyridoxamine.

Apart from such isolation of the Schiff base, its existence can be demonstrated by reduction with sodium borohydride, a relatively mild reducing reagent which reduces the aldimine to a secondary amine. This technique has been used to confirm the presence of a Schiff base intermediate in enzyme-catalysed pyridoxal-P reactions. Studies on the non-enzymic transamination of pyridoxal and α-amino-phenylacetic acid, catalysed by imidazole buffer rather than metal ions, have yielded spectroscopic evidence for the existence of two tautomeric forms of the Schiff base, an aldimine and a ketimine, and suggest that in non-enzymic systems the tautomerization from the initially formed aldimine to the ketimine may well be the rate limiting step.

The catalysis of non-enzymic reactions by imidazole is of interest in view of the report by Martinez-Carrion and coworkers (1967) that photo-oxidation of a pair of histidinyl residues in aspartate aminotransferase caused a loss in activity at a rate comparable with the rate of destruction of histidine, without any major configurational change in the enzyme. Therefore it is possible that in at least some pyridoxal-P enzymes there are histidinyl residues serving the function proposed for the metal ions in the model systems. There are also some metal-dependent pyridoxal-P enzymes; these presumably are somewhat closer to the mechanism proposed for the model systems. For example, aspartate decarboxylase in the lobster (but not in most other animal species) has an absolute requirement for

Mg^{2+} or Mn^{2+}, and pig kidney diamine oxidase is not, as might be expected, a flavo-protein, but is linked to pyridoxal-*P*, and has an absolute requirement for Cu^{2+} for maximum activity.

The tautomerization of the Schiff base aldimine in the model systems is visualized as occurring as shown in Figure 2.6. The electron-withdrawing effect of the heterocyclic nitrogen results in a withdrawal of electrons from all three of the bonds about the α-carbon (not the α-carbon–amino bond), but especially from the α-carbon–hydrogen bond, resulting in deprotonization of the aldimine, and tautomerization to the ketimine.

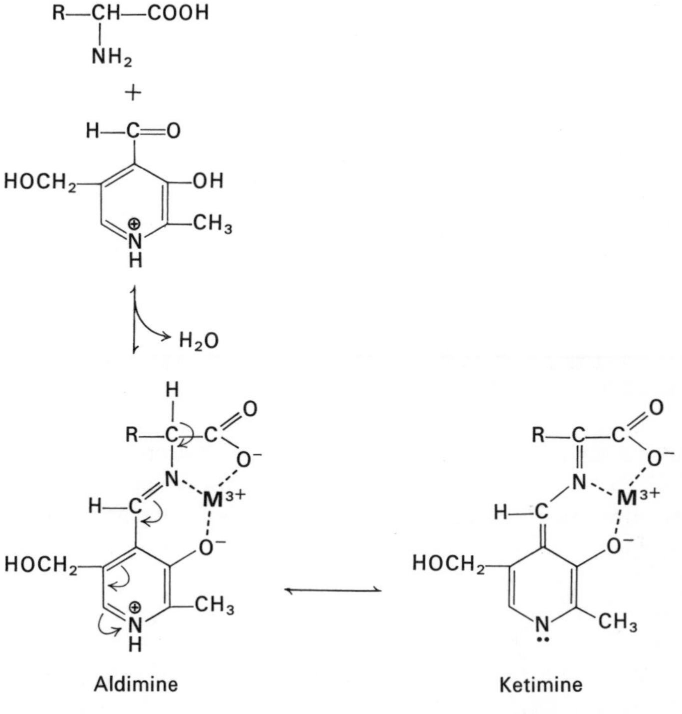

Figure 2.6. Tautomerization of the pyridoxal–amino acid Schiff base

Reprotonation of the now-symmetrical α-carbon at the site of deprotonation will result in the reverse tautomerization, and by reversing the whole sequence in Figure 2.6 will give racemization of the original amino acid.

Reprotonation of the ketimine at the 4′-carbon of the pyridoxal moiety followed by hydrolysis, results in cleavage of the α-carbon–amino bond, aminating the pyridoxal to pyridoxamine and releasing the oxo-acid, the half reaction of transamination, as shown in Figure 2.7. This pyridoxamine can then react with another oxo-acid in the reverse of the reaction sequences of Figures 2.7 and 2.6 to give the full transamination reaction.

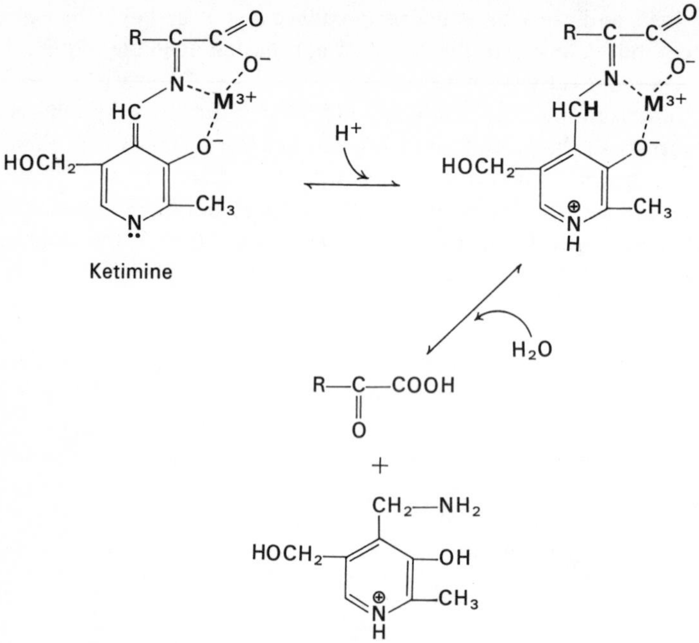

Figure 2.7. Reaction of the Schiff base ketimine to yield pyridoxamine and α-oxo-acid

The mechanism of decarboxylation is simpler. The electron shifts in the Schiff-base aldimine do not withdraw electrons from the α-carbon–hydrogen bond as in tautomerization, but from the α-carbon–carboxyl bond, releasing carbon dioxide. Hydrolysis then yields the primary amine and pyridoxal, as shown in Figure 2.8.

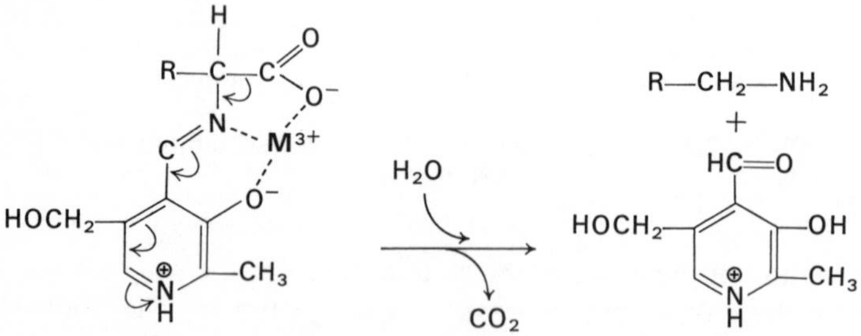

Figure 2.8. Decarboxylation of the Schiff base

The aldimine can also undergo removal of the side chain of the amino acid as in the threonine aldolase and serine hydroxymethyl transferase reactions. Instead of electrons being withdrawn from the α-carbon–carbonyl bond, as in decarboxylation, or the α-carbon–hydrogen bond as in tautomerization, they are withdrawn from the α-carbon–side-chain bond. Threonine aldolase removes the side chain as acetaldehyde, but serine hydroxymethyl transferase uses tetrahydrofolic acid as acceptor for the formyl group removed, forming N^5-formyl-tetrahydrofolate. The final product on hydrolysis of the residual Schiff base is glycine in both cases. There is considerable evidence that at least in mammalian liver these two reactions may be catalysed by the same enzyme, although in some organisms the two activities can be shown to be associated with separate proteins (see page 60).

Two other, less general, reactions of the Schiff base are the elimination reactions, an α-β elimination in the deamination of serine and threonine, and a β-γ elimination in the desulphuration of homocysteine. The deamination of serine is shown in Figure 2.9. The lone pair of electrons on the heterocyclic nitrogen of the ketimine migrates into the ring, and in the resulting electron shifts a hydroxyl ion is eliminated from the β-carbon of serine. Hydrolysis of the intermediate aldimine yields pyridoxal and α-amino acrylic acid, which spontaneously hydrolyses to pyruvate and ammonia. The deamination of threonine follows the same pathway, with the eventual production of α-oxo-butyrate.

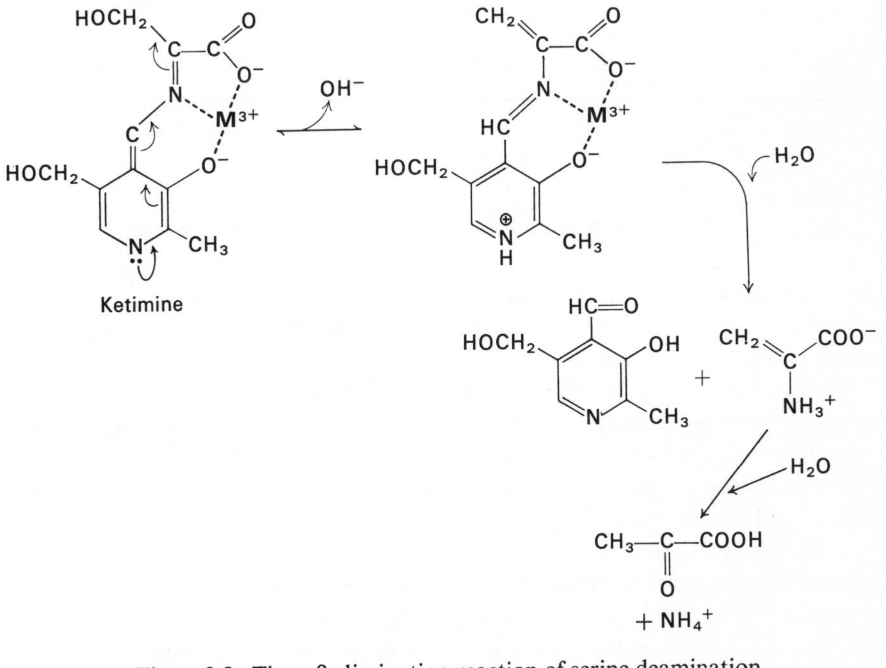

Figure 2.9. The α-β elimination reaction of serine deamination

The α-β unsaturated intermediate in the serine deamination reaction can undergo, instead of hydrolysis, nucleophilic attack by indole followed by tautomerization of the immediate addition product to an aldimine, which is then hydrolysed to tryptophan and pyridoxal. This is the tryptophan synthetase reaction. The

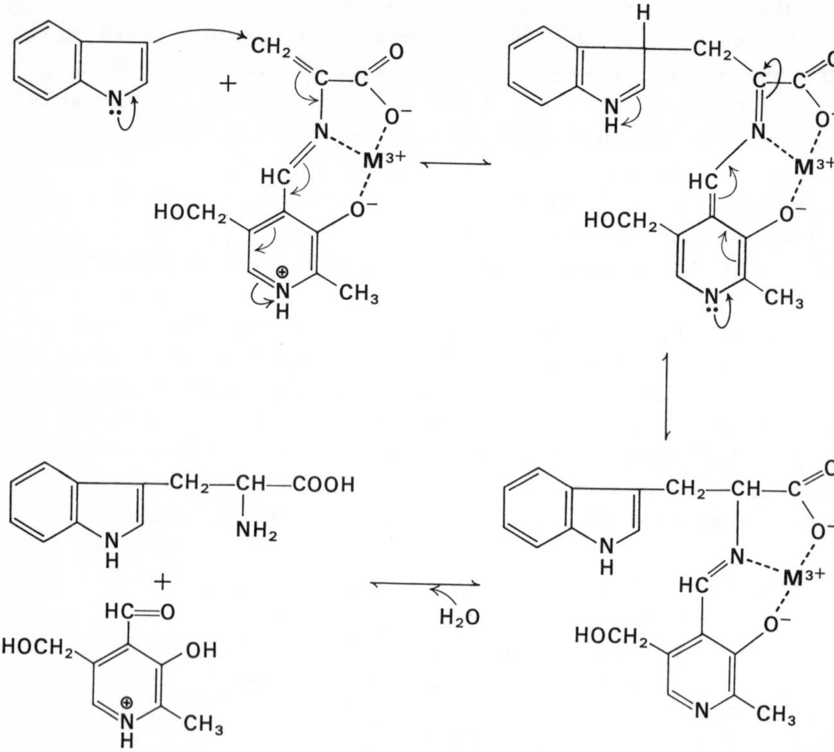

Figure 2.10. The synthesis of tryptophan from indole and serine

reverse reaction sequence is catalysed by a bacterial enzyme, tryptophanase, which cleaves tryptophan to give indole and serine. The tryptophan synthetase reaction is shown in Figure 2.10.

The β-γ elimination in the desulphuration of homocysteine is considerably more complex mechanistically; the Schiff base undergoes two tautomerizations before the elimination of hydrogen sulphide. This is followed by a further tautomerization before hydrolysis releases pyridoxal and an α-β unsaturated amino acid which spontaneously hydrolyses to ammonia and α-oxo-butyrate. An outline of this reaction sequence is shown in Figure 2.11.

Homocysteine can be shown to inhibit a number of pyridoxal-*P* dependent enzymes; the mechanism of this inhibition has been studied by Pestaña and co-workers (1971), using rat liver serine deaminase. Homocysteine inhibits the enzyme in a time-dependent process which is competitive with respect to pyridoxal-*P* but not serine. The homocysteine–pyridoxal-*P* Schiff base formed has no catalytic activity, but since it does not inhibit the recombination of the apoenzyme with pyridoxal-*P*, it presumably does not bind to the enzyme. The inhibition of a number of pyridoxal-*P* dependent enzymes by such cofactor blockage may be important in the symptomatology of homocystinuria, when

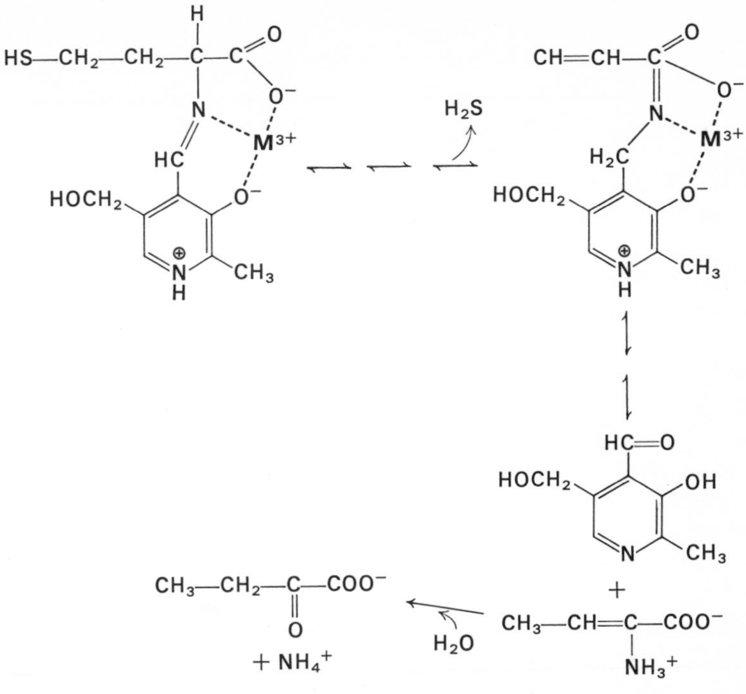

Figure 2.11. The desulphuration of homocysteine

blood levels of homocysteine and homocystine are extremely high. Increased dietary vitamin B_6 might then be indicated.

The non-enzymic model reactions differ from enzyme-catalysed reaction of pyridoxal-P with amino acids in three major respects:

(a) The enzymic reactions proceed at a very much greater rate than do the model reactions: aspartate aminotransferase has been estimated to form oxalo-acetic acid from aspartate about 10^6 times faster than the non-enzymic system. The rate constant for formation of the substrate–pyridoxal-P Schiff base is considerably faster in the enzymic systems than in the models, so the enzyme must catalyse formation of this intermediate, as well as later stages in the reaction.

(b) The enzyme reactions show a great deal of substrate specificity, as would be expected, while the model systems are almost wholly non-specific.

(c) The enzyme systems display a great deal of specificity for the reaction followed, while the model systems do not. Any amino acid reacted in a non-enzymic system with pyridoxal will undergo mixed decarboxylation, deamination and racemization, and if the substrates are suitable there may also be elimination reactions, or even non-enzymic synthesis of tryptophan. In contrast, the enzyme reactions in general follow only a single pathway, yielding almost entirely a single predictable product. An exception here is bacterial aspartate β-decarboxy-lase, which converts aspartate to alanine in a pyridoxal-P dependent reaction.

The enzyme gradually loses activity in a prolonged incubation with aspartate and activity can be restored by addition of either fresh pyridoxal-P or a suitable α-oxo-acid. Addition of radioactive pyruvate or α-oxo-glutarate to the incubation mixture results in the formation of labelled alanine or glutamate. It is thought that as well as β-decarboxylation, some of the aspartate undergoes deamination. The β-decarboxylation proceeds through a ketimine intermediate, so this is possible. The resulting pyridoxamine-P is catalytically inactive, and must either be displaced by fresh pyridoxal-P or deaminated by addition of an excess of a suitable amino acceptor.

The general reaction specificity of the enzyme systems is probably due to the maintenance of rigid geometry of the Schiff base at the catalytic site. Delocalization of the π-electrons of the Schiff base will facilitate bond cleavage only when the bond to be broken is perpendicular to the plane of the pyridoxylidine conjugated system. Therefore the geometry in which the Schiff base is bound to the enzyme will determine which bond about the α-carbon will be broken, and hence which reaction will be followed. This geometry will in turn be determined by the binding of the α-carboxyl group of the substrate as well as the binding in the aldimine of the side chain and amino group. Consistent with this is the observation that α-decarboxylases, in which the α-carboxyl group must be perpendicular to the conjugated system, display the greatest reaction specificity, and the least ability to distinguish between the D- and L-stereoisomers of the substrate. Aldolases acting on L-amino acids also show a slight aminotransferase activity towards the corresponding D-amino acid. Such steric factors will not apply in non-enzymic systems where free rotation about the α-carbon-α-amino bond of the aldimine is possible, enabling any of the other three bonds to lie perpendicular to the plane of the delocalized system.

ENZYME–COENZYME INTERACTIONS

Resolution of pyridoxamine-P containing enzymes is generally relatively simple, but removal of the cofactor from pyridoxal-P containing enzymes is more difficult. Even prolonged dialysis will remove only a small amount of the cofactor, and such activity as is lost is frequently not restored on addition of fresh pyridoxal-P, indicating that it may be due to protein denaturation rather than simply to loss of cofactor. Methods that are successful in removal of the cofactor are generally those which involve some distortion of the protein structure, such as prolonged dialysis against detergents, electrophoresis, ammonium sulphate treatment, or the action of EDTA or other metal chelating agents. There is no evidence that the action of chelating agents is due to removal of metal ions, since, with the few exceptions noted above, pyridoxal-P enzymes do not contain any metals. Rather it seems to be due to a protein deforming effect of the reagent itself.

Just as resolution of pyridoxal-P enzymes is difficult, so reconstitution of apo-pyridoxal-P enzymes is a slow process, frequently involving conformational changes in the enzyme, and with some multi-subunit enzymes there may even be a change in quaternary structure. Tryptophanase from *Bacillus alvei* contains two molecules of pyridoxal-*P* with dissociation constants (measured for reconstitution of the holoenzyme) of 1·14 and 14·4 μM respectively. The apoenzyme dissociates into subunits and it has been proposed that one of the two pyridoxal-*P* molecules has a purely structural role, while the other functions catalytically. A similar structural role has been proposed for the pyridoxal-*P* associated with glycogen phosphorylase: it has no obvious coenzyme role and sodium borohydride reduction has no effect on the activity of the enzyme. However, on removal of the pyridoxal-*P*, the apoenzyme dissociates into a number of inactive subunits. Therefore it is assumed that the role of pyridoxal-*P* in this enzyme is to maintain the quaternary structure. As much as 50% of the total body reserves of vitamin B_6 may be in muscle glycogen phosphorylase, and in avitaminosis B_6 there appears to be a release of this stored pyridoxal-*P*. Muscle phosphorylase activity falls to about 35% of the control value, parallel with the fall in muscle total vitamin B_6 content (Krebs and Fischer, 1964).

It can readily be shown that the phosphate group of pyridoxal-*P* and pyridoxamine-*P* is involved in the binding of the cofactor to the enzyme. High concentrations of inorganic phosphate will inhibit the reconstitution of many apoenzymes and this may frequently be a source of error when restoration of activity to apo-tyrosine decarboxylase is used as an assay for pyridoxal-*P*, as it frequently is, using phosphate buffers. Similarly, oestradiol and stilboestrol phosphate esters compete with pyridoxal-*P* in recombination of aspartate and kynurenine aminotransferases, although they have no effect on the holoenzymes. Pyridoxal-5′-sulphate will act as a satisfactory cofactor for bacterial tryptophanase and arginine decarboxylase, but not for a number of other enzymes that have been tested, suggesting that in general the di-anionic phosphate group is essential for binding.

There is evidence that the 2′-methyl group of pyridoxal-*P* is also bound to the enzyme, probably hydrophobically. When either other alkyl groups or hydrogen are substituted at the 2′-position there are changes in the catalytic activity, binding characteristics and circular dichroism of the resultant holoenzyme. However 2-*nor*-pyridoxal-*P*, with hydrogen at the 2′-position, will bind strongly to aspartate aminotransferase to yield an active holoenzyme. It has been proposed (Ivanov and Karpeisky, 1969) that the heterocyclic nitrogen of the cofactor is also bound to the protein, probably to a proton-donating group, on the basis of the observed lowering of the pK_a of the enzyme-bound aldimine compared with the free aldimine. A suitable group for this purpose would be a tyrosyl residue and it has been shown that there is a tyrosyl residue which is ionized in holo-aspartate aminotransferase, but not in the apoenzyme. The 3′-hydroxyl group of the coenzyme does not appear to be involved in binding. 3-Methoxy-pyridoxal-*P* will apparently reconstitute apoenzymes satisfactorily, but the holoenzyme formed is catalytically inactive, suggesting that the hydroxyl group has a catalytic role, as shown above in the model reactions.

The major difference between the model systems and enzyme-catalysed pyridoxal-*P* reactions is that in enzymes the 4′-carbonyl group of the cofactor is not free, but is bound in a Schiff base to an amino group in the protein. It is the formation of this internal (enzyme–coenzyme) aldimine which is thought to explain the relatively slow recombination of apoenzymes with pyridoxal-P. It also explains why aminotransferases are so much more readily resolved in the pyridoxamine than the pyridoxal form, since pyridoxamine cannot form such a covalent linkage to the enzyme, but will be bound only by ionic (phosphate), hydrophobic (2′-methyl) and hydrogen bond (heterocyclic nitrogen) linkages, as noted above.

Reduction of pyridoxal-P holoenzymes with sodium borohydride shows that the internal aldimine is to the ε-amino group of a lysyl residue in the protein in all cases which have been examined to date. The peptide sequence in which this lysyl residue occurs has been termed the *pyridoxyl peptide*. Studies on the pyridoxyl peptide from the β-chain of tryptophan synthetase of *E. coli* and *Pseudomonas putida* have shown that 14 of the 23 amino acids of the peptide are the same in the two bacteria, and most of the remaining changes are conservative (Maurer and Crawford, 1971). This close similarity between the amino acid sequences of the pyridoxyl peptides of these two enzymes is especially impressive since they are otherwise very different, with different total amino acid compositions, and showing no immunological cross-reactivity. Partial amino acid sequences in four other bacterial pyridoxal-P enzymes show that either lysine (in tryptophanase) or histidine (in glutamate decarboxylase and tryptophan synthetase from *E. coli* and *Ps. putida*) is immediately adjacent to the pyridoxyl-lysine on the amino side. In all four cases there are several amino acids with small side-chains to the amino side of this basic group, and amino acids with hydrophobic side-chains predominate to the carboxyl side of the lysyl residue.

The formation of the internal aldimine explains not only the more rapid formation of the coenzyme–substrate aldimine, but also the observation that the reaction of alanine racemase in tritiated water gives only 2·7 % of the theoretical incorporation of label into the product. While this might be explained as an isotope effect, it is more probable that although the formation of the coenzyme–substrate Schiff base in the model systems is a condensation, with elimination of water, this is not so when the pyridoxal-P is already bound in an internal aldimine. It is believed that the internal Schiff base is not hydrolysed to allow the pyridoxal-P to react with the substrate, but rather that the substrate directly displaces the lysyl side-chain from the aldehyde. This process has been termed *transaldimination* or trans-Schiffization. At the termination of the reaction the lysyl residue of the protein displaces the products from the cofactor, again a direct interaction, so that the process is not a direct hydrolysis and no incorporation of label from tritiated water would be expected, apart from that incorporated by ionization of the lysyl side-chain.

STAGES OF THE ASPARTATE AMINOTRANSFERASE REACTION

Ivanov and Karpeisky (1969) have proposed a three-dimensional model for the enzymic transamination of aspartate. Initially, the cofactor is bound to the enzyme at four points: the internal aldimine at the 4'-carbonyl group, and interactions with the heterocyclic nitrogen, phosphate and methyl groups, The stages of the reaction are then envisaged as follows:

(a) A non-covalent binding of the substrate amino acid to the enzyme, which is probably electrostatic. At physiological pH both the amino and carboxyl groups would be ionized.

(b) The substrate amino acid then nucleophilically attacks the internal aldimine at the C=N bond. To acquire nucleophilicity, the substrate amino acid would have to be deprotonated. This is visualized as the role of the phenolic hydroxyl group of the cofactor, which, especially if protein-bound, would be partially ionized and would therefore carry some negative charge. This group would then form a dative bond with the imino nitrogen of the internal aldimine, increasing its electrophilicity and so enhancing the nucleophilic attack by the substrate.

(c) Once formed, this coenzyme–substrate aldimine loses a proton from the α-carbon, a process which is base catalysed, possibly by the unprotonated ε-amino group of the lysyl residue which was involved in the original internal aldimine. At this stage the multi-point attachment of the cofactor to the enzyme is important in maintaining a rigid geometry as the cofactor ring rotates about its C_2–C_5 axis to bring the reacting region of the aldimine into juxtaposition with the groups in the protein which catalyse the various stages.

(d) The deprotonated aldimine is then reprotonated at carbon-4, to form the pyridoxamine-P ketimine. This proton is believed to be donated by a histidinyl residue in the protein. Hydrolysis of this complex gives the free oxo-acid (oxaloacetate) and enzyme-bound pyridoxamine-P.

NON-PYRIDOXAL-P CATALYSED BACTERIAL AMINO ACID DECARBOXYLASES

Histidine decarboxylase from *Lactobacillus* 30a does not contain any pyridoxal-P. The purified enzyme has no visible spectrum, undergoes no spectral shift when pyridoxal-P is added (although such a shift is observed when the cofactor is added to any pyridoxal-P-dependent apoenzyme), and the addition of pyridoxal-P has no effect on the activity of the enzyme.

Recsei and Snell (1970) showed that on reduction of this *Lactobacillus* enzyme with sodium borohydride in the presence of [^{14}C]histidine, there was an incorporation of radioactivity into the protein fraction as is observed with pyridoxal-P enzymes. On hydrolysis the label was present in the form of N^1-(1-carboxy-ethyl)-histidine, and the corresponding histamine derivative. When the reaction was performed in the presence of [^{14}C]histamine, the label was found only in N-carboxy-ethyl-histamine. It therefore appears that the reaction in this enzyme proceeds by combination of histidine with pyruvate in a Schiff base complex similar to that formed by pyridoxal-P-dependent enzymes. It had previously been shown that the enzyme contains five pyruvoyl residues (in the form of pyruvoyl-phenylalanine) in five of the ten polypeptide chains of the native enzyme. To date it has not been possible to separate the two types of subunit of this enzyme and reconstitute an active polymer, nor have the isolated subunits been shown to have any enzymic activity.

Riley and Snell (1970) examined the origin of the pyruvate in this enzyme by growing the bacteria in a chemically defined medium containing radioactive serine. They showed that the specific activity of the pyruvate incorporated into the protein was the same as that of serine, both in the medium and incorporated into the protein, while the specific activity of lactate and pyruvate in the medium was less than 0·01 % of that of serine. This demonstrated that the pyruvoyl residue of the protein does not arise from the intra-cellular pool of pyruvate and lactate formed from glucose but must arise from serine, possibly being incorporated as serine and subsequently undergoing deamination.

While unusual, this histidine decarboxylase from *Lactobacillus* 30a is not unique; the same enzyme from *Micrococcus* species, and several bacterial *S*-adenosyl methionine decarboxylases also contain pyruvoyl residues, serving the same function as does pyridoxal-*P* in most similar enzymes. To date, no mammalian enzyme has been demonstrated as having such a prosthetic group. In *Clostridium* SB4, the enzyme responsible for the biosynthesis of β-lysine by amino migration normally uses α-oxo-glutarate as cofactor, although in this case pyridoxal-*P* can be substituted *in vitro*.

AMINO ACID RACEMASES

It was noted above that racemization of the substrate amino acid can occur by hydrolysis of the substrate–pyridoxal-*P* Schiff base. However, while some of the bacterial amino acid racemases do appear to act in this way, in many there is evidence that as well as pyridoxal-*P* the enzyme contains a flavin. This suggests that a probable mechanism involves α-β unsaturation of the aldimine to yield a symmetrical intermediate. Reprotonation of this would yield either stereo-isomer.

In general, amino acid racemases are highly substrate specific, apart from the broad specificity racemase isolated from pseudomonads. Therefore glutamate racemase from *Lactobacillus fermentii* will not act on aspartate or alanine, and the ATP-dependent phenylalanine racemase from *Bacillus brevis* does not act on any other aromatic or neutral amino acid. This ATP-dependent racemase appears to be involved in synthesis of the peptide antibiotic Gramicidin S, and serves both to racemize phenylalanine and to activate the D-amino acid for peptide incorporation. The reaction is thought to proceed by way of formation of phenylalanyl-AMP, and the D-derivative is incorporated directly, consequently little free D-phenylalanine is normally found *in vivo* in this organism. Such a racemization and activation for incorporation catalysed by a single enzyme would explain why, in several bacterial peptide synthesizing systems where there is a D-amino acid in the peptide, the L-stereoisomer is a considerably better precursor of the peptide-bound D-amino acid than is the free D-amino acid.

In mammalian systems, there is little or no evidence of the presence of amino acid racemases, yet D-amino acids can not only be degraded, but frequently the label from radioactive D-amino acid can be recovered in proteins and other cell constituents. While some of this utilization of D-amino acids may be due to racemization by intestinal bacteria, it is probable that a considerable amount is endogenous; the symmetrical oxo-acid formed by D-amino acid oxidase activity can readily be transaminated, in a stereo-specific reaction, to the L-amino acid.

REGULATION OF THE *IN VIVO* ACTIVITY OF PYRIDOXAL-*P*-DEPENDENT ENZYMES

As with all other enzymes, the activity of pyridoxal-*P*-dependent enzymes *in vivo* can be controlled by regulation of the synthesis and degradation of the enzyme protein. However, the availability of cofactor, and the relative affinity of the apoenzyme for the cofactor also affect the activity. A number of enzymes appear to be always fully saturated with pyridoxal-*P*, and to show the same activity on assay *in vitro* whether additional cofactor is present in the incubation medium or not: examples are rat and rabbit liver cysteine sulphinic acid decarboxylase and mammalian liver and brain glutamate–pyruvate and glutamate–oxaloacetate aminotransferases. Other enzymes do not show their full potential activity *in vitro* unless further pyridoxal-*P* is added; examples are tyrosine decarboxylase from *S. faecalis*, diamino-pimelic acid decarboxylase from *E. coli*, and mammalian brain glutamic acid decarboxylase. For these enzymes, the percentage saturation of the apoenzyme with cofactor *in vivo* can be estimated by comparing the activity *in vitro* with and without added pyridoxal-*P*. In this way it has been shown that rat brain glutamate decarboxylase is normally about 60% saturated with pyridoxal-*P*. An increase in the availability of the cofactor will increase the *in vivo* activity of these enzymes which are not normally fully saturated, while those which are normally fully saturated with cofactor will not be affected. Similarly, a fall in the availability of pyridoxal-*P* will in the first instance mainly affect those enzymes which have such a low affinity for the cofactor that even at normal levels they are not fully saturated.

Hence, in vitamin B_6 deficiency, at least in the early stages, one would not expect any change in the level of those enzymes which are normally fully saturated with cofactor, while the activity of those enzymes which are not fully saturated would be expected to fall. The results obtained by various workers are somewhat in conflict with this simplistic view.

Within a few days of feeding a vitamin B_6 free diet to experimental animals, the activity of cysteine sulphinic acid decarboxylase in the liver falls markedly, and within 2 weeks there is no detectable activity of this enzyme. Therefore, presumably, the synthesis or degradation of the enzyme is regulated to some extent by the availability of dietary vitamin B_6, and in deficiency it is 'sacrificed' for pyridoxal-*P*-dependent enzymes which are more essential to the continued well-being of the animal. In the same way, muscle glycogen phosphorylase is degraded, releasing large amounts of pyridoxal-*P*. Liver cystathionase also falls, but can be restored by incubation in the presence of added pyridoxal-*P*, i.e. the apoenzyme has remained at the normal level, but the degree of cofactor saturation is lower than normal.

Bayoumi and coworkers (1972) have shown that in neonate rats from dams fed on a vitamin B_6 deficient diet, the activity of glutamate decarboxylase in the brain is very low, as would be expected. However, *in vitro* incubation in the presence of additional pyridoxal-*P* shows that the amount of apoenzyme is several times the normal level. The response to avitaminosis here appears to be the induction of massive synthesis of the enzyme protein to ensure that as much pyridoxal-*P* as possible is sequestered by the brain decarboxylase. The product of glutamate decarboxylation, γ-aminobutyric acid, is a neurotransmitter, and its continued production is obviously essential to the well-being of the animal. Under the same conditions, the activity of brain DOPA decarboxylase, the enzyme responsible for the formation of dopamine (and hence noradrenaline) and serotonin, also essential as neurotransmitters, is unchanged. DOPA decarboxylase is normally fully saturated with cofactor and appears to be present in the brain in greater amounts than needed, certainly the decarboxylation step is not rate-limiting in the synthesis of these amines.

Injection of massive doses of vitamin B_6 into rats not only increases the percentage saturation of brain glutamate decarboxylase and other enzymes which are not normally fully saturated with cofactor, but also greatly increases the activity of liver tyrosine aminotransferase. This increase in activity is due not only to an increase in the percentage saturation of the apoenzyme with pyridoxal-*P*, but also to increased synthesis of new apoenzyme. The response can be blocked with protein synthesis inhibitors.

Apart from redistribution of pyridoxal-*P* from less essential to more essential enzymes in vitamin B_6 deficiency, there is evidence that factors which induce the synthesis of pyridoxal-*P*-dependent enzymes may also cause a redistribution of the vitamin between enzymes. Thus, Lefauconnier and coworkers (1973) have shown that administration of cortisone over a prolonged period leads to an increase in the activity of liver tyrosine and alanine aminotransferases, and serine deaminase, without any increase in the total liver pool of vitamin B_6. They also showed, as this observation would require, that there is a fall in the activities of homoserine dehydratase and cysteine sulphinic acid decarboxylase, both of which enzymes are known to lose their activity readily under conditions of deficiency.

Katunuma and coworkers (1971a) showed that in the small intestine and skeletal muscle of the rat there is a specific protease which degrades the apoenzymes of a number of pyridoxal-*P*-dependent enzymes. This enzyme did not react with any of a number of non-pyridoxal-*P*-dependent enzymes tested, and it did not attack the holoenzymes of the apoenzymes which were substrates. Katunuma *et al.* also showed that the activity of the enzyme increased 10–20-fold in vitamin B_6 deficiency. In a later paper (Afting *et al.*, 1972), they demonstrated that a similar enzyme from yeast was equally active in degrading apo-ornithine decarboxylase from yeast or rat liver, suggesting that the 'inactivase' was not species specific, but rather that it sought out the amino-acid sequence of the catalytic site of pyridoxal-P-dependent enzymes, the pyridoxyl-peptide. They proposed a two-fold role for such enzymes, both to make pyridoxal-P available for other enzymes in periods of deficiency, and to make available the amino acids from enzyme degradation during what may also be a period of general starvation. A functionally similar but distinct enzyme has been isolated from the intestine of niacin-deficient rats which degrades NAD-dependent apoenzymes (Katunuma et al., 1971b).

Thus, as well as regulation of the activity of pyridoxal-P-dependent enzymes by the availability of cofactor, and possible induction of new enzyme protein in response to variation in the supply of cofactor, it appears that in times of vitamin B_6 deficiency, apoenzymes may be specifically degraded to make their coenzymes available for more essential reactions.

VITAMIN B_6 DEPENDENCY

Vitamin B_6 deficiency is almost unknown in adult man, although there are several reports of convulsions in children due to infant formula foods deficient in the vitamin. Deficiency can be induced in experimental animals, when the symptoms include dermatitis, fatty infiltration of the liver, and, most characteristically, epileptiform convulsions. These convulsions appear to be due to a reduction in the rate of formation of γ-aminobutyrate in the brain.

There are reports of spontaneous convulsions in children that have responded to massive doses of vitamin B_6 (200–600 mg/day, compared with a recommended daily intake of 1·5–2 mg/day). Frimpter and coworkers (1969) listed a number of conditions which responded to massive doses of vitamin B_6 in the same way; they called them vitamin B_6-dependency syndromes. In general each patient showed only one of the following symptoms: B_6-dependent convulsions, B_6-responsive anaemia (due to defective haem synthesis, see page 67), xanthurenic aciduria or cystathioninuria. Had the condition been due to a generalized avitaminosis B_6 then several or all of these signs would have been expected.

Mudd (1971) has pointed out that no disease syndrome in man has been attributed to defective metabolism of vitamin B_6, and the known B_6-dependency syndromes are in any case more specific than would be expected were they due to such a metabolic failure. Xanthurenic aciduria can be attributed to a deficit of kynureninase (a pyridoxal-P-dependent enzyme, see page 172. Biopsy samples from a number of patients showed that although the unsupplemented activity of the enzyme was low, supplementation in vitro with large amounts of pyridoxal-P raised the activity to that of normal controls, in whom there was only a slight increase in kynureninase activity on assay in the presence of added cofactor. These results suggest that the dependency syndromes may be due to the presence of an abnormal enzyme in which the apoenzyme–coenzyme interaction is abnormal. Whether this is due to an altered affinity of the apoenzyme for pyridoxal-P, or to a slower rate of reaction between the two is difficult to determine. Such a mutant apoenzyme might also be less stable than the normal type, and more susceptible to degradation.

In vitamin B_6-responsive homocystinuria where cystathionine synthetase is defective, massive doses of vitamin B_6 alleviate the symptoms but do not raise the activity of the enzyme to the control level. The activity in biopsy samples from untreated patients is about 1–2% of control; after treatment this rises to about 3–4% of control, a rise which appears to be adequate for normal homocysteine metabolism. Heterozygotes for the disease, who would be expected to have levels of the enzyme intermediate between the normal and the affected subjects, can cope adequately with a test dose of methionine, suggesting that there is normally a vast excess capacity for cystathionine synthesis.

A similar condition can be seen in some bacterial mutants. A histidine-requiring strain of *Salmonella typhimurium* can synthesize adequate amounts of the amino acid if it is provided with very large amounts of pyridoxal-*P* in the growth medium. The defective enzyme is imidazole acetol phosphate aminotransferase, which does not bind pyridoxal-*P* adequately unless very large amounts are present. Synthesis of the enzyme is derepressed in this mutant, so the defect does not lie in failure to produce the enzyme, but in the production of an aberrant protein. The K_m of this mutant enzyme for its substrates is normal, but the concentration of pyridoxal-*P* required for half-maximal activity (not strictly a measure only of the affinity of the apoenzyme for the cofactor) is raised in the mutant from a normal value of 0·1 to 5 μM. The intracellular vitamin B_6 level in this mutant is normal. (Henderson and Snell, 1971). Other pyridoxal-*P*-dependent enzymes in bacteria which have been observed to show a similar phenomenon include: threonine deaminase (leading to a requirement for isoleucine) in *E. coli* and *S. typhimurium* mutants, and diamino-pimelate decarboxylase (lysine-requiring strain) and phosphoserine aminotransferase (serine-requiring strain) in *E. coli*. A tryptophan-requiring strain of the mould *Neurospora crassa* similarly has a defective tryptophan synthetase which requires very high concentrations of pyridoxal-*P* for satisfactory activity.

Further reading

Adams, E. (1972). Amino acid racemases and epimerases. In *The Enzymes*, Vol. 6, pp. 479–507. Academic Press, London and New York.

Fasella, P. M. (1967). Pyridoxal phosphate. *Ann. Rev. Biochem.*, **36**, 185–210.

Fasella, P. M. and Turano, C. (1970). Functional groups of aspartate aminotransferase. *Vit. and Horm.*, **28**, 157–194.

Hammes, G. G. and Fasella, P. (1963). The mechanisms of enzymic transamination, pp. 185–196; Snell, E. E. (1963). Non-enzymic reactions of pyridoxal and their significance, pp. 1–12. *Chemical and biological aspects of pyridoxal catalysis* (Snell, E. E., Fasella, P. M., Braunstein, A. and Rossi-Fanelli, A., Eds). Pergamon Press, Oxford and New York.

References cited in the text are listed in the bibliography

CHAPTER 3

GLYCINE, SERINE, THREONINE AND THE 'ONE-CARBON' POOL

Glycine is a non-essential amino acid, readily synthesized in all organisms from common metabolic intermediates. Apart from its role in protein synthesis, it is also important as a precursor in purine, porphyrin and creatine biosynthesis, and in mammalian liver in the detoxication of foreign compounds taken in with the diet. Benzoic acid derivatives are detoxicated by conjugation with glycine to form hippuric acids which are then excreted in the urine. Although glycine is readily synthesized, it is possible, by ingesting very large amounts of benzoic acids, to outstrip the body's synthetic capacity, and so render the body dependent on exogenous sources of glycine, i.e., to make glycine an apparently essential amino acid, at least for the period of ingestion of the toxin. The enzyme phenyl-serine aldolase, which, as shown below, catalyses the cleavage of phenylserine to glycine and benzaldehyde, probably functions *in vivo* mainly in the reverse direction, forming relatively non-toxic phenylserine derivatives for excretion from dietary benzaldehydes.

Both serine and threonine have hydrophilic side-chains and therefore contribute to the hydrophilicity of proteins when they are in exposed regions of the chain. The hydroxyl groups of both are readily available for phosphorylation in many proteins, notably the enzymes which are activated or inhibited by protein kinase systems, and a number of mitochondrial and central nervous system membrane proteins.

Serine also has a role in many hydrolytic reactions catalysed by the so-called 'serine hydrolases', which have a reactive seryl residue in the catalytic site. Inactivation of these enzymes by di-isopropylfluorophosphonate (DFP) is by attachment of a di-isopropylfluoro group onto the hydroxyl group of such a reactive seryl residue; the immediate toxicity of DFP is because choline esterase, an important enzyme in the regulation of normal levels of acetyl choline at neuro-muscular junctions, is a 'serine hydrolase'.

Threonine is an essential amino acid. Its catabolism is discussed in this chapter because the pathways are similar to those involved in the degradation of serine and glycine. However, the bacterial and plant pathway for the biosynthesis of threonine is the same as that used for isoleucine synthesis, and therefore the biosynthesis of threonine is discussed in Chapter 5, together with the other amino acids derived from aspartate.

METABOLIC SOURCES OF GLYCINE

By aminotransfer

Glycine can be readily formed and degraded by transamination to or from glyoxylic acid, which can arise from the pentose phosphate pathway of carbohydrate metabolism, from isocitrate cleavage (the isocitrate lyase reaction) in organisms which have the enzymes for the glyoxylate shunt, and from the oxidation of ascorbic acid (vitamin C).

Two separate glycine aminotransferases have been identified in mammalian liver preparations, one linked to glutamate and α-oxo-glutarate and the other to alanine and pyruvate as the amino donor and acceptor. Both of these enzymes appear to function almost solely in the direction of glycine synthesis from any available glyoxylate, and not at all in the direction of glycine catabolism.

The aldolase reactions

In mammalian liver, the activity of threonine aldolase is low, and therefore the direct cleavage of threonine to glycine and acetaldehyde is probably of minor importance. However, in some bacteria (notably *C. pasteurianum*), which lack the enzymes of serine synthesis by the phosphoserine pathway, there is little surplus serine available for synthesis of glycine, and threonine aldolase cleavage is probably the major source of glycine. In these organisms, the label from [^{14}C]threonine can be recovered in both serine and glycine, so serine is probably synthesized from glycine, while in most other organisms the reaction pathway is in the reverse direction, with a net flow of carbon atoms from serine to glycine.

Although they are similar in many respects, and probably follow the same reaction pathways, threonine and phenylserine aldolases are separate enzymes in most preparations which have been examined to date. The reactions catalysed by the aldolases which give rise to glycine are shown in Figure 3.1. Threonine aldolase in most species acts more rapidly on L-allo-threonine than on L-threonine, suggesting that epimerization at the β-carbon may be an essential prerequisite for the reaction of threonine with the enzyme. This is borne out by the observation that threonine aldolase is freely reversible, and the product of the condensation of glycine and acetaldehyde is L-allo-threonine. Although in rat liver, threonine and allo-threonine aldolase activities appear to be associated with the same protein, in sheep liver they are clearly distinct; the ratio of threonine to allo-threonine activity does not remain constant through purification. Furthermore, some inhibitors affect the two activities differentially. This, however, is not necessarily evidence of the presence of separate enzymes, since separate substrate affinity sites on the same enzyme could also be differentially inhibited. In *C. pasteurianum* there is a threonine aldolase which is wholly without allo-threonine aldolase activity.

In the rat, threonine aldolase has been shown to be the same protein as serine hydroxymethyltransferase, although in sheep liver the two activities are associated with separate proteins. Serine aldol cleavage does not give rise to free formaldehyde. As well as pyridoxal-*P*, the enzyme requires tetrahydrofolic acid, and the

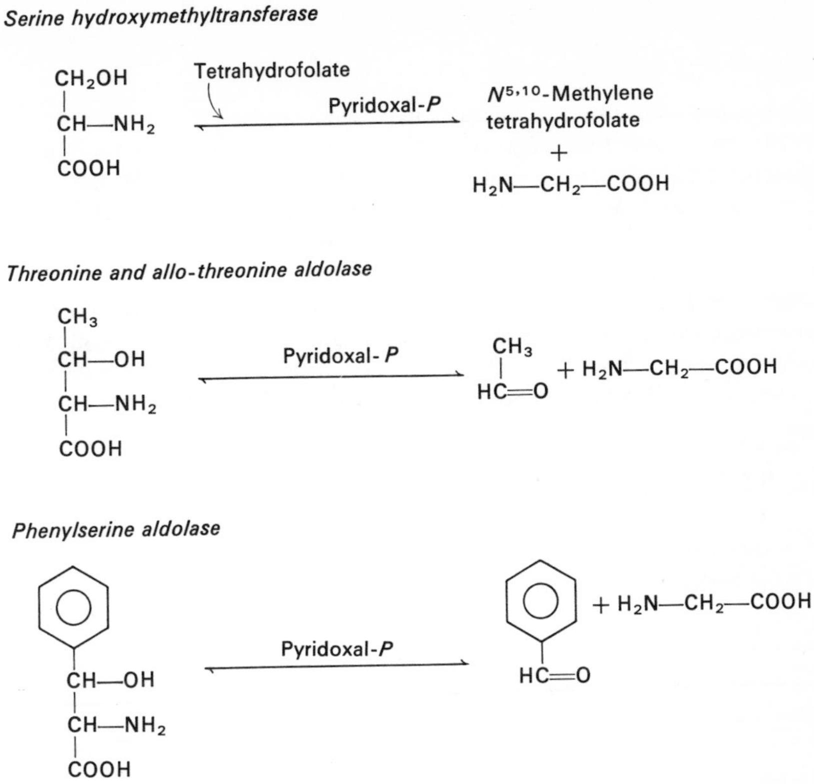

Serine hydroxymethyltransferase

Threonine and allo-threonine aldolase

Phenylserine aldolase

Figure 3.1. Aldolase reactions for glycine synthesis

product of the reaction is $N^{5,10}$-methylene tetrahydrofolate, an important intermediate in the metabolism of one-carbon compounds, as will be described below. In most species, the aldol cleavage of serine, catalysed by serine hydroxy-methyltransferase, appears to be both the major metabolic source of glycine and the major pathway of serine catabolism.

All three of these aldolase reactions to yield glycine appear to proceed by way of the same mechanism. The substrate forms a Schiff base with pyridoxal-P at the catalytic site of the enzyme, and the α-carbon-side-chain bond is cleaved by the resulting electron shifts before hydrolysis of the residual glycine–pyridoxal-P Schiff base.

Carboxylation of serine

Glycine can also arise from serine as the result of a carboxylation reaction, in which carbon dioxide and ammonia react with 1 mol of serine to yield 2 mol of glycine, This reaction is catalysed by the multi-enzyme complex known as the glycine cleavage system, described below, which requires tetrahydrofolic acid, pyridoxal-P and NAD.

THE CATABOLISM OF GLYCINE

Deamination

Although glycine aminotransferases in mammalian systems appear to function almost entirely in the direction of glycine synthesis from glyoxylate, both liver and kidney have a flavoprotein glycine oxidase which appears to be distinct from the general D- and L-amino acid oxidases. These last two enzymes generally act only very poorly on glycine. The possible metabolic fates of the glyoxylate formed by this reaction in liver are shown in Figure 3.2. Direct oxidation yields carbon dioxide and formaldehyde, and at concentrations greater than about 5 mM, xanthine oxidase can act to yield oxalic acid. Apart from its general toxicity, oxalate is involved in the formation of kidney stones. However, it is not clear whether the oxalic acid involved here is of endogenous or exogenous origin.

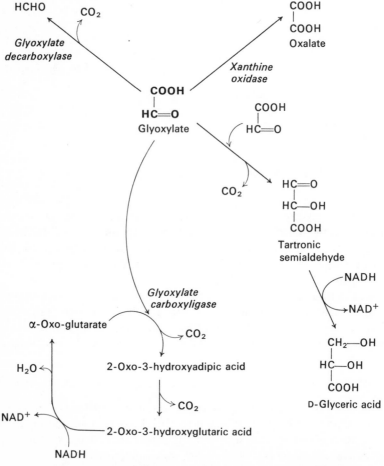

Figure 3.2. The metabolic fates of glyoxylate in mammalian liver

A condensation of two molecules of glyoxylate is catalysed by the enzyme glyoxylate carboxyligase. Carbon dioxide is eliminated in this thiamin-pyrophosphate-dependent reaction, and the resultant tartronic semialdehyde is normally reduced to D-glyceric acid. Glyoxylate carboxyligase will also catalyse the condensation of glyoxylate with α-oxo-glutarate, forming 2-oxo-3-hydroxyadipate. Again carbon dioxide is eliminated in the condensation. Oxo-hydroxyadipic acid loses carbon dioxide to yield 2-oxo-3-hydroxyglutarate, which can be reduced in an NADH-dependent reaction to α-oxo-glutarate, thus providing a cyclic pathway for the catabolism of glyoxylate. This cycle is especially active in bacteria, but is also thought to function in mammalian liver.

As noted above, glycine aminotransferase in mammalian liver appear to function mainly as a drain on the available glyoxylate, and it appears that the main mammalian pathway for glyoxylate metabolism is reamination to glycine. Thus, a combination of glycine oxidase, producing glyoxylate, and glycine aminotransferase, converting that glyoxylate back to glycine, will function as a pathway for the transdeamination of any amino acids which are linked to glutamate or alanine, the amino donors for the glycine aminotransferase reaction. Certainly if, as much of the available evidence suggests, the main function *in vivo* of glutamate dehydrogenase is in the reductive amination of α-oxo-glutarate to glutamate and not deamination, there is a clear role for a cycle such as that shown in Figure 3.3, using glycine and glyoxylate catalytically in the transdeamination of amino acids.

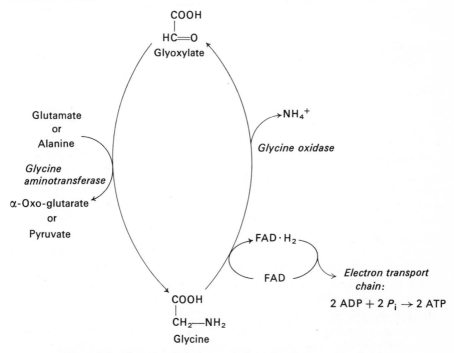

Figure 3.3. The role of glycine and glyoxylate in transdeamination

The amino-acetone pathway

Glycine can condense with acetyl-SCoA, with the elimination of carbon dioxide, to form amino-acetone. This reaction has been demonstrated in a number of bacteria, in mammalian erythrocytes and liver mitochondria. Malonyl-SCoA will also act as a substrate in this reaction; it presumably undergoes a preliminary decarboxylation to acetyl-SCoA before condensation.

Amino-acetone also arises directly from threonine in an NAD-dependent oxidation. The presumed enzyme-bound intermediate, 2-amino-3-oxo-butyrate, decarboxylates spontaneously. Although the formation of amino-acetone may be only a minor pathway of glycine catabolism, in most organisms it appears to be the major route of threonine degradation.

The catabolism of amino-acetone is shown in Figure 3.4. The deamination to methyl glyoxal (2-oxo-propanal) can occur either by aminotransfer, or by an oxidative mechanism. The oxidative reaction is believed to be catalysed by monoamine oxidase, since the clinically used monoamine oxidase inhibitors inhibit the reaction *in vitro*. In mammals and some bacteria, methyl glyoxal is then reduced directly to pyruvate. In other bacteria, the reaction proceeds through intermediate formation of D-lactate, catalysed by glyoxylase. D-Lactate can then be oxidized to pyruvate either by the action of a direct D-lactate dehydrogenase, or by the action of lactate racemase followed by the more common L-lactate dehydrogenase.

The glycine cleavage system

Glycine can undergo a direct enzymic cleavage whereby the carbon atom of the carboxyl group is released as carbon dioxide. There is almost no release of carbon dioxide from the methylene group, which is incorporated into serine by reaction with a second molecule of glycine. The reaction requires pyridoxal-P, tetrahydrofolic acid and NAD^+. In preparations from bird liver, where this reaction was first demonstrated, almost no radioactivity from glycine labelled in either carbon atom is incorporated into glyoxylate, suggesting that deamination is unimportant as a pathway for glycine catabolism in birds. The sequence of reactions involved in glycine cleavage is shown in Figure 3.5.

Yoshida and Kikuchi (1969) showed that in at least one case of hyper-glycinaemia in a human patient the primary lesion was a deficit of the glycine cleavage system in the liver. They therefore proposed that quantitatively the most important pathway of glycine catabolism in human liver was direct cleavage, releasing carbon dioxide and ammonia. The methylene group of glycine forms methylene tetrahydrofolic acid, which can react with a further molecule of glycine to form serine. This is the reverse of the serine hydroxymethyltransferase reaction shown in Figure 3.1.

It appears that in man the main pathway of serine metabolism is cleavage by the action of hydroxymethyltransferase to form glycine and methylene tetrahydrofolic acid. The glycine thus formed is further degraded, by direct cleavage, to methylene tetrahydrofolic acid, carbon dioxide and ammonia. Thus,

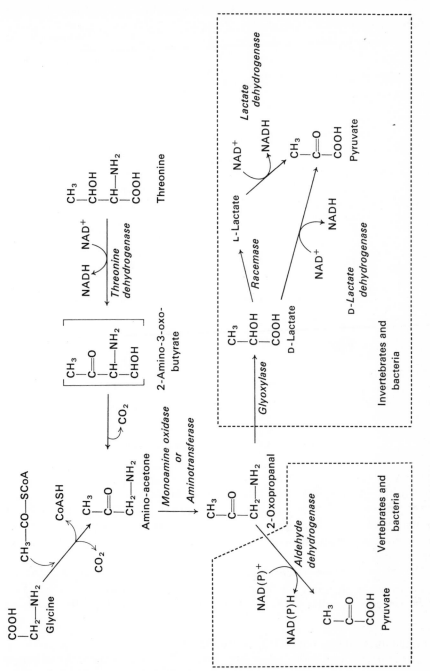

Figure 3.4. The amino-acetone pathway for glycine and threonine catabolism

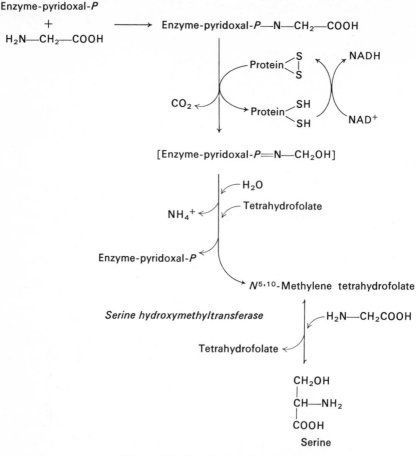

Figure 3.5. The glycine cleavage system

the net yield from 1 mol of serine catabolized in human liver is 2 mol of methylene tetrahydrofolic acid, and 1 mol each of carbon dioxide and ammonia. Although the enzymes are present in human liver, it is unlikely that there is any significant formation of serine from glycine; the major pathway appears to be the one described, the formation of glycine from serine and subsequent cleavage of that glycine.

The glycine cleavage system has been separated into two distinct components: a multi-enzyme complex, which has not been further fragmented to date, and a hydrogen carrier protein. The multi-enzyme complex catalyses the following steps:

(a) the formation of a glycine–pyridoxal-P Schiff base;

(b) A lipoamide dehydrogenase-like activity, in which a protein disulphide bridge is reduced by the Schiff base to two sulphydryl groups. The Schiff base loses carbon dioxide in this process. The disulphydryl protein then transfers the two protons to the hydrogen carrier protein, being restored to the disulphide form. The hydrogen transfer protein reacts with NAD^+;

(c) Reaction of the decarboxylated Schiff base with tetrahydrofolic acid to form methylene tetrahydrofolate.

The stages of this reaction are shown in Figure 3.5.

Both enzymes of the glycine cleavage system, and serine hydroxymethyl transferase, are associated with the inner mitochondrial membrane in rat liver. While the hydroxymethyltransferase and the hydrogen carrier protein can be solubilized readily, the multi-enzyme complex cannot.

Porphyrin synthesis

The four nitrogen atoms of the porphyrins (the tetrapyrrole pigments, including haem and the chlorophylls) all arise from glycine. The pathway of porphyrin synthesis is shown in Figure 3.6; the first step is the condensation of glycine and succinyl-SCoA to form δ-amino-laevulinic acid (δ-ALA). This reaction is catalysed by δ-ALA synthetase, a pyridoxal-*P*-dependent enzyme. The reaction is believed to proceed by way of α-amino-β-oxo-adipic acid, which then decarboxylates spontaneously to δ-ALA. It is not certain whether this intermediate occurs freely in solution, or is decarboxylated while still enzyme-bound.

Two molecules of δ-ALA condense to form porphobilinogen, a reaction catalysed by δ-ALA dehydrase. A reaction catalysed by porphobilinogen deaminase and uroporphyrinogen III cosynthetase results in the condensation of four molecules of porphobilinogen to form uroporphyrinogen III, the parent compound of the porphyrins.

There is some evidence that δ-ALA may be deaminated, by a specific δ-ALA aminotransferase, to γ-δ-di-oxovaleric acid. This intermediate can then lose its δ-carbon (that derived from the methylene carbon of glycine) to reform succinate. It is therefore possible that formation of δ-ALA, and its subsequent deamination, may represent a minor pathway of glycine catabolism. However, in most systems which have been investigated, the equilibrium of δ-ALA aminotransferase is in the direction of formation of δ-ALA from di-oxo-valerate rather than in the direction of δ-ALA degradation. This may be an important route of porphyrin synthesis in some tissues, since although the other enzymes required are widely distributed, few tissues contain δ-ALA synthetase. The aminotransferase is also widely distributed. However, those cells which synthesize large amounts of porphyrins (for example, animal reticulocytes, and the photosynthetic bacteria), have high activities of δ-ALA synthetase.

The various forms of porphyria are all associated with the excretion of large amounts of porphyrins in the urine. It is assumed that this arises because of a defect in the normal regulation of δ-ALA synthetase. Soon after barbiturates came into clinical use, it was noted that many of them caused porphyria in some patients. This appears to be mediated by additional stress on an already marginally stressed regulatory system, and thus the drug acts by precipitating a latent condition. Studies of animals with experimentally-induced porphyria have used a number of different barbiturates, but most workers now use allyl-isoprop-

68

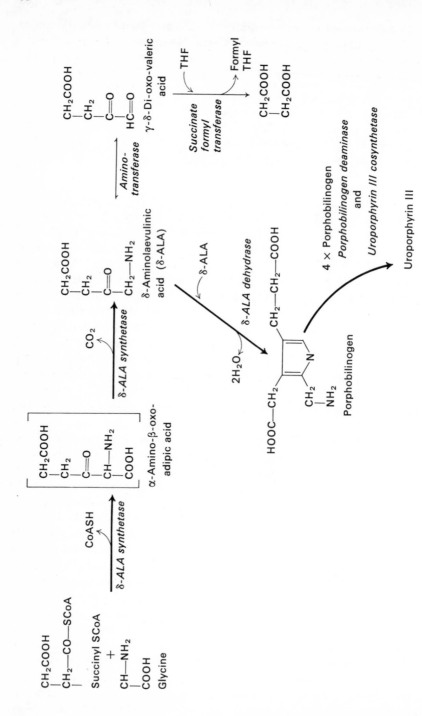

Figure 3.6. Porphyrin biosynthesis

acetamide, which does not have any sedative action. This drug acts by inducing *de novo* synthesis of δ-ALA synthetase. The induced enzyme, and its mRNA, have extremely short half lives; that for the enzyme is between 67 and 72 minutes, This suggests that control of porphyrin synthesis normally depends on very close control of the activity of δ-ALA synthetase, by *de novo* enzyme synthesis.

Although the biochemistry of the experimental drug-induced porphyrias in animals is very similar to human porphyria, the clinical picture is very different. The physical signs of porphyria, paralysis and tachycardia, are not seen in the animal model. There is no way of assessing whether the psychiatric disturbances of human porphyria are also shown by experimental animals.

THE DEAMINATION OF SERINE AND THREONINE

It was noted above that the major pathway for serine degradation under normal circumstances is through serine hydroxymethyltransferase and the glycine cleavage system. Quantitatively the most important route of threonine catabolism is the amino-acetone pathway shown in Figure 3.4, although threonine can also undergo aldol cleavage to yield glycine. Both threonine and serine can also be deaminated non-oxidatively by the serine and threonine deaminase or dehydratase reactions. In most species it is thought that a single enzyme catalyses the reaction with both substrates, and with allo-threonine the rate is about 20% of that observed with threonine. However, there is some evidence that in mammalian liver there are two separate proteins, one which is specific for threonine and allo-threonine and is inactivated by prolonged incubation with serine, and another which has a dual specificity, showing a constant ratio of serine/threonine activity of 1·4 through purification.

Two forms of serine deaminase can be separated from rat liver preparations. They differ only in that the more electronegative isoenzyme has one lysyl residue fewer, and one or two prolyl residues more than the more electropositive form. The electronegative isoenzyme is induced by glucagon administration, while the other isoenzyme is induced by glucocorticoids.

Yoshida and Kikuchi (1970) showed, mainly on kinetic grounds, that deamination was a minor pathway of serine metabolism in mammalian liver. In the rat, the K_m of serine hydroxymethyltransferase is 0·5 mM, that of serine deaminase is estimated at between 50 and 70 mM, while the normal liver concentration of serine is only 2·0–2·5 mM. It is therefore unlikely that under normal conditions a significant proportion of serine catabolism would be by way of deamination. However, as well as the induction of this enzyme by gluconeogenic hormones, as noted above, feeding a high protein diet to rats will increase the activity of serine deaminase several-fold. Thus, when there is a requirement for production of pyruvate for gluconeogenesis, serine deaminase activity is increased to overcome the barrier imposed by its relatively low affinity for the substrate.

The mechanism of the deamination of serine to pyruvate is shown in Figure 2.8; the deamination of threonine to 2-oxo-butyrate follows the same pathway. Purified serine and threonine deaminases do not show any cystathionine synthetase activity, although it was formerly believed that this was a secondary activity of the enzyme.

Bacterial threonine deaminases differ greatly from their mammalian counterparts. Two different types of primarily catabolic deaminase have been reported in different organisms, and in organisms which are capable of the synthesis of isoleucine from threonine there is a separate ('biosynthetic') threonine deaminase associated with this pathway. The biosynthetic threonine deaminases are considered on page 132, together with the biosynthesis of threonine and isoleucine.

When *E. coli* is grown in the absence of glucose, the catabolic threonine deaminase is induced by threonine or serine in the growth medium, so that the amino acids are acting as prime sources of carbon. This is akin to the induction of the mammalian deaminase under conditions where gluconeogenesis is needed. The *E. coli* enzyme is activated by 5′-AMP (and to a lesser extent also by GMP, CMP and dAMP); it is probably a key regulatory step in the anaerobic metabolism of this organism, providing oxo-acids to be reduced in the regeneration of NAD^+ from NADH. The activation by 5′-AMP is of a mixed type; the activator lowers the K_m of the enzyme for serine and threonine by a factor of about five, and at the same time increases the V_{max} about ten-fold. This activation appears to be by the formation of a dimer of the enzyme.

The other type of bacterial catabolic threonine deaminase is found in the *Clostridia*. It is stimulated by ADP but not by AMP; a ten-fold increase in substrate conversion is achieved by lowering of K_m, without any effect on V_{max}. This type of enzyme has a sigmoid substrate/velocity curve, which becomes hyperbolic in the presence of the activator, while the *E. coli* type of deaminase has a sigmoid substrate/velocity curve in the presence or absence of the activator. There is no change in the molecular weight of the clostridial enzyme on activation.

THE BIOSYNTHESIS OF SERINE

Two pathways are known for the biosynthesis of serine from intermediates of carbohydrate metabolism (D-glyceric acid and 2- and 3-phosphoglyceric acids). One produces serine directly by transamination of hydroxypyruvate, and the other, generally known as the 'phosphorylated' pathway, produces phosphoserine starting from 3-phosphoglycerate. Both pathways are found in the liver and kidney of most vertebrates, and in the mould *N. crassa*, The relative importance of the two pathways differs with species. In dog, rat and frog liver, serine is synthesized from non-phosphorylated intermediates, while in the livers of most other vertebrates, and in the kidneys and brains of all vertebrates examined, the phosphoserine pathway predominates. In most micro-organisms, the enzymes of the phosphorylated pathway are present in greater amounts, but in pseudomonads and some strains of *E. coli*, the non-phosphorylated pathway is more important.

Pseudomonas strain MA can use a variety of one-carbon compounds (methanol, methylamine and formic acid) as sole sources of carbon, initially forming serine by reversal of the hydroxymethyltransferase reaction. This serine is then either

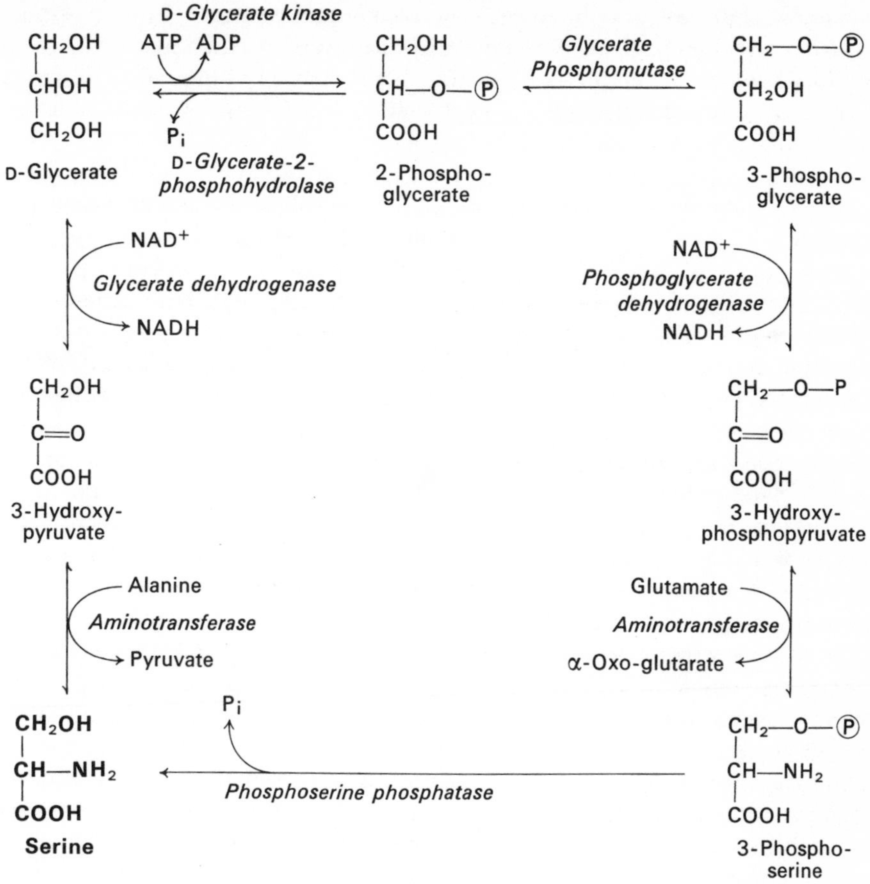

Figure 3.7. Serine biosynthetic pathways

deaminated to pyruvate, or, by reversal of the non-phosphorylated pathway of serine biosynthesis, converted to 3-phosphoglycerate. The same organism, when grown on succinate, forms serine via the phosphoserine pathway. These two pathways of serine biosynthesis are shown in Figure 3.7.

In both vertebrates and bacteria, the availability of serine controls the activity of the serine biosynthetic pathways. In mammals fed on a low-protein diet, the enzymes of the phosphoserine pathway are present in greater amounts than in animals maintained on a diet richer in protein. In bacteria, serine inhibits 3-phosphoglycerate dehydrogenase, the first enzyme unique to the serine biosynthetic pathway. Serine binds at two sites on the molecule, inducing conformational changes in the protein. This inhibition is non-competitive with respect to the immediate product, 3-phospho-hydroxypyruvate, and uncompetitive with respect to 3-phosphoglycerate and NADH. In both mammalian liver and bacteria, the equilibrium of this reaction is such that it does not favour serine synthesis, but favours the formation of phosphoglycerate from phospho-hydroxypyruvate. In *E. coli* the activity for the reverse reaction may be as much as 40 times that of the forward reaction. Thus, as well as inhibition by serine *per se*, any accumulation of serine or precursors in the (freely reversible) pathway, will lead to a rapid cessation of further phosphoglycerate utilization.

In mammalian liver, the preferred point of regulation of the phosphorylated pathway is the final step, the phosphoserine phosphatase reaction. When this enzyme is inhibited by serine, the remainder of the pathway will tend to proceed towards the resynthesis of phosphoglycerate because of the preferred position of the equilibrium of phosphoglycerate dehydrogenase. Serine appears to inhibit the phosphatase non-competitively, displacing water from the catalytic site, rather than simply by product accumulation or by an allosteric effect. Mammalian cells in culture show repression of both phosphoserine phosphatase and phosphoglycerate dehydrogenase when grown in a serine-rich medium: when the cells are cultured in a low serine medium the enzyme levels rise to normal. Although phosphoserine phosphatase will catalyse an exchange reaction between [^{14}C]serine and phosphoserine, to form some [^{14}C]phosphoserine, there is no evidence that any net phosphorylation of serine can be achieved by this enzyme so that although all steps except the last are freely reversible, the phosphorylated pathway cannot be used for the catabolism of serine.

In those systems where serine inhibits phosphoglycerate dehydrogenase, the enzyme is considerably more sensitive to D-serine than to the L-isomer. It has been suggested that the D-serine produced by the silk moth larva immediately before pupation may serve mainly as a potent inhibitor of further serine synthesis at a time when the organism will not require a great deal of *de novo* amino acid synthesis, and may well need to degrade protein for energy. The D-serine appears to be formed by racemization of L-serine, not by a separate pathway. Although serine in this insect will incorporate a significant amount of label from [^{14}C]-glucose, there is no significant incorporation of label from [^{14}C]glycine, suggesting that reversal of serine hydroxymethyltransferase is of little importance in serine synthesis.

Glyceric acid and 3-phosphoglycerate are readily interconverted; both glycerate-2-phosphomutase and glycerate kinase are found in mammalian liver in relatively large amounts. Mammalian glycerate phosphomutase requires the presence of small amounts of 2,3-diphosphoglycerate, either as a cofactor or as an intermediate in the reaction.

THE METABOLISM OF ONE-CARBON COMPOUNDS

Methylation is important in the biosynthesis of many compounds, and is also a major pathway of inactivation of many biologically active materials (for example the catecholamines, see page 167). It can be shown that if [*methyl*-^{14}C]-methionine is given to an animal, the label is recovered in the methyl groups of adrenaline, thymidine, lecithin, and many other compounds. However, under normal conditions, the dietary intake of methionine is not adequate to account for all the methyl groups introduced into metabolic products; other sources of one-carbon fragments must be used to maintain the methionine pool.

It was shown above that both serine and glycine give rise to methylene tetra-hydrofolate on degradation, and that these two amino acids are major con-tributors to the pool of one-carbon compounds in the cell used for methylation reactions. Most methyl transferases use either coenzyme B_{12} or S-adenosyl methionine (SAM) as the immediate methyl donor. There are few examples of methylation reactions using folate derivatives directly, apart from reversal of reactions which use tetrahydrofolate as a one-carbon acceptor.

Figure 3.8 shows the structure of tetrahydrofolic acid (THF). The molecule consists of a reduced pteridine nucleus linked at C-9 to p-amino-benzoic acid, which in turn is linked by peptide linkage to the α-amino group of glutamate.

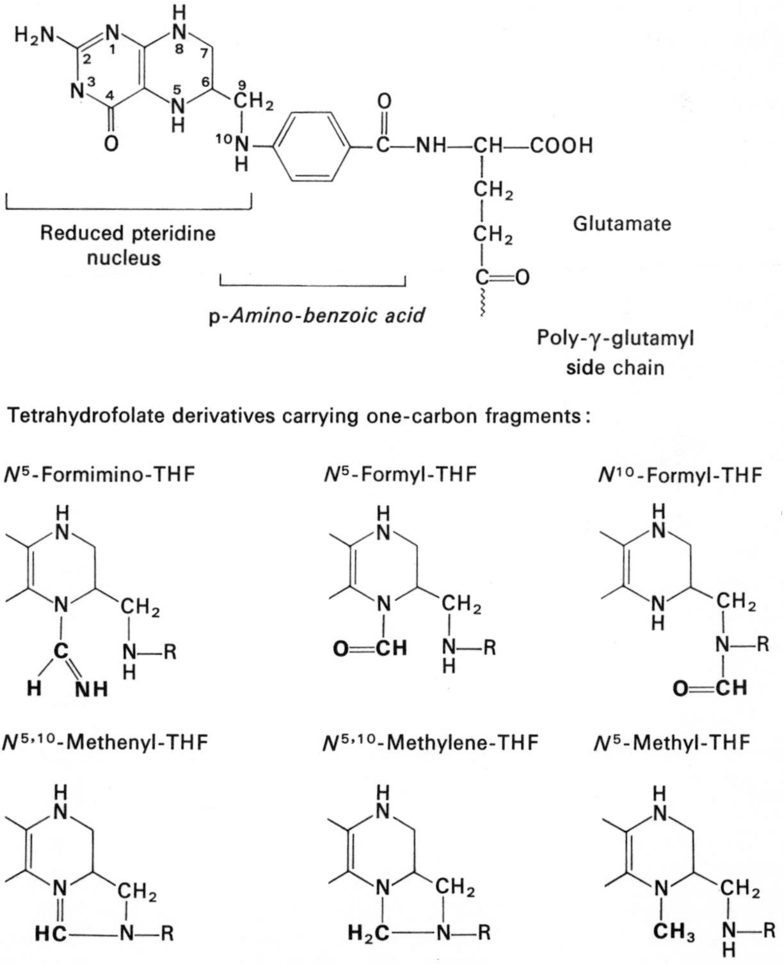

Tetrahydrofolate derivatives carrying one-carbon fragments:

Figure 3.8. Tetrahydrofolic acid

There are several poly-γ-glutamyl derivatives of this basic pteroyl-glutamate, with up to seven glutamyl residues linked to each other by γ-glutamyl peptide bonds. There appears to be little or no species dependence in the various poly-γ-glutamyl folates. Several different forms may be present in the same organism.

One-carbon fragments can be accepted at a number of different sites on THF, at the level of oxidation of formic acid, formaldehyde or methanol. At the formic acid level, formyl residues attach to THF at N-5 or N-10, to produce formyl-THF, or as a methenyl group linking N-5 and N-10. A formimino group can also attach at N-5; this is important in the catabolism of histidine (see page 148). Which of these sites of incorporation is used depends on the enzyme catalysing the transfer, but the products are readily interconvertible. Formaldehyde attaches to THF only as $N^{5,10}$-methylene-THF, and methanol adds a methyl group at N-5. It is this last derivative, N^5-methyl-THF, which is used for transfer of one-carbon units to other carriers. N^{10}-Formyl-THF is converted to N^5-formyl-THF in an ATP-dependent reaction, the other derivatives are simply reduced to the methyl level.

Methyl-THF functions primarily to methylate homocysteine to methionine, so that the role of THF in the metabolism of one-carbon compounds is one of

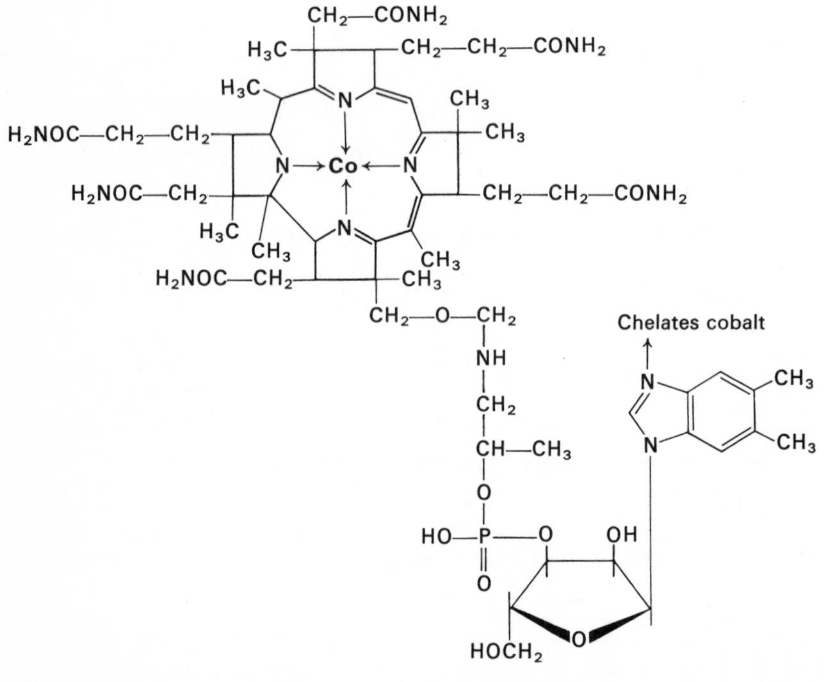

Figure 3.9. Vitamin B_{12}—cobalamin. Four chelation sites on the cobalt atom are occupied by nitrogen of the corrinoid ring. Position 5 of the cobalt is occupied by the imidazole nitrogen of the nucleotide, and the sixth position can be occupied by a methyl group (methyl cobalamin), a hydroxyl ion (hydroxo-cobalamin) or a cyanide ion (cyano-cobalamin)

collecting one-carbon fragments from a variety of reactions at several different levels of oxidation, and reducing them to the methyl level for transfer to the methyl pool, mainly represented by methionine and its S-adenosyl derivative. The methyl group of methionine is activated for methyl transfer by S-adenosylation, and formation of the sulphonium ion enhances the chemical leaving properties of the methyl group. The other common carrier of methyl groups is coenzyme B_{12}, shown in Figure 3.9. Coenzyme B_{12} is methylated by direct reaction with S-adenosyl methionine, as shown in Figure 3.10.

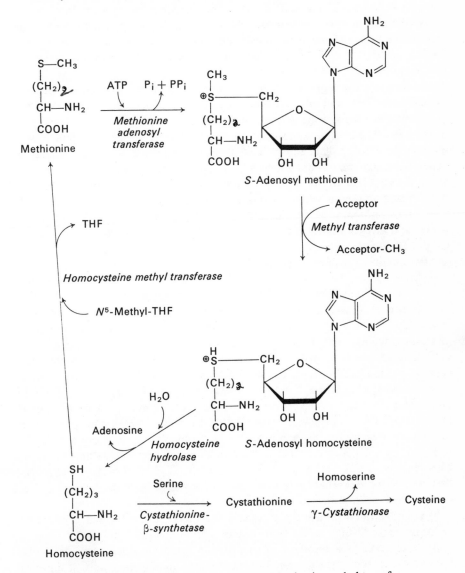

Figure 3.10. The role of S-adenosyl methionine in methyl transfer

The adenosylation of methionine is catalysed by a specific methionine S-adenosyltransferase; ATP is the adenosyl donor, and inorganic phosphate and pyrophosphate are released in the reaction. Tri-polyphosphate is thought to be an enzyme-bound intermediate, and the enzyme *in vitro* shows tri-polyphosphatase activity. The specificity of the transferase is such that while methionine and its ethyl homologue, ethionine, are substrates, the next higher and lower homologues, homomethionine and S-methyl cysteine, are not. The D-isomers of methionine and ethionine are not substrates either although the selenium analogues, seleno-methionine and seleno-ethionine, are adenosylated. Methionine adenosyltransferase is uncompetitively inhibited by its product, S-adenosyl methionine. The enzyme shows great specificity for the nucleoside donor, and apart from ATP, only UTP, to a very limited extent, and only in some systems, acts as donor.

In mammals, the highest concentration of methionine adenosyltransferase is found in the liver, and while pancreas and kidney also have moderate activity, in other tissues the specific activity of this enzyme is only about one tenth that in the liver. The enzyme appears to be repressed by androgens. In female rats the specific activity of adenosyltransferase in the liver is about twice that in males. Castrated male animals have a liver specific activity of the enzyme which is about the same as that in females, but administration of testosterone will abolish this. Presumably as a result of this greater activity of methionine adenosyltransferase, ethionine is considerably more toxic to female animals than to males, and after administration of ethionine to female rats, ethyl analogues of choline (the methylated phospholipid base) can be identified.

After methyl transfer from SAM, the resultant S-adenosyl homocysteine undergoes deadenylation to homocysteine. Homocysteine can then undergo one of two metabolic fates: it can be condensed with serine to form cystathionine (and thence by trans-sulphuration, to cysteine, see page 128) or be remethylated in a reaction which uses N^5-methyl-THF as methyl donor, and coenzyme B_{12} as an intermediate methyl carrier. In general, S-adenosyl homocysteine must be deadenylated before remethylation; there are few systems known which will catalyse the methylation of S-adenosyl-homocysteine directly to SAM. Homocysteine methyltransferase is activated by SAM; the mechanism is apparently an initial methylation of the coenzyme to methyl coenzyme B_{12}. After this initial methylation, the coenzyme is remethylated by methyl-THF. The proportion of homocysteine undergoing condensation to form cystathionine or methylation to methionine depends on the relative abundance of methionine and cysteine; when animals are fed on a cysteine-rich diet, the activity of cystathionine synthetase is reduced so that more homocysteine is converted back to methionine, the so-called methionine-sparing effect of cysteine.

In a number of bacteria and plants, S-methyl methionine is formed, accounting for as much as 40–80% of the non-protein methionine pool in some plants and appears to serve as a reservoir of one-carbon fragments for remethylation of homocysteine. It is formed from SAM and methionine, presumably at times of plentiful methionine availability, when homocysteine can be degraded rather than remethylated.

Among other methyl transfer reactions, there is one which has been associated with an enzyme so far identified only in the pituitary gland of a number of animals, which catalyses the transfer of a methyl group from SAM to water, forming methanol. This reaction thus explains the origin, although not the purpose, of the methanol which has been identified in human breath.

As well as its catalytic role in methyl transfer, methionine is a net donor of methyl groups of considerable importance in the body. It has been demonstrated that feeding a rat with large amounts of methionine leads to an increase in the hepatic pool of SAM. However, it is unlikely that this action as a net methyl donor will explain the observation of Pollin and coworkers (1961), who found that when some schizophrenic patients were given large doses of methionine they underwent a marked exacerbation of their symptoms for a period. Although this experiment has been cited as evidence for the occurrence of abnormal methylation in schizophrenia, the same authors showed that feeding comparable doses of serine or glycine, also important methyl donors, had no effect on the patients.

In man and other mammals, where folic acid is a vitamin, there is evidence that it is formylated in the process of transport across the intestine. This has been demonstrated both *in vitro*, using everted gut sacs, and *in vivo* (Perry and Chanarin, 1973). Both formyl folate and formyl-THF were found on the serosal side of gut sacs when folate was placed on the mucosal side. There is evidence that these are reduced in the liver to N^5-methyl-THF before being circulated throughout the body. The source of the formyl residues has not yet been identified.

THE PHOSPHOLIPID BASES

Phospholipids have the general structure shown in Figure 3.11. Two of the three hydroxyl groups of glycerol are esterified with fatty acids, while the third is linked, through a phosphate diester, to either a polyhydric alcohol or a nitrogenous base. The alcohols include glycerol, diglycerol (in cardiolipin, a major

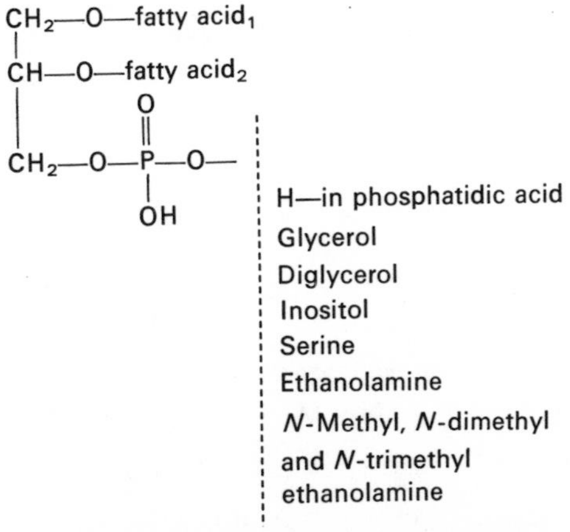

```
CH2—O—fatty acid1
|
CH—O—fatty acid2
|        O
|        ‖
CH2—O—P—O—
         |
         OH
```
H—in phosphatidic acid
Glycerol
Diglycerol
Inositol
Serine
Ethanolamine
N-Methyl, *N*-dimethyl
and *N*-trimethyl
ethanolamine

Figure 3.11. Phospholipid structure

constituent of mitochondrial membranes) and inositol, while the nitrogenous bases are derived from serine.

The precursor of phospholipid synthesis is the phosphatidic acid, where the R-group in Figure 3.11 is hydrogen. All the nitrogen-containing phospholipids are formed from phosphatidyl serine. Decarboxylation of the serine residue gives phosphatidyl ethanolamine (cephalin), and successive methylations of the amino group of cephalin give the relatively rare mono- and di-methyl derivatives, and the ubiquitous trimethyl derivative, phosphatidyl choline, or lecithin. All of these methylations use SAM as the methyl donor.

Many of the enzymes of phospholipid metabolism are mitochondrial, and have been little studied as they are not readily solubilized. The stages in lecithin catabolism have been elucidated: free choline is liberated, and is then metabolized as shown in Figure 3.12. Choline undergoes two dehydrogenations to betaine (N-trimethylglycine), which is then demethylated, the first methyl group being removed in a reaction involving direct methylation of homocysteine to

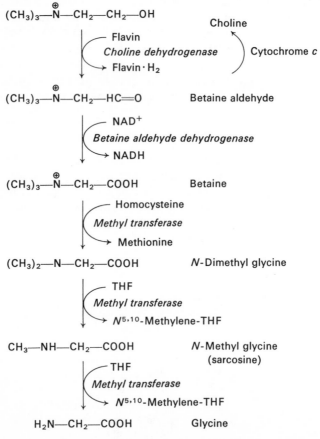

Figure 3.12. The catabolism of choline

methionine, and the remaining two in THF-dependent reactions, forming methylene-THF. Choline dehydrogenase is an unusual enzyme in that it is a flavoprotein which interacts directly with cytochrome c; *in vitro* it can also use a variety of synthetic dyes as electron acceptors.

The THF-dependent demethylations of dimethylglycine and sarcosine (methylglycine) are not direct methyl transfers; the methyl group is first oxidized to the level of formaldehyde, followed by the formation of $N^{5,10}$-methylene-THF. The two enzymes are similar but distinct. Both are flavoproteins containing non-haem iron, and both can be separated into two components, one interacting with the substrate and THF, and the other an electron-transferring flavoprotein containing FAD.

One possible effect of avitaminosis B_6 in mammals is a deficiency of serine in the brain due to reduced activity of phosphoserine aminotransferase. If this occurs *in utero* or during early life, then serious defects of myelination of the central nervous system would be expected to occur since the myelin sheath of nerves is largely nitrogen-containing phospholipid. Unlike a deficiency of the amino-acid derived neurotransmitters, which can also occur in vitamin B_6 deficiency, defective myelination is irreversible and any defect would be permanent.

Further reading

Goodwin, T. W. (Ed.) (1968). Porphyrins and related compounds. *Biochemical Society Symposia*, **28**, Academic Press, London and New York.

Greenberg, D. M. (1963). Biological methylation. *Adv. Enzymol.*, **25**, 395–432.

Lombardini, J. B. and Talalay, P. (1971). Formation, functions and regulatory importance of *S*-adenosyl methionine. *Adv. Enz. Reg.*, **9**, 349–384.

Stadtman, T. C. (1971). Vitamin B_{12}. *Science*, **171**, 859–867.

Yoshida, T. and Kikuchi, G. (1970). Major pathways of glycine and serine catabolism in rat liver. *Arch. Biochem. Biophys.*, **139**, 380–392.

Zaman, Z., Jordan, P. M. and Akhtar, M. (1973). Mechanism and stereochemistry of the δ-aminolaevulinic acid synthetase reaction. *Biochem. J.*, **135**, 257–263.

References cited in the text are listed in the bibliography

CHAPTER 4

AMINO ACIDS SYNTHESIZED FROM GLUTAMATE: PROLINE, ORNITHINE AND ARGININE

The central role of glutamate in the incorporation of inorganic nitrogen into amino acids has already been discussed on page 11. Many aminotransferases are linked to glutamate and α-oxo-glutarate, so that in many ways the α-amino group of glutamate is central to amino acid nitrogen metabolism.

Glutamine, the γ-amide of glutamate, is also important in the metabolism of ammonia, as was shown on page 15. As well as this, glutamine is a nitrogen donor in many reactions, for example, the nitrogen of amino sugars arises from glutamine, by amidotransfer to fructose-6-P.

Glutamate is also the metabolic source of the carbon skeletons of proline and the urea cycle amino acids, ornithine, citrulline and arginine.

GLUTAMINE SYNTHETASE

Glutamine is formed from glutamate by a relatively simple energy-requiring reaction, in which ammonia acts as the nitrogen donor. Because of the central role of glutamine in the control of nitrogen metabolism, especially in bacteria, glutamine synthetase is subject to careful regulation.

The enzyme from *E. coli* has been studied in some detail; it is subject to control both by induction and repression mechanisms, and by feed-back inhibition of the formed enzyme by a number of compounds which require glutamine in their synthesis. Many of the glutamine-requiring reactions of micro-organisms can use ammonia instead if there is a sufficient concentration, and when the organisms are grown on ammonia-rich media there is a considerable repression of glutamine synthetase. This is especially clear in *Bacillus* and *Saccharomyces* species, where there is an eight-fold increase in glutamine synthetase activity when the organisms are grown on ammonia-poor media. In *E. coli* this effect is less clear-cut because of interconversion of active and less active forms of the enzyme.

E. coli glutamine synthetase has a molecular weight of 592,000, and consists of 12 identical subunits, arranged as two hexamers. Removal of divalent ions from the preparation causes a 'relaxation' of the enzyme to an inactive form which is susceptible to disaggregation; manganese ions allow reaggregation and a partial restoration of activity to this relaxed form. The active (taut) form of the enzyme exists in two extreme forms: enzyme I has no covalently-bound AMP, and requires Mg^{2+} for activity, while enzyme II has 12 covalently-bound AMP residues, and requires Mn^{2+}. There are also intermediate, partially adenylated, forms of the enzyme. The fully adenylated form (II) of the enzyme has a low

V_{max}, and a pH optimum of about 6·8, while the deadenylated form has a pH optimum about 7·6, and a V_{max} four times that of form II. Under growth conditions where ammonia is a limiting factor, the glutamine synthetase is almost wholly deadenylated, while under conditions of high ammonia availability the less active, fully adenylated form of the enzyme is synthesized. Apart from regulation of synthetase activity by induction and repression, and synthesis of more or less active forms of the enzyme, there is also interconversion of the adenylated and deadenylated enzyme with changes in the culture medium. While it is known that glutamine synthetase adenylase is activated by glutamine, and inhibited by glutamate, the controls acting on the deadenylase are less clear (Stadtman et al., 1968; Shapiro and Stadtman, 1970).

As well as substrate binding sites, each of the 12 subunits of glutamine synthetase has binding sites for feed-back inhibitors. Histidine, tryptophan and CTP inhibit only the adenylated form of the enzyme, while alanine and glycine have most effect on the deadenylated form, but are also moderately inhibitory towards the adenylated form. AMP paradoxically inhibits the deadenylated enzyme, but activates the fully adenylated form.

Glutamine synthetase from all species examined can also use hydroxylamine (NH_2OH) instead of ammonia as donor, forming γ-glutamyl hydroxamate. The enzyme also catalyses a γ-glutamyl transfer, forming the hydroxamate from hydroxylamine and glutamine in the presence of ADP and phosphate.

The rate of reaction with D-glutamate for glutamine synthesis is about one third that observed with L-glutamate. However, when the second substrate is hydroxylamine, the reaction proceeds at the same rate with either stereoisomer of glutamate. In the absence of either ammonia or hydroxylamine, the enzyme will catalyse the cyclization of glutamate to pyrrolidone carboxylic acid (5-oxo-proline). This reaction also proceeds at the same rate with either stereoisomer of the substrate, and it has been suggested that the first step of the glutamine synthetase reaction is the formation of γ-glutamyl phosphate, by a non-stereospecific mechanism. This intermediate would readily cyclize to 5-oxo-proline, or react with hydroxylamine to form the hydroxamate non-enzymically. The reaction of the γ-glutamyl phosphate with ammonia to form glutamine is postulated to be stereo-specific (Meister, 1968).

THE INTERCONVERSION OF GLUTAMATE AND PROLINE

Glutamate is oxidized to glutamic-γ-semialdehyde by an NAD-dependent enzyme. The semialdehyde spontaneously cyclizes to Δ^1-pyrroline-5-carboxylate, losing a molecule of water in the process. Δ^1-Pyrroline-5-carboxylate is reduced by a specific reductase to proline. The reductases from different species have different cofactor requirements; for example, that from rat liver preferentially uses NADH, while that from calf liver uses NADPH, as do many fungal enzymes.

As can be seen from Figure 4.1, the enzymes involved in the formation of proline from glutamate do not function in the reverse direction under physio-

82

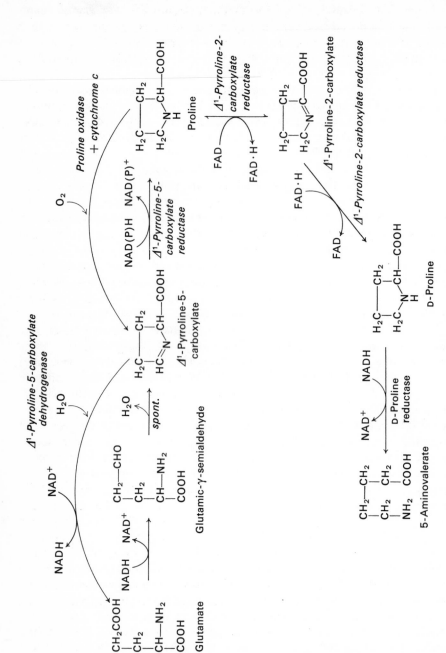

Figure 4.1. The interconversion of glutamate and proline

logical conditions. Although oxidation of glutamate yields the semialdehyde, this is not a substrate for reduction to either glutamate or proline. Studies with substrate analogues have shown that both reductions specifically require the ring-closed condensation product, Δ^1-pyrroline-5-carboxylate.

The major pathway for the catabolism of proline is oxidation to glutamate. Proline is oxidized by a specific proline oxidase, which is closely associated with the electron transport chain, and interacts directly with cytochrome c. Unlike Δ^1-pyrroline-5-carboxylate reductase, which is the NAD(P)-linked enzyme associated with the formation of proline from glutamate, proline oxidase is an oxygenase.

The synthesis of the two enzymes catalysing the interconversion of proline and Δ^1-pyrroline-5-carboxylate is controlled by opposing factors. Proline oxidase in bacteria is induced by growth on a proline-rich medium, while the reductase is repressed under these conditions. It is fully derepressed under conditions of low proline availability. The oxidation of Δ^1-pyrroline-5-carboxylate to glutamate is also catalysed by a distinct enzyme, Δ^1-pyrroline-5-carboxylate dehydrogenase, which is essentially irreversible, and clearly distinct from the enzyme which catalyses the reduction of glutamate to the semialdehyde, as noted above.

In anaerobic organisms, proline is not degraded by the reversal of the synthetic pathway as it is in aerobic organisms, but by racemization to D-proline, followed by reduction to 5-aminovalerate, as shown in Figure 4.1. The racemization can occur in two ways; presumably in strict anaerobes it is catalysed by a racemase, but in other organisms the reaction involves an FAD-linked oxidase, forming Δ^1-pyrroline-2-carboxylate as intermediate. This is then reduced to D-proline by a specific Δ^1-pyrroline-2-carboxylate reductase, which is also FAD linked. D-Proline is then reduced to 5-aminovalerate by D-proline reductase, an NAD-dependent enzyme which has a pyruvate prosthetic group. It is thought that the reaction proceeds by way of formation of an addition complex between the carbonyl group of the pyruvate and the imino nitrogen of the proline, thus facilitating a reductive cleavage, using a dithiol group in the enzyme as the immediate proton donor.

Hydroxyproline is found only in connective tissue proteins, and as will be shown later, it is not generally incorporated into these proteins *per se* but as proline, which is subsequently hydroxylated in peptide linkage. Thus, when protein synthesis is inhibited, for example by puromycin, most hydroyproline synthesis ceases. However, there is still some formation of hydroxyproline, which can be shown not to have arisen from collagen breakdown. It is thought that traces of free hydroxyproline may arise as a result of reversal of the mammalian pathway of hydroxyproline catabolism, shown in Figure 4.2. Although the pathway is initially similar to that of proline degradation, the enzymes involved in hydroxyproline catabolism are distinct from those of proline oxidation.

Efron (1965) reported studies on familial hyperprolinaemia which included, among other signs, deafness and slight mental retardation. Although blood proline in these patients was very high, and proline was excreted in the urine, hydroxyproline excretion was normal, and the blood levels of hydroxyproline

84

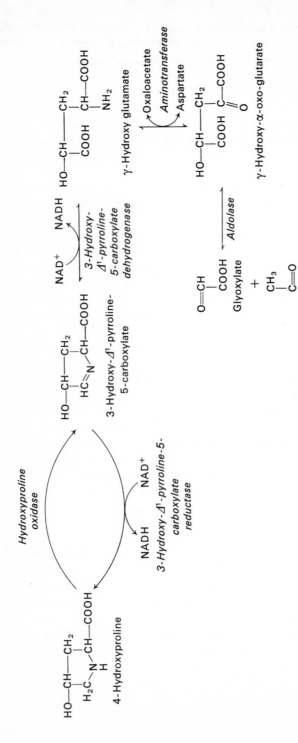

Figure 4.2. The catabolism of 4-hydroxyproline in animal tissue

were low, indicating that the defective enzymes of the proline catabolic pathway were not required for hydroxyproline catabolism. In one of the families studied, as well as hyperprolinaemia and prolinuria, there was some Δ^1-pyrroline-5-carboxylic aciduria, suggesting that the defective enzyme was Δ^1-pyrroline-5-carboxylate dehydrogenase. In the other family there was no Δ^1-pyrroline-5-carboxylate in the urine, suggesting that the defect lay in the oxidation of proline by proline oxidase.

Investigation of cases of hydroxyprolinaemia showed that proline catabolism was normal, and that the defect probably lay in specific enzymes of hydroxyproline catabolism. More hydroxyproline was excreted as the free amino acid in these patients than in normal subjects. Most of the hydroxyproline from collagen catabolism is normally excreted as small peptides: 50% of the urinary hydroxyproline is found as prolyl and hydroxyprolyl dipeptides, a further 10% as glycyl-prolyl-hydroxyproline, and less than 10% as larger peptides. Little free hydroxyproline normally appears in the urine, since it is readily resorbed from the glomerular filtrate, so that hydroxyprolinuria may reflect renal damage as well as a metabolic defect. Since in these patients there were no abnormalities of collagen metabolism, it was suggested that the excess hydroxyproline must arise from some other source (Efron et al., 1965 and 1968).

The urinary excretion of hydroxyprolyl peptides, but not generally of free hydroxyproline, is considerably increased when collagen turnover is high, either during periods of rapid growth or when tissue is being resorbed, for example post partum. There is also an increase in the excretion of hydroxyprolyl peptides in severe protein-energy malnutrition, and it has been suggested that this may provide the basis of a method of screening for under-nutrition before there are any obvious clinical signs.

The final enzyme of mammalian hydroxyproline catabolism is an aldolase, which cleaves γ-hydroxy-α-oxo-glutarate to yield pyruvate and glyoxylate. This enzyme is freely reversible under physiological conditions, and will catalyse the formation of hydroxy-oxo-glutarate from glyoxylate and pyruvate. Since, as shown in Figure 4.2, the other enzymes of hydroxyproline catabolism are also reversible (or can be by-passed, as in the case of the interconversion of hydroxyproline and Δ^1-pyrroline-3-hydroxy-5-carboxylate), it is therefore possible to synthesize hydroxyproline from common metabolic intermediates. Under normal conditions, this reaction sequence would not be expected to be of very great importance, but it could account for much of the imino acid observed in the blood and urine of patients suffering from hydroxyprolinaemia.

ORNITHINE, CITRULLINE AND ARGININE

Arginine synthesis

Ornithine, citrulline and arginine are all intermediates of the urea synthesis cycle, shown in Figure 1.9, and it is hardly surprising that the pathway for arginine biosynthesis is the same as that for urea synthesis. Hence, the first stage of arginine biosynthesis must be the formation of ornithine.

The first step in the synthesis of ornithine is the formation of N-acetyl gluta-mate. In most organisms this is achieved by acetyl transfer from acetyl-SCoA, and the main feed-back regulation of the pathway is exerted at this stage. N-Acetyl glutamate synthetase is sensitive to inhibition by arginine, and synthesis of the enzyme is also repressed by arginine in bacteria.

In some organisms, N-acetyl glutamate is formed by acetyl transfer from N-acetyl ornithine, formed at a later stage in the pathway, in a reaction catalysed by ornithine acetyl transferase. In this case, feed-back regulation of the bio-synthesis of arginine acts at the next step, the phosphorylation of N-acetyl glutamate, catalysed by N-acetyl-γ-glutamokinase. The γ-phosphate product of this reaction can then be oxidized to the γ-semialdehyde. Because the amino group is acetylated, this cannot cyclize as does glutamic-γ-semialdehyde, but is a substrate for aminotransfer to yield N-acetyl ornithine. In those organisms where N-acetyl glutamate is formed by transfer from acetyl-SCoA, the deacetyla-tion of N-acetyl ornithine is not catalysed by ornithine acetyltransferase, but by acetyl ornithinase and proceeds by a simple hydrolysis to yield ornithine and acetate. This sequence of reactions involved in the synthesis of ornithine from glutamate is shown in Figure 4.3.

Ornithine is converted to citrulline, and thence (through argininosuccinic acid) to arginine, by the same sequence of reactions as those involved in the urea synthesis cycle, shown in Figure 1.9 (page 23).

Although only the first enzyme of the pathway is inhibited by arginine, all eight enzymes required for arginine formation can be shown to be coordinately repressed by arginine in many micro-organisms. The genetics of this coordinate repression have not been wholly clarified. In *E. coli*, the genes for four of the enzymes, N-acetyl glutamokinase, N-acetyl glutamate semialdehyde dehydro-genase, acetyl ornithinase and argininosuccinase, are closely linked, while the other four and the regulator gene for the pathway, are widely scattered throughout the genome. In mammals, no repression by excess arginine of the enzymes converting ornithine to arginine would be expected since these enzymes, together with arginase, form part of the urea synthesis cycle, as well as being used for the net synthesis of arginine for protein synthesis and other requirements.

Muscle phosphagens

The store of ATP in muscle tissue from most species is very small, and there is a considerable time lag between the onset of maximal muscle effort and an increase in energy-yielding metabolism which will allow rephosphorylation of ADP to ATP. Muscle therefore contains a phosphagen, a phosphorylated compound which can be used to rephosphorylate ADP at times of great exertion. It is itself rephosphorylated when there is sufficient ATP production from energy-yielding metabolism.

In many invertebrates, the muscle phosphagen is arginine-P, and in the lobster (*Homarus vulgaris*) arginine phosphotransferase, the enzyme which catalyses the exchange of phosphate between arginine-P and ADP, can account for as much as 13% of the total soluble protein of muscle. In the earthworm, the muscle

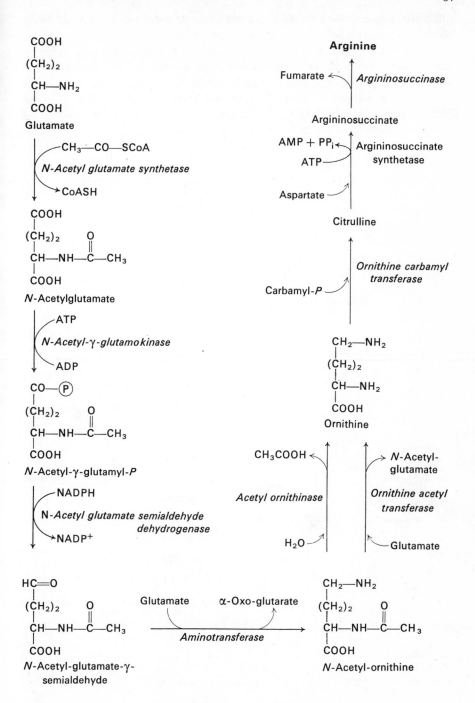

Figure 4.3. Arginine biosynthesis

phosphagen is guanidine-*P*, while marine annelids use creatine-*P*, as do verte-brates.

Mammals can use dietary creatine *per se*, but most of the body's large stores of creatine are synthesized in the liver from arginine via the pathway shown in Figure 4.4. Arginine donates its guanido group to glycine, to form guanido-acetic acid, in a reaction essentially the same as the hydrolysis of arginine to form urea and ornithine. Guanidoacetic acid is methylated to creatine in an *S*-adenosyl methionine-dependent reaction.

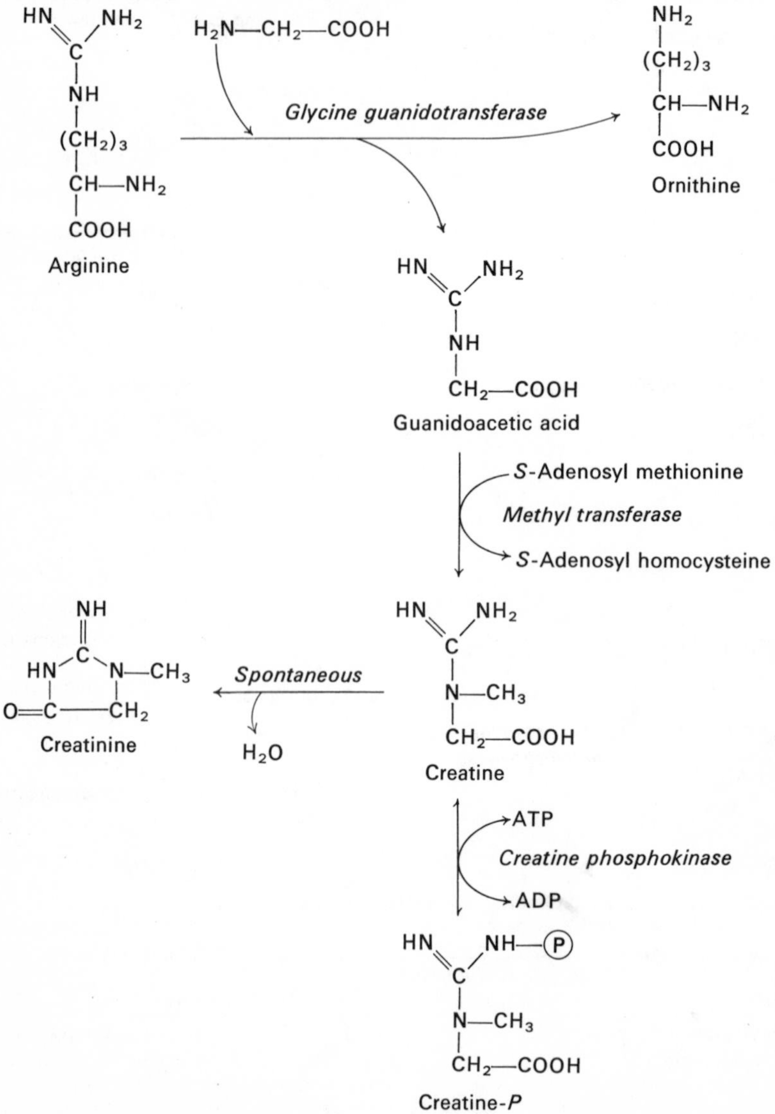

Figure 4.4 Creatine and creatinine biosynthesis

There does not appear to be a pathway for the catabolism of creatine in mammals. Wastage is almost entirely by way of a spontaneous cyclization to creatinine, the anhydride of creatine which cannot be further used, and is excreted in the urine. Since creatinine in the urine arises solely from the spontaneous cyclization of muscle creatine, the excretion rate is relatively constant for any individual. The amount excreted depends on the muscle mass of the body more than on any other factor, although vigorous excercise will increase urinary creatinine for several days. Because of this relative constancy, creatinine is frequently determined in urine as an index of the completeness of collection of a sample, and the concentrations of urine constituents are frequently quoted per mg of creatinine rather than per litre of urine. However, there is sufficient variation in creatinine excretion to cast doubt on the utility of this practice.

Creatine is found in the urine only when there is muscle wastage in adults although in growing children some creatinuria is normal. Creatinuria also occurs in females after menstruation, when the increased uterine muscle is broken down.

Creatine phosphokinase, the enzyme which catalyses the interchange of phosphate between creatine-P and ADP, has been widely studied. This is partly because there are several isoenzymes of the phosphotransferase which can be distinguished by electrophoresis or by study of their reaction kinetics. The different isoenzymes are found in different tissues, and measurement of serum creatine phosphokinase activity is a sensitive index of muscle disease, or, when the myocardial isoenzyme is found, of myocardial infarct.

Mammalian creatine phosphokinase has random reaction kinetics; either ATP or creatine can bind to the enzyme first, and the binding of either substrate aids the binding of the other. There is no evidence of any phosphorylated enzyme intermediate. Some crustacean arginine phosphotransferases are kinetically similar to the mammalian enzyme, while others have been shown to form a phosphorylated enzyme intermediate. Enzymes of the latter type will catalyse phosphate exchange between ATP and ADP, while enzymes which are not phosphorylated during the reaction will not.

Arginine catabolism

In most organisms, the main route of arginine catabolism is by way of hydrolysis to ornithine. This ornithine can then transfer the δ-amino group to a suitable acceptor, forming glutamic-γ-semialdehyde which can be oxidized to glutamate as described above.

Arginine can undergo an α-decarboxylation in some bacteria, yielding the primary amine, agmatine. This is a precursor of the diamine putrescine; hydrolysis of agmatine releases urea and the diamine. However, the normal route of putrescine synthesis in most systems, as noted below, is the decarboxylation of ornithine.

In organisms which do not have arginase activity, and are therefore unable to catabolize arginine by way of ornithine, arginine is oxidatively decarboxylated to yield γ-guanidobutyramide. This is the first reaction of the sequence shown

90

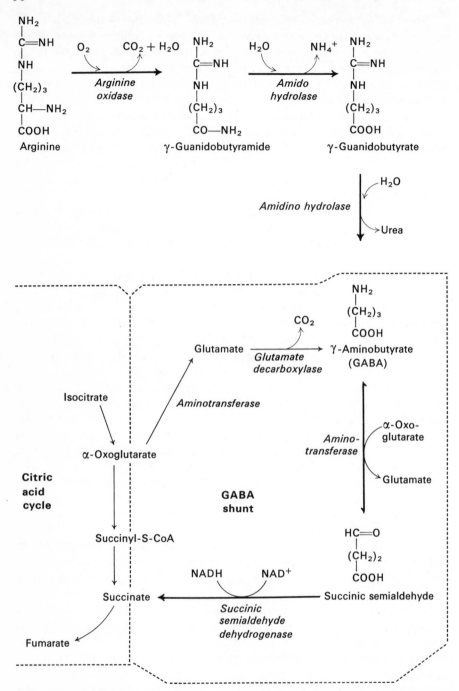

Figure 4.5. The γ-guanidobutyramide pathway of arginine catabolism

in Figure 4.5. Arginine oxidase is an oxygenase, and is specific for arginine and its next higher and lower homologues, homo-arginine and canavanine. After hydrolysis of guanidobutyramide to remove the amide group as ammonia, γ-guanidobutyrate undergoes a further hydrolysis, releasing the formamidine group as urea. Although the reaction is very similar, γ-guanidobutyrate amidino-hydrolase is distinct from arginase, and neither enzyme acts to any significant extent on the substrate for the other.

The product of this amidino-hydrolase is γ-aminobutyric acid (GABA), which can be catabolized by transamination to succinic semialdehyde, and then

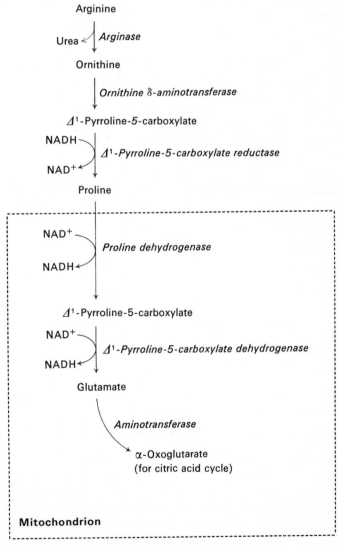

Figure 4.6. The role of arginase in insect flight muscle

by dehydrogenation to succinate. GABA is important in the central nervous system, where it is believed to function as a neurotransmitter (see page 190). Synthesis of GABA in the nervous system is not by the pathway shown here from arginine, but by decarboxylation of glutamic acid, catalysed by glutamate decarboxylase. The glutamate is formed by transamination of α-oxo-glutarate from the citric acid cycle pool, possibly catalysed by the same aminotransferase as later degrades GABA to succinic semialdehyde. The formation of GABA thus provides an alternative pathway for the conversion of α-oxo-glutarate to succinate. It is believed that in the mammalian central nervous system, a considerable proportion of the substrate flux through the citrate cycle in fact passes through this GABA shunt rather than through the more conventional pathway of oxidative decarboxylation to yield succinyl-SCoA.

In insects, ornithine δ-aminotransferase and Δ^1-pyrroline-5-carboxylate reductase are both cytoplasmic enzymes, while in all other animals the transaminase is located inside the mitochondrion. Also, although not ureotelic, insects have an active arginase. During the development of the silk moth, arginase develops at the time of the emergence of the winged imago, mainly in the flight muscle cytoplasm. It has been shown that the insect flight muscle mitochondrial membrane is impermeable to glutamate, but permeable to proline, and therefore the scheme shown in Figure 4.6 has been proposed as a mechanism for mitochondrial substrate uptake. Proline enters the mitochondrion, where it can be converted to α-oxo-glutarate by the action of proline dehydrogenase, to form Δ^1-pyrroline-5-carboxylate, which is then oxidized to glutamate. In the cytosol, proline is formed from Δ^1-pyrroline-5-carboxylate by reduction, so that as well as acting as a source of carbon for the citrate cycle, this mechanism provides a means for re-oxidation of cytoplasmic NADH and transfer into the mitochondrion of its protons. The cytoplasmic Δ^1-pyrroline-5-carboxylate is presumed to be formed mainly from arginine.

THE DIAMINES AND POLYAMINES

The trivial nomenclature of the polyamines and diamines, whose structures are shown in Figure 4.7, arose as a result of their original discovery. Spermine and spermidine were first observed by Leeuwenhoek in 1677 as phosphate crystals in a sample of semen, although they were not identified for some 200 years. The two commonly occurring diamines, putrescine and cadaverine, were so named because they were first found in putrefying matter as a result of bacterial decomposition.

The distribution of these compounds is not so limited as their names might suggest; polyamines are found in almost all cells, frequently in large amounts. In *Azotobacter vinelandii*, as much as 22% of the non-protein nitrogen (4% of the total cellular nitrogen) is present as spermidine and putrescine. In general, Gram-negative bacteria contain large amounts of polyamines, while Gram-positive organisms contain very small amounts. However, the polyamine content of an individual organism may vary widely depending on the culture conditions,

The diamines

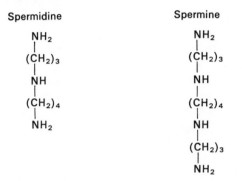

1,3-Diaminopropane

$$NH_2$$
$$|$$
$$(CH_2)_3$$
$$|$$
$$NH_2$$

1,4-Diaminobutane
(putrescine)

$$NH_2$$
$$|$$
$$(CH_2)_4$$
$$|$$
$$NH_2$$

1,5-Diaminopentane
(cadaverine)

$$NH_2$$
$$|$$
$$(CH_2)_5$$
$$|$$
$$NH_2$$

The polyamines

Spermidine

$$NH_2$$
$$|$$
$$(CH_2)_3$$
$$|$$
$$NH$$
$$|$$
$$(CH_2)_4$$
$$|$$
$$NH_2$$

Spermine

$$NH_2$$
$$|$$
$$(CH_2)_3$$
$$|$$
$$NH$$
$$|$$
$$(CH_2)_4$$
$$|$$
$$NH$$
$$|$$
$$(CH_2)_3$$
$$|$$
$$NH_2$$

Figure 4.7. The diamines and polyamines

especially pH and age. Therefore, older cultures, with a more depleted food supply, have lower levels of polyamines than the same organisms in a younger culture.

Bacteria can take up exogenous polyamines to a great extent and there appear to be two mechanisms involved: both active uptake into the cells and passive adsorption onto the cell membrane. This latter can be demonstrated *in vitro* with bacterial membrane preparations. Adsorbed polyamines can exchange with other amines, or be removed from the membrane by washing in a medium of high ionic strength. It has been suggested (Tabor and Tabor, 1966) that this membrane adsorption of polyamines may be connected with resistance to osmotic shock.

Ames and Dubin (1960) showed that some bacteriophages also have high polyamine levels. Phages of the T_{even} series contain enough spermidine and putrescine to neutralize about 40% of the total nucleic acid phosphate. The T_{odd} series phages have very much less polyamine, and the function of neutralizing the nucleic acid phosphate appears to be carried out mainly by Mg^{2+} and Ca^{2+} ions. A similar interchangeability between metal ions and polyamines is seen in plants, where putrescine synthesis is greatly increased in potassium deficiency.

In mammals, polyamines are found in all tissues. While human plasma contains no polyamines (presumably because it contains an active amine oxidase) the cell fraction of human blood is relatively rich in spermidine (0·96 mg/l blood) and spermine (1·3 mg/l). The ratio of these two compounds is not constant from one individual to another. In general, three mammalian tissues have been used for studies of polyamine metabolism: the prostate gland, which synthesizes the polyamines found in semen; the liver, and the central nervous system where Shimizu and coworkers (1964) showed that spermine is mainly asociated with the cell bodies in the grey matter, and spermidine with the fibres in the white matter and peripheral nerves.

As well as their general function as cations, polyamines appear to be specifically associated with RNA *in vivo*, and can be shown to associate with DNA *in vitro*, protecting it from thermal denaturation. The association is ionic, but the amines cannot generally be removed either by addition of further polyamine or by incubation in media of high ionic strength.

Pearce and Schanberg (1969) have shown that spermidine (and histamine, which, for many purposes can be included with the polyamines) is maximal in foetal rat brain at about 17 days of gestation, declining sharply just before birth, and then rising to a post-natal peak at 5–10 days, before falling to the lower adult level at weaning. This developmental pattern is very different from that shown by the biogenic (neurotransmitter) amines, and correlates well with the two 'growth spurts' of brain development: the prenatal increase in neuronal cellularity and the postnatal development of glial cells. Brain RNA synthesis shows an absolute requirement for spermidine, and Singh and Sung (1972) showed that spermidine stimulated brain RNA polymerase II (forming mRNA) considerably more than RNA polymerase I (forming rRNA). This activation of RNA polymerase by polyamines appears to be because the polyamines complex with the nascent RNA chain, thus preventing product inhibition of the polymerase. Activation is not seen when the polymerase is primed by synthetic or denatured single-stranded DNA, because the nascent RNA anneals with the primer, and is prevented from either associating with polyamines or inhibiting the enzyme. In bacteria, polyamines have been shown to stabilize the $70S$ ribosome, a function which can also be served by metal ions, suggesting that the major function of the polyamines is to neutralize the negative charges of the phosphate groups of ribosomal RNA.

It is well established that after partial hepatectomy, or other stimulus to growth, the synthesis of polyamines is greatly increased by induction of ornithine decarboxylase, the rate-limiting enzyme of the pathway of polyamine synthesis (see below). This effect appears to be mediated by growth hormone, and it has been shown that administration of growth hormone leads to the induction of ornithine decarboxylase; the elevation of enzyme activity persists throughout the period of tissue regeneration. As soon as 1 h after partial hepatectomy, a three-fold increase in the decarboxylase activity can be observed, and a maximal increase in activity of 25–70-fold is shown about 16 h after surgery. In general, the degree of enzyme induction is proportional to the extent of damage to the liver, although not necessarily to the rate of tissue regeneration subsequently observed.

Cross-circulation experiments between partially hepatectomized and normal animals have shown an increase in the activity of ornithine decarboxylase in the liver of the normal partner, again suggesting a hormonal factor which could be growth hormone. A thermostable factor, which cannot therefore be growth hormone, has been isolated from foetal calf serum and shown to stimulate ornithine decarboxylase activity. This compound is not present in adult serum.

The biosynthesis of polyamines

Two possible routes for the formation of putrescine are shown in Figure 4.8. In mammals, the decarboxylation of ornithine appears to be the only source of putrescine, and this reaction is rate-limiting for biosynthesis of all the polyamines. Ornithine decarboxylase has a very short half-life, so that sensitive control of polyamine synthesis is possible by alteration in the rate of synthesis of the enzyme.

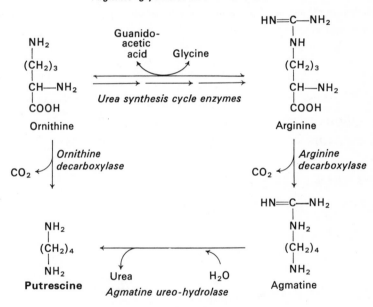

Figure 4.8. The biosynthesis of putrescine

In *E. coli*, there are two separate ornithine decarboxylases. The first to be discovered is inducible when the organism is grown on ornithine-rich media, and appears to be mainly catabolic; the activity of this enzyme in organisms grown on minimal culture medium would certainly not account for the observed synthesis of polyamines. In 1965, Morris and Pardee demonstrated the presence of a second, constitutive enzyme which they called the biosynthetic ornithine decarboxylase. Arginine decarboxylase in *E. coli* also shows separate catabolic and biosynthetic isoenzymes.

Morris and Pardee (1966) proposed two distinct pathways of putrescine biosynthesis in *E. coli*, one directly from ornithine, as in mammals, and the other from arginine by decarboxylation to agmatine, followed by removal of urea from agmatine to yield putrescine. This latter pathway would be energetically less efficient than the direct pathway from ornithine, and they suggested that it is used mainly when an accumulation of arginine inhibits the synthesis of ornithine from glutamate or proline. The arginine which has accumulated can be used to ensure continued production of putrescine. In plants, the arginine decarboxylase pathway may be the major source of putrescine at all times; potassium deficient plants show an accumulation of agmatine as well as of putrescine. There is no evidence that agmatine is formed to any significant extent in animals.

Cadaverine (1,5-diaminopentane) is synthesized by the decarboxylation of lysine, in a reaction parallel to ornithine decarboxylation, and 1,3-diamino-propane can arise either by decarboxylation of 1,3-diaminobutyrate, or, more importantly, in bacteria as one of the products of spermidine catabolism (see below).

As shown in Figure 4.9, spermidine is synthesized from putrescine by transfer of a propylamine group. A further propylamine transfer converts spermidine to

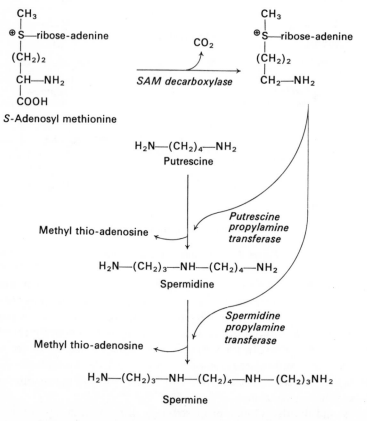

Figure 4.9. The biosynthesis of spermidine and spermine

spermine. In both cases, the propylamine group is derived from 3-methyl-thiopropylamine sulphonium adenosine, the decarboxylation product of S-adenosyl methionine.

S-Adenosyl methionine decarboxylase is activated by putrescine, and therefore, indirectly, by any factor which increases ornithine decarboxylase activity. In bacteria, S-adenosyl methionine decarboxylase does not contain pyridoxal-P, although the mammalian enzyme does, and it is assumed that the pyruvoyl residue in the enzyme catalyses the reaction in the same way as that in some bacterial histidine decarboxylases (see page 53).

In mammalian liver, a multi-enzyme complex catalyses the decarboxylation of S-adenosyl methionine, and propylamine transfer to putrescine to yield, successively, spermidine and then spermine. This complex has been resolved, and it has been shown that there are two separate propylamine transferases, one forming spermidine, and the other forming spermine.

The other product from decarboxylated S-adenosyl methionine after propyl-amine transfer is methyl thio-adenosine. In yeasts, this can be used for synthesis of S-adenosyl methionine, but in other micro-organisms, and in mammals, it is degraded by deadenylation.

Catabolism of the polyamines

The turn-over of polyamines appears to be fairly slow in mammals; within 12 h of administration of ^{14}C-labelled spermidine to experimental animals about 8% of the label is recovered in expired carbon dioxide, and a further 7% in the urine. Less of the label from radioactive spermine is recovered in the same time.

The urinary radioactivity after administration of [^{14}C]spermidine or [^{14}C]-spermine is mainly in various conjugates, which only release the polyamine on acid hydrolysis. It is assumed that these are γ-glutamate conjugates because it has been shown that both polyamines and diamines can replace the amide group of glutamine. This replacement reaction is catalysed by transglutaminase in free solution, and by a separate amidotransferase when the glutamine is incorporated in protein. The amidotransferase catalyses the exchange of the amide group of glutamine with a variety of polyamines, and lysine. It appears to be distinct from the enzyme which catalyses the protein incorporation of mescaline and other psychoactive amines, and it shows a broad specificity for the acceptor protein.

Polyamines can be inactivated by N-acylation, especially in bacteria, but the main route of degradation is oxidative. Bacterial polyamine oxidases can be divided into two classes according to the point of attack on the substrate. In most organisms, the initial step in spermidine degradation is attack to the butyl-amine side of the central imino group, yielding 1,3-diaminopropane and γ-amino-butyraldehyde:

$$H_2N—(CH_2)_3—NH—(CH_2)_4—NH_2 \rightarrow$$
$$H_2N—(CH_2)_3—NH_2 + OCH—(CH_2)_3—NH_2$$

The γ-aminobutyraldehyde spontaneously dehydrates, and cyclizes to form Δ^1-pyrroline. This can be metabolized by way of γ-aminobutyric acid to the citrate cycle intermediate, succinate.

In *Mycobacterium* and *Pseudomonas* species, the point of attack by polyamine oxidase is to the propylamine side of the central imino group of spermidine, yielding putrescine and aminopropionaldehyde:

$$H_2N—(CH_2)_3—NH—(CH_2)_4—NH_2 \rightarrow$$
$$H_2N—(CH_2)_2—CHO + H_2N—(CH_2)_4—NH_2$$

Aminopropionaldehyde can be catabolized by way of β-alanine.

Polyamine oxidase action on spermine yields initially aminopropionaldehyde and spermidine. The onward metabolism of the spermidine depends on the type of oxidase.

Diamine oxidases are widely distributed in nature. Putrescine is oxidized to γ-aminobutyraldehyde, which then dehydrates and cyclizes to Δ^1-pyrroline, as described above, while cadaverine yields Δ^1-piperidine, by way of δ-amino-butyraldehyde. A large number of other diamines, both naturally occurring and synthesized, are also substrates for diamine oxidase. It is possible that mammalian diamine oxidase is the same enzyme as histaminase. Diamine oxidase is distinct from monoamine oxidase (MAO), which acts only on primary mono-amines; it is not affected by clinically used MAO inhibitors.

An apparently-distinct enzyme in mammalian serum, a cupro-protein, cata-lyses oxidation of polyamines by way of oxidation of the amino group to an aldehyde, followed by β-elimination of acrolein. Thus, spermine is oxidized initially to spermidine and acrolein, and further oxidation of spermidine leads to the formation of putrescine and another molecule of acrolein.

SPECIALIZED AMINO ACIDS IN CONNECTIVE TISSUE

The main connective tissue protein is collagen, an insoluble protein found in all multi-cellular animals. It represents about 30% of the total body protein of an adult man, about 6% of the total body weight. Collagen is an extremely inelastic protein, and cannot be stretched by application of a force equivalent to 10^4 times its own weight, so that in tendon attachment the force of muscle con-traction is transmitted almost wholly undiminished.

In adult mammals turnover of collagen is very slow; a half-life in excess of 300 days has been estimated. There is also a small amount of collagen with a much shorter half-life. This appears to represent the residue of two further pools of collagen left over from the foetal and neonate mammal, with half-lives of 1 and 5 days.

The collagen molecule is highly asymmetric; its molecular weight is about 360,000, and it has a length of 300 nm with a diameter of only 1·4 nm. It is a trimer, with two α-chains and one $α_1$-chain joined by intra-molecular cross-links. The fibrils in connective tissue are formed by inter-molecular cross-linkage of trimers; the dimer is a poor substrate for fibril formation, and the monomer rarely forms any fibrils.

Collagen and elastin, the other main protein of connective tissue, contain hydroxyproline. This amino acid is not found to any significant extent in any other protein. Another amino acid found only in connective tissue proteins is δ-hydroxylysine. The structures of these amino acids are shown in Figure 4.10.

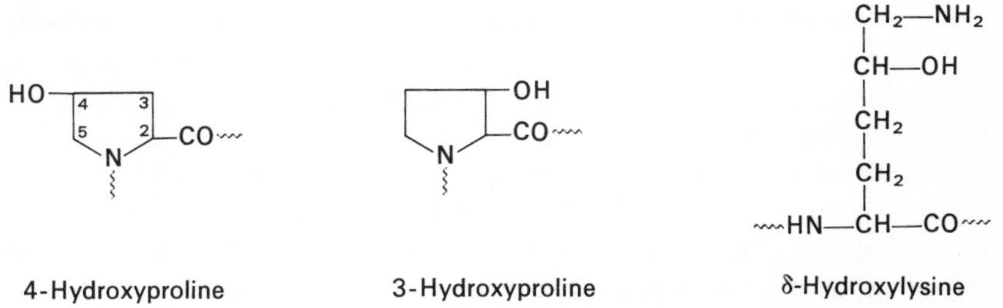

4-Hydroxyproline   3-Hydroxyproline δ-Hydroxylysine

Figure 4.10. Hydroxylated amino acids in collagen and elastin

There are two types of collagen: that found in the intercellular matrix, known as interstitial collagen, and that found in the basement membranes of epithelia. Basement membrane collagen contains more hydroxyproline and hydroxylysine than does interstitial collagen. Much of the proline of basement membrane collagen is hydroxylated at the 3-position, rather than the more usual 4-position.

Apart from the hydroxy-amino acids, the general amino acid composition of collagen is very unusual. One third of the amino acids are glycyl residues, and of the remainder 22% are prolyl or hydroxyprolyl residues. A further 11% are glutamyl residues. In interstitial collagen there is very little tyrosine, and no tryptophan or cysteine. This means that the cross-links of mature collagen cannot be disulphide bridges. However, in basement membrane collagen, there are between four and ten cysteinyl residues per 1000 amino acids, so that disulphide bridges are possible in this protein.

In interstitial collagen, there is about 0·5% carbohydrate associated with the protein; in basement membrane collagen this can be as much as 10%. In both cases, the carbohydrate is either galactose or glucosyl-galactose linked to the hydroxyl group of hydroxylysine. The sequence of amino acids about the hydroxylysyl residue determines whether or not it is glycosylated, and this glycosylation appears to be essential for extrusion of collagen into the extracellular matrix.

The other major connective tissue protein is elastin, found in the *ligamentum nuchae* of the neck, the region of the aorta near the heart, and as a minor constituent of most other vertebrate connective tissue. It consists of cross-linked, randomly-coiled protein chains, giving it a great deal of elasticity and compressibility. Elastin contains only 2–4% hydroxyproline, compared with as much as 13% in interstitial collagen. Until 1969 it was thought that the hydroxyproline found in hydrolysates of elastin was due to contamination of the protein with collagen rather than to the presence of this amino acid in elastin.

Bentley and Hanson (1969), in demonstrating the presence of hydroxyproline in elastin, also showed that free hydroxyproline was incorporated into elastin. Although there is known to be a hydroxyprolyl-tRNA, there is overwhelming evidence that collagen synthesis does not proceed by incorporation of preformed hydroxyproline into the protein, but by hydroxylation at the stage of a formed polypeptide chain. Such incorporation of labelled hydroxyproline into collagen as was observed by earlier workers has been demonstrated as being due to de-hydroxylation of the radioactive material, followed by incorporation into protein of the proline so formed and its subsequent hydroxylation in peptide linkage. However, in elastin it was shown that the specific activity of radioactive hydroxy-proline incorporated was such as to preclude any mixing with the tissue pool of proline, and therefore it is assumed that there is a genuine incorporation of hydroxyproline *per se* into elastin. This might function as a mechanism to ensure the continuation of elastin synthesis, in the event of a disturbance of hydroxylation, by allowing the utilization of hydroxyproline released by collagen degradation.

The normal catabolism of collagen is not well understood: collagen resists most proteases, but collagenases have been isolated from tadpole tail during metamorphosis, and from human bone and synovial membrane in rheumatoid diseases, as well as from a number of bacteria.

Procollagen prolyl and lysyl hydroxylases

Two separate enzymes are involved in the hydroxylation of lysyl and prolyl residues in procollagen. Pinell and coworkers (1972) showed that in an inherited disease involving hydroxylysine deficiency in collagen, normal amounts of hydroxyproline were formed in skin collagen. The two enzymes were separated by Miller (1971), who showed that purified lysyl hydroxylase had no activity towards prolyl residues, although purified prolyl hydroxylase showed slight activity towards lysyl residues, at concentrations of enzyme about 100-fold greater than required for activity towards prolyl residues. Neither enzyme will act to any detectable extent on free amino acids, and although some tripeptides which include the substrate amino acid are hydroxylated, at least a hexapeptide is required for maximal activity. Thus, $(Ile-Lys-Gly)_2$ is hydroxylated 10 times faster than Ile-Lys-Gly. The enzymes are usually assayed by release of ^3H from tritiated lysine or proline incorporated into synthetic substrates or into procol-lagen synthesized in tissue culture under anaerobic or other inhibitory conditions. Although they are readily separated by chromatography on DEAE–Sephadex, the two enzymes appear to be very similar in reaction characteristics. Prolyl hydroxylase has been most studied; there is no evidence to suggest that lysyl hydroxylase differs in any major respect. The enzyme does not act on free proline, or on small prolyl peptides, and while individual α-chains are substrates, the cross-linked dimers and trimers are only poorly hydroxylated *in vitro*. Although it is possible, under conditions of hydroxylation inhibition, to obtain under-hydroxylated procollagen fibres free from ribosomes, it appears that hydroxyla-tion normally occurs while the nascent polypeptide chain is still attached to the ribosome.

Rhoads and Udenfriend (1968) demonstrated that α-oxo-glutarate was decarboxylated simultaneously and stoichiometrically with the hydroxylation of proline. The requirement for α-oxo-glutarate for activity is absolute: pyruvate, oxaloacetate and other oxo-acids will not substitute. This reaction is clearly distinct from the α-oxo-glutarate dehydrogenase reaction found intra-mitochondrially; thiamin, coenzyme A, NAD and lipoic acid have all been shown to have no effect on the activity of this system. Since 1968, this coupling of hydroxy-

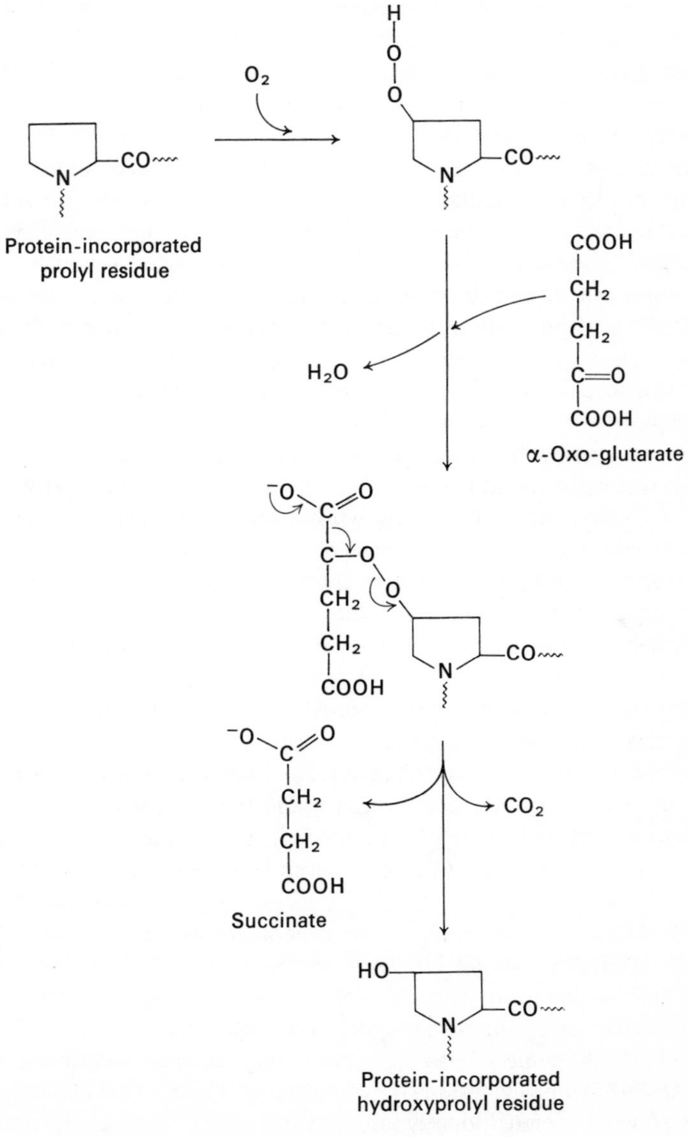

Figure 4.11. The reaction of procollagen prolyl hydroxylase

lation to the decarboxylation of α-oxo-glutarate has been observed with several other enzymes, including γ-butyrobetaine hydroxylase in carnitine biosynthesis and the hydroxylation of thymine to 7-hydroxymethyl uracil, as well as procollagen lysyl hydroxylase. Since the reaction also uses molecular oxygen, these enzymes represent a new class of mixed function oxidases.

Cardinale and coworkers (1971) demonstrated that $^{18}O_2$ was incorporated into both the hydroxyproline and succinate formed by prolyl hydroxylase, and proposed that the reaction proceeds by way of formation of a peroxide at the 4-position of proline, followed by a nucleophilic attack by α-oxo-glutarate, as shown in Figure 4.11.

The hydroxylase also contains non-haem iron, apparently loosely bound to sulphydryl groups, which can be removed readily during purification. The function of ascorbate (vitamin C), believed for many years to be a cofactor for this enzyme, may be mainly to maintain these sulphydryl groups in a reduced state, and to aid in the removal of any potentially inhibitory hydrogen peroxide formed in side reactions. The role of ascorbate is problematical. It is replaceable, in that a number of other reduced ene-diol compounds or reduced pteridines will substitute *in vitro*, but in scurvy (prolonged vitamin C deficiency) there are clear lesions of collagen synthesis, although loss of lysine and proline hydroxylating ability has not been demonstrated. There is no evidence that under-hydroxylated collagen is formed in scorbutic animals, although there may be considerably more degradation of newly formed collagen than normal.

It has been suggested that there may be two separate pools of collagen synthesis. That associated with wound healing can be demonstrated to be severely affected by vitamin C deficiency, and tissue synthesized in response to wounding in scorbutic guinea pigs is grossly deficient in collagen. However, growth of young guinea pigs and regeneration of liver after partial hepatectomy proceed with more or less normal collagen synthesis even in severely scorbutic animals, suggesting that collagen synthesis for growth may be relatively independent of ascorbate. It is noteworthy that scurvy can be cured or prevented with a daily intake of 5–10 mg of vitamin C, but to promote proper wound healing as much as 20 mg per day is required.

Intra-molecular cross-links in collagen from scorbutic guinea pigs are normal, but the inter-molecular links are defective, and the scorbutic collagen is more soluble than normal. The role of vitamin C in hydroxylation in general, with special reference to collagen synthesis has been reviewed by Barnes and Kodicek (1972).

After hydroxylation, the procollagen monomers are glycosylated. Specific procollagen UDP-glucose and UDP-galactose transferases have been isolated. Galactose is transferred to specific hydroxylysyl residues; the specificity of transfer is determined by the sequence of amino acyl residues about the hydroxylysyl residues, in the same way as the surrounding sequence determines whether or not a given lysyl or prolyl residue is hydroxylated. The glycosylated procollagen monomer is then associated loosely into a trimer which is secreted into the intercellular matrix.

Goldberg and coworkers (1972), working with cultured human fibroblasts, showed that the procollagen trimer was linked by disulphide bridges at the time of secretion, and that subsequently the amino-terminal region, containing the cysteinyl residues, was removed by proteolysis. The protease involved has been shown not to be a 'serine hydrolase', although, *in vitro*, limited tryptic digestion has the same effect. At this time, the conformation of the trimer is maintained by non-covalent bonds; the intra- and inter-molecular links are formed after removal of the terminal cysteine-containing peptide.

Cross-linkage in collagen and elastin

Although both basement membrane collagen and elastin contain small amounts of cysteine, which could be used for the formation of inter-chain links, interstitial collagen does not, and any covalent links must therefore be of a different kind. It can be shown that lysine is involved in the formation of cross-link compounds in both collagen and elastin, for example by incorporation of radioactive lysine into compounds which are not susceptible to acid hydrolysis or enzymic proteolysis. Inhibition of cross-linking is found in lathyrism. This is a condition in which collagen is more soluble than normal, and elastin less elastic. The cause of death is usually rupture of the aorta in the elastin-rich region near the heart. A number of compounds will induce a lathyritic condition (i.e. are lathyrogens), including β-aminopropionitrile, the toxic principle of the sweet pea, *Lathyrus odoratus*, from which the disease derives its name. Copper deficiency in experimental animals also leads to development of lathyrism.

The first step in collagen cross-linkage is the oxidation of the lysyl residue at position 9 from the amino terminal of soluble procollagen trimer by lysyl oxidase. This reaction can be shown to be inhibited by β-aminopropionitrile, and the failure of cross-linking in copper deficiency has been interpreted as suggesting a role for copper in lysyl oxidase, although this has not been clearly demonstrated. The product of this reaction is the ε-aldehyde of lysine, allysine (α-amino-adipic δ-semialdehyde). The specificity of attack of the oxidase on this lysyl residue is, presumably, determined by the unusual amino acid sequence around the amino terminal of procollagen. There is very little glycine, although in the rest of the molecule every third residue is glycine, and there are two tyrosyl residues. Also, there is no helical structure of any kind in this region of the chain.

The initial formation of the cross-link compound, a Schiff base between allysine and the ε-amino group of another lysyl residue, $\Delta^{6,7}$-dehydro-lysino-norleucine, may be non-enzymic. It can be shown that penicillamine, although not an inhibitor of lysyl oxidase, will inhibit the formation of cross-links, and on removal of the inhibitor there is immediate formation of dehydro-lysinonor-leucine (see Figure 4.12), and precipitation of insoluble collagen fibres. After sodium borohydride reduction of collagen, the cross-links are recovered as lysinonorleucine by hydrogenation of the Schiff base.

In foetal calf cartilage, there are cross-links formed from δ-hydroxylysine. In late uterine and early post-natal life, the synthesis of this compound gradually ceases, and the new cross-links are formed from lysyl rather than hydroxylysyl

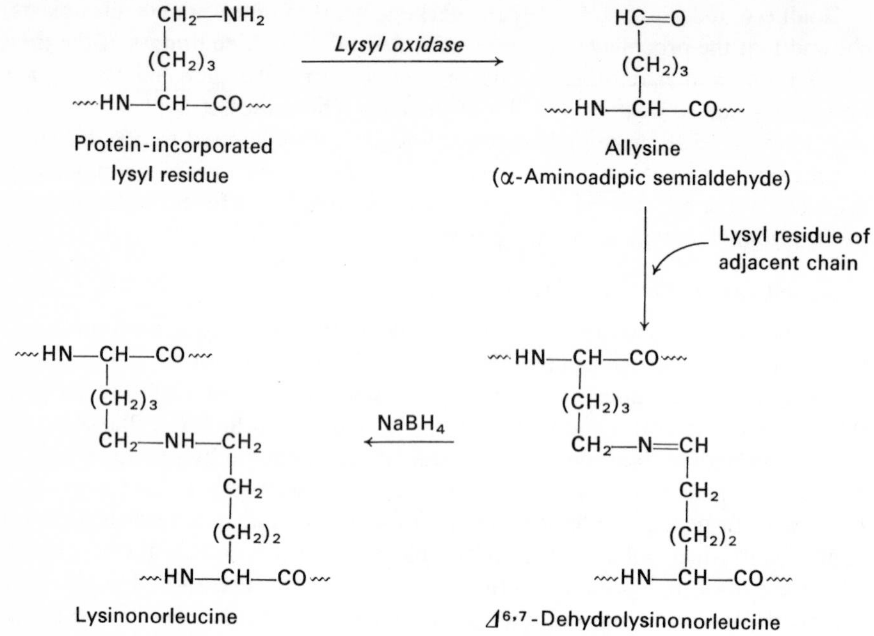

CH₂—NH₂ structure:

$$CH_2\text{—}NH_2$$
$$|$$
$$(CH_2)_3$$
$$|$$
$$\sim\sim HN\text{—}CH\text{—}CO\sim\sim$$

Protein-incorporated
lysyl residue

Lysyl oxidase →

$$HC{=}O$$
$$|$$
$$(CH_2)_3$$
$$|$$
$$\sim\sim HN\text{—}CH\text{—}CO\sim\sim$$

Allysine
(α-Aminoadipic semialdehyde)

Lysyl residue of
adjacent chain

$$\sim\sim HN\text{—}CH\text{—}CO\sim\sim$$
$$|$$
$$(CH_2)_3$$
$$|$$
$$CH_2\text{—}NH\text{—}CH_2$$
$$|$$
$$CH_2$$
$$|$$
$$(CH_2)_2$$
$$|$$
$$\sim\sim HN\text{—}CH\text{—}CO\sim\sim$$

Lysinonorleucine

← NaBH₄

$$\sim\sim HN\text{—}CH\text{—}CO\sim\sim$$
$$|$$
$$(CH_2)_3$$
$$|$$
$$CH_2\text{—}N{=}CH$$
$$|$$
$$CH_2$$
$$|$$
$$(CH_2)_2$$
$$|$$
$$\sim\sim HN\text{—}CH\text{—}CO\sim\sim$$

$\Delta^{6,7}$-Dehydrolysinonorleucine

$\Delta^{6,7}$-Dehydro-hydroxylysino-hydroxynorleucine, formed from
δ-hydroxylysyl residues, can undergo an internal rearrangement, as:

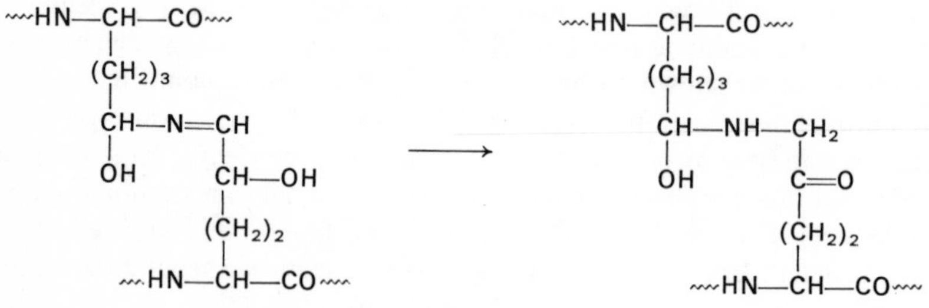

$$\sim\sim HN\text{—}CH\text{—}CO\sim\sim$$
$$|$$
$$(CH_2)_3$$
$$|$$
$$CH\text{—}N{=}CH$$
$$|\qquad\quad|$$
$$OH\qquad CH\text{—}OH$$
$$|$$
$$(CH_2)_2$$
$$|$$
$$\sim\sim HN\text{—}CH\text{—}CO\sim\sim$$

→

$$\sim\sim HN\text{—}CH\text{—}CO\sim\sim$$
$$|$$
$$(CH_2)_3$$
$$|$$
$$CH\text{—}NH\text{—}CH_2$$
$$|\qquad\qquad|$$
$$OH\qquad\quad C{=}O$$
$$|$$
$$(CH_2)_2$$
$$|$$
$$\sim\sim HN\text{—}CH\text{—}CO\sim\sim$$

Figure 4.12. The formation of lysinonorleucine based cross-links in connective tissue

residues. However, when cross-links are formed from hydroxylysine, the condensation product, dehydro-hydroxylsino-hydroxynorleucine, can undergo an internal redox reaction, similar to the enol–keto tautomerization. The resulting keto compound is considerably more stable than is dehydro-lysinonorleucine.

Elastin is considerably more cross-linked than collagen, some 5–16 lysyl residues per 1000 amino acids being involved in formation of links. As well as dehydro-lysinonorleucine, and possibly also the reduced derivative, lysinonorleucine, elastin has more complex cross-linkage compounds, involving four lysyl residues in the formation of desmosine and isodesmosine. Thus, as many as four peptide chains can be linked at each desmosine. Figure 4.13 shows the pathway of desmosine formation but little is known of the mechanism. It can be

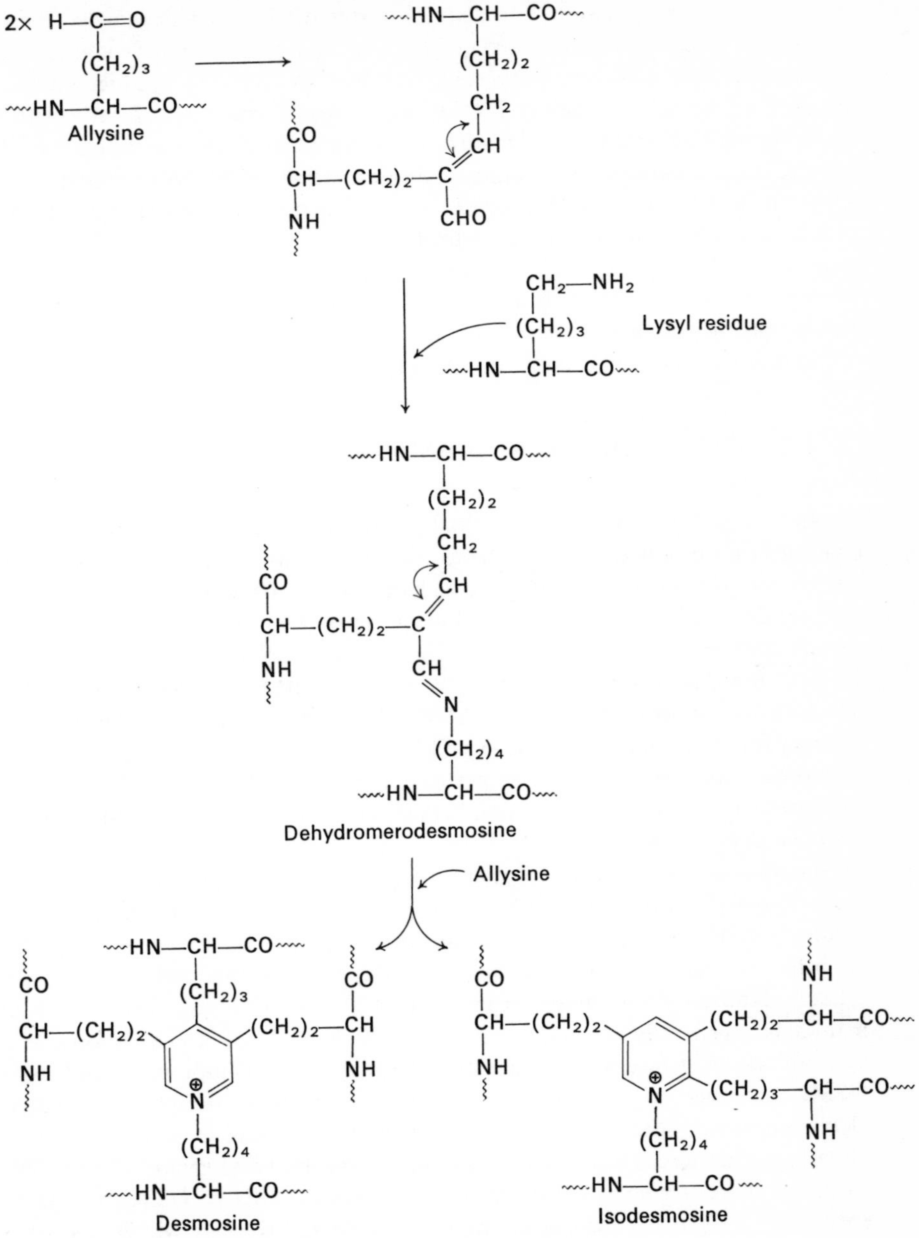

Figure 4.13. The desmosines

shown that while labels from four molecules of radioactive lysine are incorporated, only one ε-amino group is retained, and since the process is inhibited by
β-aminopropionitrile and other lathyrogens, it probably involves the formation
of the aldehyde, allysine. Starcher and coworkers (1967) isolated a compound

from elastin after reduction with sodium borohydride which they called mero-desmosine; it corresponds to the reduced condensation product of one lysyl residue with two allysines. They suggested that two allysine residues undergo an aldol condensation, the product of which then forms a Schiff base with a lysyl residue. This Schiff base, dehydro-merodesmosine, could then be chemically reduced to the isolated compound, merodesmosine. Dehydro-merodesmosine is then believed to react with a further allysine residue to form either desmosine or isodesmosine. Whether the dehydro-lysinonorleucine found in elastin represents a cross-link *per se*, or an intermediate in the formation of the desmosines is unclear, but larger amounts of dehydro-lysinonorleucine, desmosine and isodesmosine are found in mature elastin than in elastin from young animals. The amount of free lysine in elastin falls on maturation.

GLUTATHIONE AND AMINO ACID TRANSPORT

The tripeptide glutathione (γ-glutamyl-cysteinyl-glycine) is found in large amounts in animal tissues, plants and micro-organisms. In the rat liver, the concentration of glutathione can be as high as 4–5 mM, despite the presence of an active γ-glutamyl transpeptidase which degrades it to glutamate and cysteinyl-glycine. Glutathione is synthesized by two enzymes, γ-glutamyl-cysteine synthetase and glutathione synthetase. The former enzyme accounts for about 2·5% of the total soluble protein of the kidney. Both synthetases utilize ATP, and both are subject to inhibition by ADP. It has been estimated that the available capacity for glutathione synthesis in rat kidney would account for the production of several grams of the tripeptide per day, the same order of magnitude as the estimated capacity for its destruction in the same organ. Glutathione biosynthesis is shown in Figure 4.14.

Glutathione has been used for many years *in vitro* as a reductant, to maintain the sulphydryl groups of a number of enzymes in the reduced state. Under oxidizing conditions, the tripeptide can form a disulphide-linked hexapeptide; glutathione is generally abbreviated to GSH, and the oxidized form is then GSSG. Oxidized glutathione can be reduced by a specific reductase, which in mammals is generally NAD-dependent, although in *E. coli* it is a flavoprotein. Glutathione reductase will not act on other disulphide compounds, and even GSSG analogues, such as oxidized γ-glutamyl-cysteine, or β-aspartyl-cysteinyl-glycine (aspartothione) are not substrates. However, there is no evidence that glutathione has any action *in vivo* in maintaining sulphydryl groups of enzymes. In plants there is a specific system for oxidation of GSH to GSSG, linked to reduction of dehydro-ascorbate, an irreversible reaction in which dehydro-ascorbate is reduced to ascorbate while two molecules of GSH are oxidized to GSSG. It is assumed that this reaction is involved with the use of ascorbate as a terminal electron acceptor in some plant systems, but there is little experimental evidence. One of the few examples of an *in vivo* requirement for glutathione in a mammalian system is in the catabolism of phenylalanine and tyrosine; maleyl-acetoacetate isomerase has an absolute requirement for GSH as a cofactor in the reaction (see page 162).

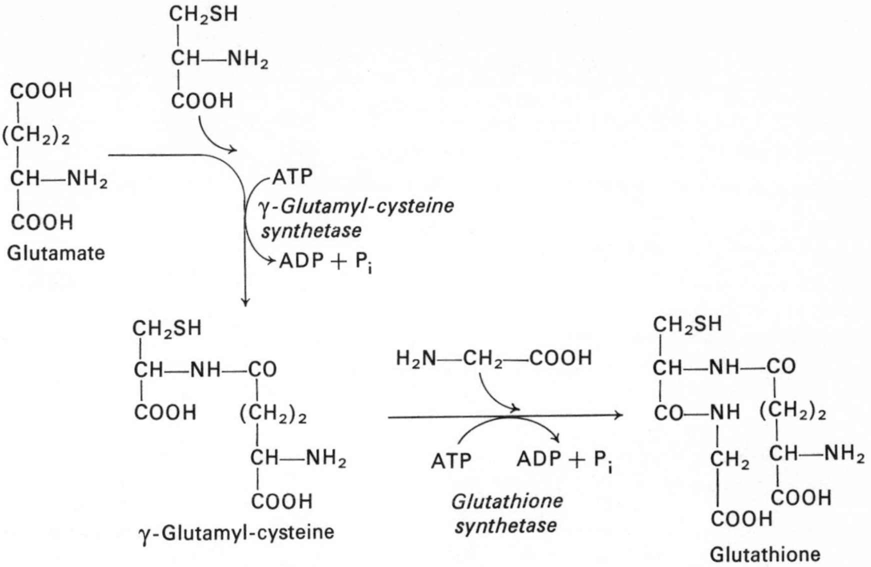

CH₂SH
|
CH—NH₂
|
COOH

COOH
|
(CH₂)₂
|
CH—NH₂
|
COOH
Glutamate

ATP
γ-Glutamyl-cysteine
synthetase
ADP + Pᵢ

CH₂SH
|
CH—NH—CO
| |
COOH   (CH₂)₂
              |
              CH—NH₂
              |
              COOH
γ-Glutamyl-cysteine

H₂N—CH₂—COOH

ATP   ADP + Pᵢ

Glutathione
synthetase

CH₂SH
|
CH—NH—CO
| |
CO—NH (CH₂)₂
| |
CH₂   CH—NH₂
| |
COOH   COOH
Glutathione

Figure 4.14. The biosynthesis of glutathione

Meister and coworkers (reviewed by Meister, 1973) have proposed a role for glutathione in the membrane transport of amino acids. The role of ATP in metabolite transport generally is unclear. A number of proposed mechanisms have postulated contractile or otherwise mobile carriers in membranes, which bind the metabolite at one side, and then use ATP in movement across to the other face of the membrane where they release the metabolite. Evidence for such proteins is scant, and a more general formulation of the role of ATP in transport is that the carrier is either chemically or conformationally modified in transport, and the role of ATP is in reformation of the active carrier.

Meister's hypothesis involves glutathione and membrane-bound γ-glutamyl transpeptidase in amino acid transport. All the common protein amino acids except proline are substrates for γ-glutamyl transpeptidase, forming γ-glutamyl-amino acid dipeptide and cysteinyl-glycine. The enzyme is tightly attached to the membrane lipo-protein, and in the rat kidney has been histochemically located in the brush border of the proximal convoluted tubule, the region associated with the resorption of amino acids from the glomerular filtrate. It accounts for as much as 1·5% of the total brush border protein. Amino acid resorption is a highly efficient process and compared with the high concentrations of amino acids in the blood there is little aminoaciduria under normal conditions.

The kidney also contains very large amounts of a soluble enzyme, γ-glutamyl cyclotransferase, which cleaves γ-glutamyl-dipeptides to form the free amino acid and 5-oxoproline (pyrrolidone carboxylic acid or pyroglutamic acid, the cyclic anhydride of glutamate). Thus, amino acids taken into the cell by formation at the membrane of γ-glutamyl peptides can be released intra-cellularly as free amino acids. It was the discovery of a further enzyme, 5-oxoprolinase,

108

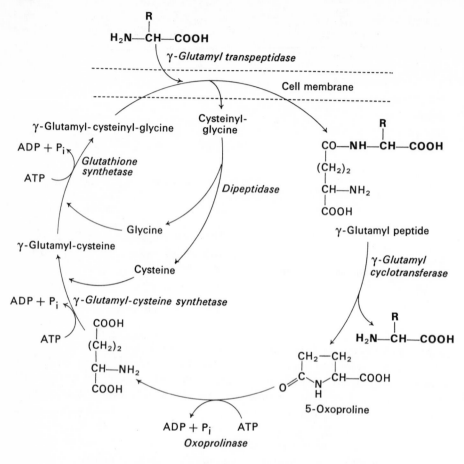

Figure 4.15. The γ-glutamyl cycle in amino acid transport

which allowed formulation of the cycle shown in Figure 4.15, the γ-glutamyl cycle for amino acid transport. Oxoprolinase rehydrates oxoproline to glutamate, in an ATP-linked reaction, so that the combined actions of the cyclotransferase and oxoprolinase represent a hitherto unknown type of enzyme reaction, an ATP-dependent cleavage of a peptide bond.

Overall, the following series of reactions requires three molecules of ATP for the transport of one molecule of amino acid: (a) the synthesis of one molecule of glutathione; (b) cleavage to form cysteinyl-glycine (which is subsequently split by a dipeptidase to yield free cysteine and glycine) and a γ-glutamyl dipeptide, followed by (c) formation of the free amino acid and 5-oxoproline, and (d) resynthesis of glutathione. Thus, a role for ATP in amino acid transport has been demonstrated, which involves synthesis of a carrier molecule that cycles intracellularly, and a membrane-associated enzyme which catalyses the attachment of the extracellular amino acid to the intracellular carrier.

It has been suggested that γ-glutamyl transpeptidase is located adjacent to a pore in the membrane which is also an amino acid binding site, with groups specific for attachment of α-amino and α-carboxyl groups. When an amino acid approaches this pore, it is 'trapped' by electrostatic interactions, and cannot cross to the inner face of the membrane. The free γ-carboxyl group of glutamate (released in the initial step of the transpeptidase reaction) then approaches the amino group of the trapped amino acid, forming a γ-glutamyl peptide, which is no longer held by the membrane receptor group, but can enter the cell.

Although preparations of the transpeptidase *in vitro* exhibit a low specificity using all of the common protein amino acids (but not the imino acids, proline and hydroxyproline), it is possible that *in vivo* the membrane amino acid binding sites have further points of attachment, apart from the carboxyl and amino group affinity sites. Thus, amino acids of similar chemical properties are generally mutually competitive for transport into cells. There is a great deal of evidence from studies on both kidney and blood–brain barrier amino acid transport, that the neutral amino acids (including alanine, the branched-chain amino acids, phenylalanine, tyrosine and tryptophan) are all carried by the same mechanism, and any one in excess will compete with the others for uptake. A similar system has been proposed for the basic amino acids (lysine, ornithine, arginine and possibly also cysteine), and another for the dicarboxylic amino acids (glutamate and aspartate). Proline is not a substrate for the transpeptidase, and being an imino acid it does not have free amino and carboxyl groups which could associate with a membrane affinity site. The non-metabolizable amino acid, α-amino-isobutyric acid, is also not a substrate for γ-glutamyl transpeptidase, and it is possible that these two amino acids, and glycine, which competes with proline for uptake but not with the neutral amino acids, may share a separate transport mechanism, not related to the γ-glutamyl cycle.

Mercapturic acid formation

Glutathione is also important in mammals in the detoxication of a variety of ingested compounds, by the formation of mercapturic acids. The stages in mercapturic acid formation from dichloronitrobenzene are shown in Figure 4.16. Initially, the foreign compound is conjugated with the sulphydryl group of the cysteinyl residue of glutathione, a reaction catalysed by glutathione-*S*-transferase. Several enzymes catalyse this reaction, with different specificities for the foreign material. Aryl and alkyl *S*-transferase catalyse the replacement of nitro and halogen groups on aromatic and alkyl compounds respectively, aralkyl *S*-transferase displaces aralkyl groups and esters, and a number of α-β unsaturated compounds, including esters and vinyl and cyclic ketones, can also be conjugated.

Details of the enzymology of further steps of mercapturic acid synthesis are less clear. The γ-glutamyl link of the conjugated peptide is broken, then the glycine moiety is released by peptidase action, and finally, prior to excretion, the *S*-substituted cysteine is *N*-acetylated. It is possible that cleavage of the γ-glutamyl link is catalysed by the same γ-glutamyl transpeptidase as is involved

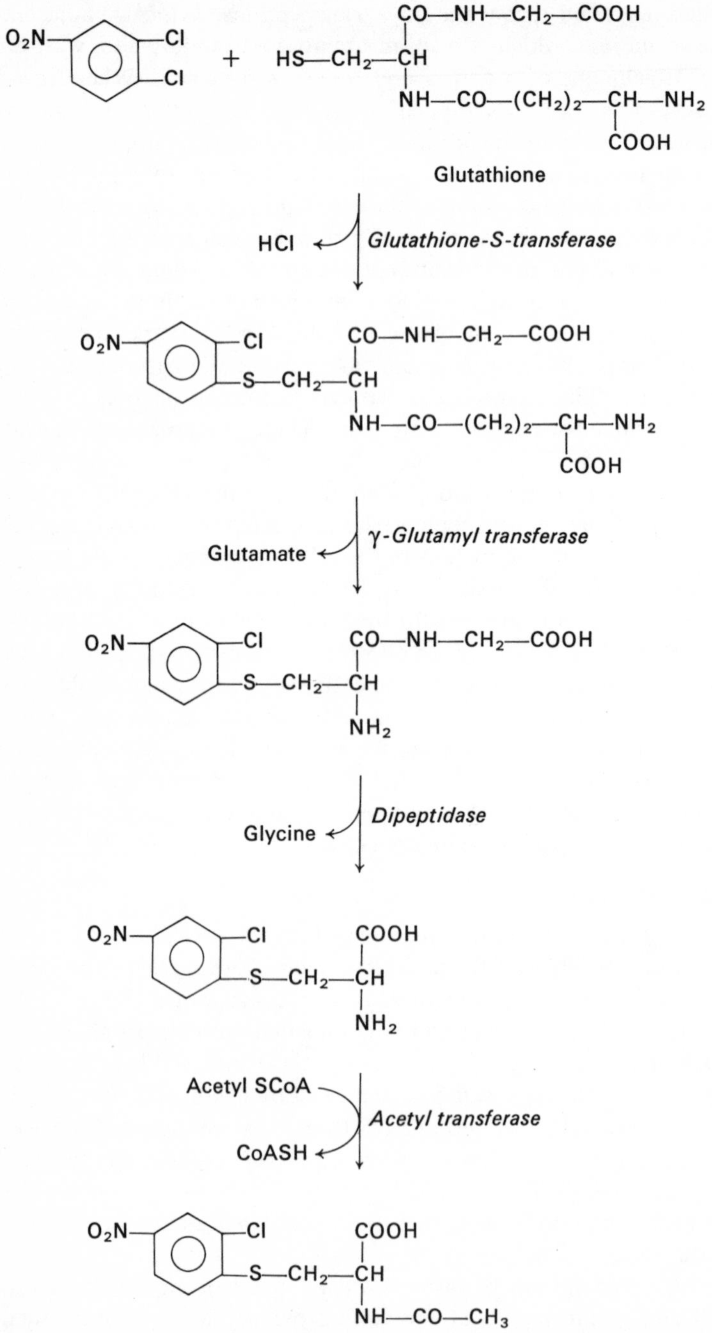

110

Figure 4.16. Mercapturic acid biosynthesis

in the γ-glutamyl cycle. γ-Glutamyl transpeptidase is associated with liver micro-somal membranes where much drug metabolism occurs, and administration of drugs such as barbiturates, which are known to induce a number of microsomal proteins, leads to an increase in liver γ-glutamyl transpeptidase, and release of the enzyme into the blood. Measurement of serum γ-glutamyl transpeptidase activity can be used as an index of liver microsomal activity, but a number of other factors are also involved, including release together with other enzymes, in cases of liver disease or damage.

Further reading

Boyland, E. and Chasseaud, L. F. (1969). The role of glutathione and glutathione-sulphotransferases in mercapturic acid biosynthesis. *Adv. Enzymol.*, **32**, 173–219.
Francis, G., John, R. and Thomas, J. (1973). Biosynthetic pathway of desmosines in elastin. *Biochem. J.*, **136**, 45–55.
Grant, M. E. and Prockop, D. J. (1972). The biosynthesis of collagen. *New Engl. J. Med.*, **286**, 194–199; 242–249; 291–300.
Meister, A. (1968). On the synthesis and utilisation of glutamine. *Harvey Lect.*, **63**, 139–178.
Stadtman, E. R., Shapiro, B. M., Kingdom, H. S., Woolfolk, C. A. and Hubbard, J. S. (1968). Cellular regulation of glutamine synthesis in *E. coli. Adv. Enz. Reg.*, **6**, 257–289.
Tabor, H. and Tabor, C. W. (1972). Biosynthesis and metabolism of 1,4-diaminobutane, spermidine, spermine and related amines. *Adv. Enzymol.*, **36**, 203–269.

References cited in the text are listed in the bibliography

CHAPTER 5

AMINO ACIDS SYNTHESIZED FROM ASPARTATE: LYSINE, METHIONINE (AND CYSTEINE), THREONINE AND ISOLEUCINE (AND LEUCINE AND VALINE)

Aspartate is readily synthesized by transamination of oxaloacetate, an intermediate of the citrate cycle; the formation of the amide, asparagine, was discussed on page 15. Alanine is formed from aspartate in a number of organisms by β-decarboxylation, and a common pathway from aspartate is used by microorganisms and plants for the synthesis of threonine, isoleucine and methionine. In plants and bacteria, lysine is also formed from aspartate, although yeasts and fungi use a different pathway. These pathways are not found in higher organisms, and so all of these amino acids (except alanine) are essential to mammals.

The other branched-chain amino acids, leucine and valine, are synthesized by pathways which closely follow that for isoleucine formation. All three are catabolized by parallel pathways, and they are therefore also considered in this chapter.

THE COMMON METABOLIC PATHWAY

The regulation of any branched metabolic pathway is a complex process, and a common biosynthetic pathway such as that shown in Figure 5.1 has an extremely intricate and interesting pattern of regulation. As would be expected, each amino acid inhibits the first step unique to its own biosynthesis. Thus, lysine inhibits the conversion of aspartic semialdehyde to dihydro-dipicolinic acid, methionine inhibits the O-succinylation of homoserine, and isoleucine inhibits the biosynthetic threonine deaminase. In each case these appear to be simple feed-back inhibitions.

The first reaction of the common pathway is the phosphorylation of aspartate to β-aspartyl phosphate, an ATP-dependent reaction catalysed by aspartokinase. In E. coli, there are three isoenzymes of aspartokinase: aspartokinase I is inhibited by threonine, aspartokinase II is repressed by methionine, and aspartokinase III is both inhibited and repressed by lysine. Methionine has no effect on preformed aspartokinase. The synthesis of isoenzyme I (the form which is inhibited by threonine) is not repressed by threonine, although a large excess of isoleucine does repress synthesis of this isoenzyme.

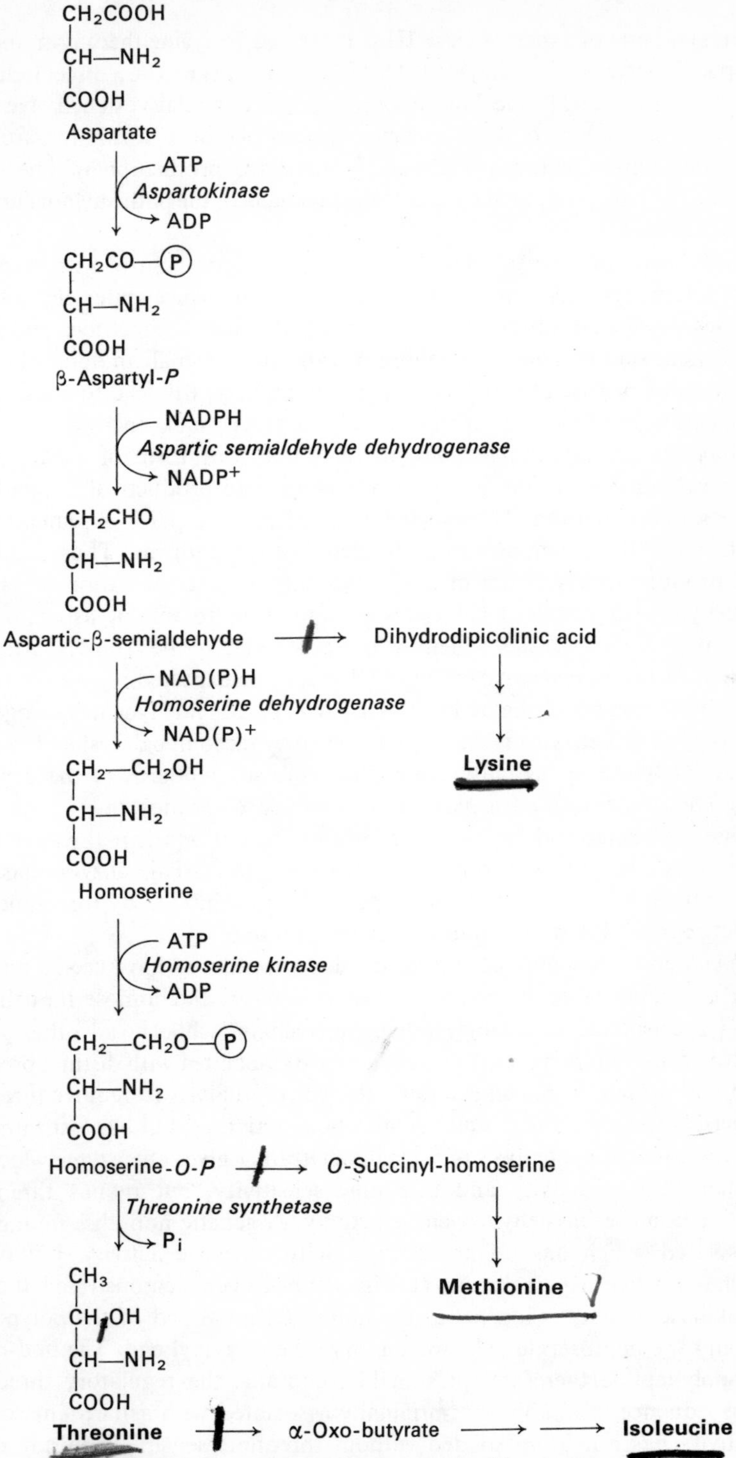

CH$_2$COOH

CH—NH$_2$

COOH

Aspartate

⎡ ATP
⎢ *Aspartokinase*
⎣ ADP

CH$_2$CO—(P)

CH—NH$_2$

COOH

β-Aspartyl-*P*

⎡ NADPH
⎢ *Aspartic semialdehyde dehydrogenase*
⎣ NADP$^+$

CH$_2$CHO

CH—NH$_2$

COOH

Aspartic-β-semialdehyde ⟶ Dihydrodipicolinic acid

⎡ NAD(P)H
⎢ *Homoserine dehydrogenase*
⎣ NAD(P)$^+$

↓

Lysine

CH$_2$—CH$_2$OH

CH—NH$_2$

COOH

Homoserine

⎡ ATP
⎢ *Homoserine kinase*
⎣ ADP

CH$_2$—CH$_2$O—(P)

CH—NH$_2$

COOH

Homoserine-*O-P* ⟶ *O*-Succinyl-homoserine

⎡ *Threonine synthetase*
⎣ P$_i$

↓

Methionine

CH$_3$

CH$_2$OH

CH—NH$_2$

COOH

Threonine ⟶ α-Oxo-butyrate ⟶ ⟶ **Isoleucine**

Figure 5.1. Amino acids synthesized from asparate

When synthesis of aspartokinase III is repressed by lysine there is an increase in the specific activity of isoenzyme I. This does not appear to be a direct induction of enzyme synthesis by lysine, but rather a response to a relative deficit of aspartyl phosphate when only two of the enzymes responsible for its formation are being synthesized. This is compensated for by increased production of one of the isoenzymes which is regulated by one of the products of the pathway not currently present in excess.

The inhibition of aspartokinase I by threonine is competitive with respect to aspartate, although this is not likely to have any significance under physiological conditions. Lysine inhibition of aspartokinase III is non-competitive, and at low levels of lysine (not in themselves inhibitory) addition of small amounts of leucine and isoleucine, neither of which is normally inhibitory, will lead to considerable inhibition. The physiological significance of this synergism is unclear.

In *Rhodopseudomonas spheroides*, there is only one form of aspartokinase which is not sensitive to inhibition by any of the end products of the pathway, singly or in combination. The enzyme is inhibited by aspartic β-semialdehyde, the last intermediate common to all branches of the pathway. Thus, inhibition by end-product accumulation of enzymes catalysing the utilization of aspartic semialdehyde will result in sufficient accumulation to inhibit aspartokinase. In organisms such as yeasts which do not synthesize lysine from aspartate, no equivalent of the *E. coli* aspartokinase III would be expected.

The second enzyme of the pathway is aspartic β-semialdehyde dehydrogenase. The activity of this enzyme is unaffected *in vitro* by threonine or lysine. However, an excess of lysine in the culture medium represses synthesis of the dehydrogenase. The conversion of aspartic semialdehyde to homoserine, common to threonine, isoleucine and methionine synthesis but not on the pathway of lysine formation, is catalysed by homoserine dehydrogenase. This enzyme has been shown to have two isoenzymes, one repressed and inhibited by threonine, and the other repressed, but not inhibited, by methionine.

In *E. coli* and other *Enterobacteriaciae*, there appears to have been a measure of gene fusion, since threonine-sensitive aspartokinase I and homoserine dehydrogenase I are isolated as a single polypeptide chain, while in all other genera that have been examined these two activities are associated with distinct proteins. The normal protein in *E. coli* is a tetramer, but on dialysis to remove threonine it dissociates to a monomer, which retains both activities, but has lost threonine sensitivity. Limited proteolysis of the native tetramer gives an enzyme which has lost aspartokinase activity and threonine sensitivity, but retains threonine-insensitive homoserine dehydrogenase activity. A genetic nonsense mutant has been isolated which has no homoserine dehydrogenase activity, but retains threonine-sensitive aspartokinase activity. It has been demonstrated that the aspartokinase activity is located at the amino terminal end of the polypeptide chain, and the homoserine dehydrogenase at the carboxyl end. The mid-region of the polypeptide therefore, presumably, contains the regulatory threonine-binding sequence, probably that originally associated with aspartokinase since this activity has not been isolated without threonine sensitivity in any of the manipulations noted above. It is probable that the threonine-sensitivity-conferring region originally associated with homoserine dehydrogenase has been lost in the process of gene fusion. There is evidence that a considerable portion of at least one of the two separate polypeptides must have been lost in fusion, since the molecular weight of the *E. coli* double enzyme is considerably less than the sum of the molecular weights of the individual enzymes in other species.

Thus, in *E. coli* the activity of the enzymes common to the biosynthesis of all the amino acids synthesized from aspartate by this pathway is regulated by a combination of feed-back inhibition and end-product repression on families of isoenzymes catalysing key reactions. In other organisms the pattern of regulation is less complex.

Threonine synthetase, which catalyses the formation of threonine from homoserine-O-phosphate, is inhibited by accumulation of isoleucine, but only to a small extent by its product, threonine. It is a pyridoxal-P dependent enzyme, and it can be shown that the oxygen introduced at the β-carbon, and the hydrogen atoms introduced at the α- and γ-carbons come from water. It has been proposed that the homoserine–pyridoxal-P Schiff base loses phosphate, and the resultant α–β unsaturated intermediate is hydrated prior to hydrolysis of the complex to yield threonine.

LYSINE

Bacterial biosynthesis—the diaminopimelate pathway

In bacteria, algae, lower fungi and most green plants, lysine is synthesized through the pathway shown in Figure 5.2. The conversion of aspartate to aspartic semialdehyde and the regulation of the pathway, have been discussed above.

The first reaction unique to the biosynthesis of lysine is the condensation of aspartic semialdehyde with pyruvate to form 2,3-dihydrodipicolinic acid, a reaction catalysed by dihydrodipicolinate synthetase. The reaction proceeds in two stages, an aldol condensation between the oxo-group of aspartic semialdehyde and the pyruvate, followed by ring closure and elimination of a further molecule of water formed from the oxo-group of the pyruvate moiety and the hydrogen of the aspartic semialdehyde amino group. The synthetase is highly specific for both substrates; neither glutamic nor succinic semialdehyde can substitute for aspartic semialdehyde, and no other oxo-acid can be used in place of pyruvate. The equilibrium strongly favours cyclization, so in practice this reaction is not readily reversible. As was noted above, the synthetase is strongly inhibited by lysine.

After reduction of dihydrodipicolinate to Δ^1-piperidine-dicarboxylate, the ring is opened hydrolytically, and the amino group is succinylated, to yield N-succinyl-ε-oxo-α-amino pimelic acid. The ring opening and succinyl transfer are successive steps catalysed by the same enzyme, Δ^1-piperidine dicarboxylate succinylase. The purpose of this N-substitution is the same as that of acetylation in the biosynthesis of ornithine (see page 86), namely to prevent cyclization by condensation between the ε-oxo and α-amino groups before a second amino group can be added.

116

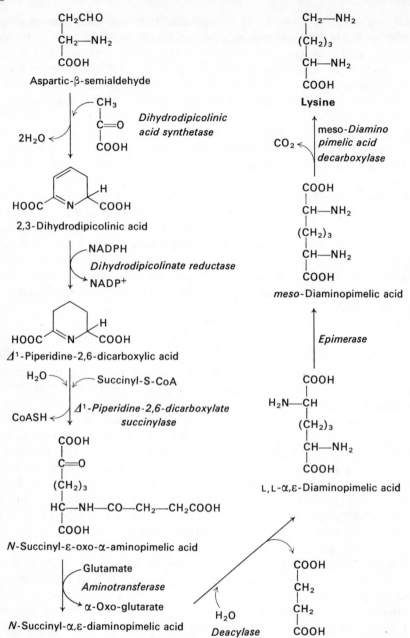

Figure 5.2. Bacterial biosynthesis of lysine—the diaminopimelic acid pathway

The second amino group is added by aminotransfer from glutamate, catalysed by a specific aminotransferase which has been shown to be distinct from *N*-acetyl ornithine aminotransferase. Although the reaction can proceed in either direction, the enzyme is strongly inhibited by an excess of α-oxo-glutarate, so that lysine synthesis will be inhibited at times of low nitrogen availability, when the α-oxo-glutarate/glutamate ratio is shifted towards the oxo-acid.

Deacylation of the resultant N-succinyl diaminopimelate is catalysed by a specific deacylase, again distinct from the similar enzyme involved in ornithine biosynthesis. N-Acetyl-diaminopimelate is not a substrate for this enzyme, which specifically requires the N-succinyl derivative. The product of the deacylase is L,L-diaminopimelate, which is not a substrate for the subsequent decarboxy-lase, and so must undergo epimerization to *meso*-diaminopimelate, in which the α-carbon has L-configuration, and the ε-carbon D-configuration. In *E. coli*, partially purified preparations of *meso*-diaminopimelate epimerase have been shown to be pyridoxal-P dependent; they can be inactivated by reaction with hydrazines and other pyridoxal-P reacting compounds. In preparations from *B. megaterium* it has not been possible to demonstrate any role of pyridoxal-P in the epimerase, suggesting that in this organism the reaction must have a different mechanism.

meso-Diaminopimelate is decarboxylated to L-lysine, a reaction catalysed by an enzyme which is distinct from L-α-lysine decarboxylase, the enzyme which produces the diamine cadaverine. *meso*-Diaminopimelate decarboxylase is the only D-amino acid decarboxylase reported to date. Like most L-amino acid decarboxylases, it is pyridoxal-P dependent, and in *E. coli* mutants, defective forms of the enzyme have been isolated which have an impaired affinity for pyridoxal-P; these strains are therefore lysine-dependent unless grown in high concentrations of pyridoxal-P.

In some Gram-positive bacteria, *meso*-diaminopimelate is itself an end-product of the pathway, since it is required for cell wall synthesis. In *B. stearothermophilus*, a specific *meso*-diaminopimelate-sensitive aspartokinase has been isolated, and shown to be antigenically distinct from the threonine and lysine sensitive enzymes of this organism. In such sporulative Gram-positive organisms as *B. stearo-thermophilus*, dihydrodipicolinic acid is also an important intermediate, since it can give rise to dipicolinic acid, which is required for synthesis of the sporulation capsule.

Lysine biosynthesis in yeasts and fungi—the α-amino-adipic acid pathway

In yeasts and higher fungi, and in some green algae, the pathway of lysine biosynthesis is that shown in Figure 5.3; the carbon source is α-oxo-glutarate, and hence glutamate, rather than aspartate as in other organisms. The first enzyme of the pathway, homocitrate synthetase, is repressed by lysine, but is not inhibited, except at unphysiologically high levels of the end-product. Feedback inhibition of lysine biosynthesis does occur, but has not been localized with more precision than as being at some stage after the formation of α-amino-adipic acid (Tucci and Ceci, 1972). The second enzyme of the pathway, homoaconitase, is also repressed by lysine.

The initial steps of the pathway, the formation of homocitric acid by condensa-tion between α-oxo-glutarate and acetyl-SCoA, the formation of homo-isocitric

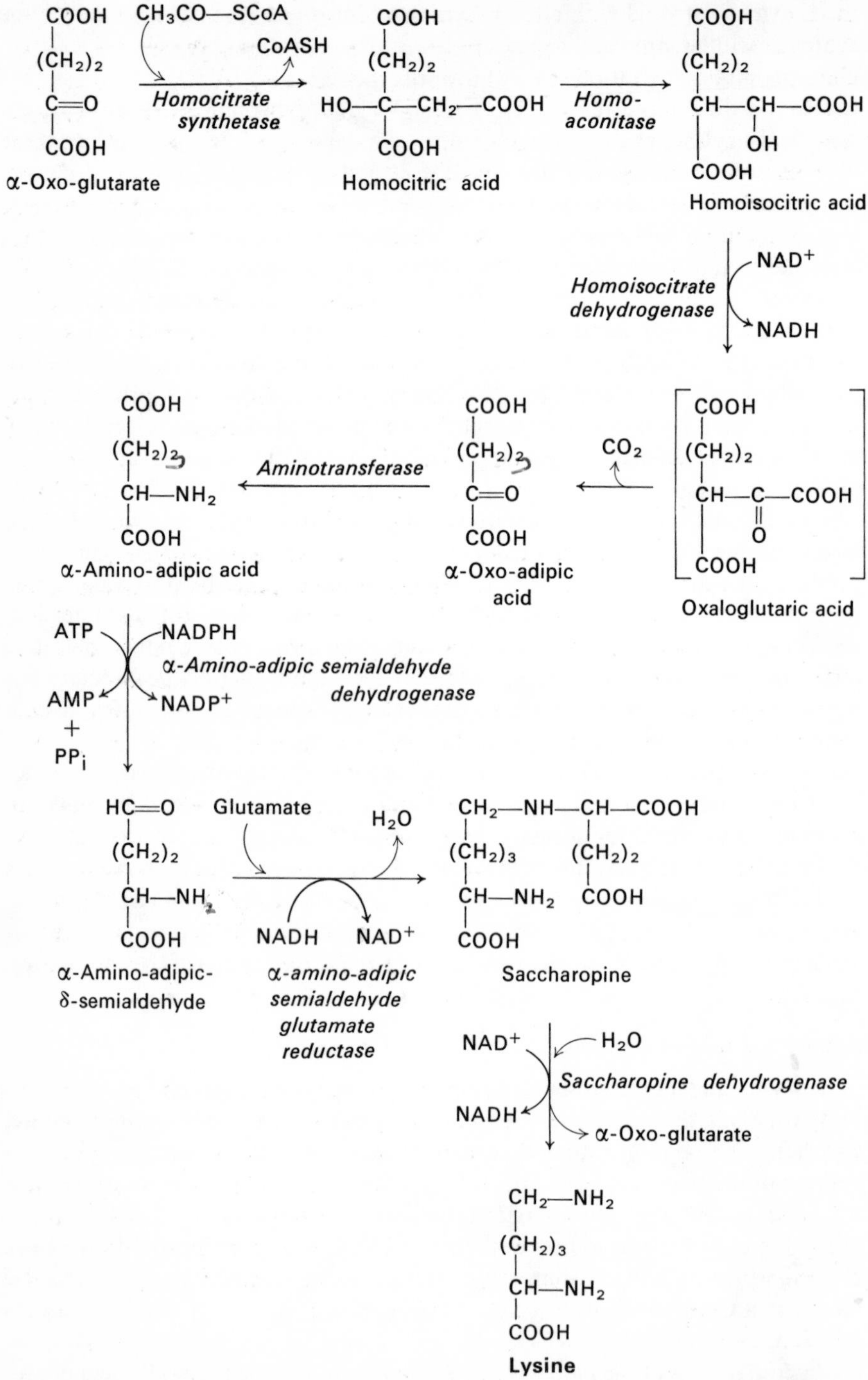

COOH CH_3CO—SCoA

$(CH_2)_2$ CoASH

C=O   *Homocitrate synthetase*

COOH

α-Oxo-glutarate

COOH

$(CH_2)_2$

HO—C—CH_2—COOH

COOH

Homocitric acid

Homo-aconitase

COOH

$(CH_2)_2$

CH—CH—COOH

     OH

COOH

Homoisocitric acid

Homoisocitrate dehydrogenase NAD^+ NADH

COOH

$(CH_2)_2$

CH—NH$_2$

COOH

α-Amino-adipic acid

Aminotransferase

COOH

$(CH_2)_2$

C=O

COOH

α-Oxo-adipic acid

CO_2

$\left[\begin{array}{l} COOH \\ (CH_2)_2 \\ CH-\underset{\underset{O}{\|}}{C}-COOH \\ COOH \end{array}\right]$

Oxaloglutaric acid

ATP   NADPH

α-Amino-adipic semialdehyde dehydrogenase

AMP $NADP^+$

+

PP$_i$

HC=O   Glutamate H_2O

$(CH_2)_2$

CH—NH$_2$

COOH

α-Amino-adipic-δ-semialdehyde

NADH NAD^+

α-amino-adipic semialdehyde glutamate reductase

CH_2—NH—CH—COOH

$(CH_2)_3$ $(CH_2)_2$

CH—NH$_2$ COOH

COOH

Saccharopine

NAD^+ H_2O

Saccharopine dehydrogenase

NADH   α-Oxo-glutarate

CH_2—NH$_2$

$(CH_2)_3$

CH—NH$_2$

COOH

Lysine

Figure 5.3. Fungal biosynthesis of lysine—the α-amino adipic acid pathway

acid, and its oxidation to α-oxo-adipic acid, are parallel to the reactions of the citrate cycle between the formation of citrate and α-oxo-glutarate. However, the enzymes have been shown to be distinct in the two pathways. In view of the similarity of the two pathways, it is interesting to note that the absolute configuration of homo-isocitrate formed in the biosynthesis of lysine, and isocitrate formed in the citrate cycle, are opposite. Presumably this prevents any (highly undesirable) cross inhibition between the two pathways, since homo-isocitrate and isocitrate might be expected to compete for the same catalytic site if they had the same configuration.

Like the reaction of aconitase, the interconversion of homocitrate and homo-isocitrate is believed to proceed by way of dehydration to enzyme-bound homo-aconitate, followed by rehydration to homo-isocitrate. Although other cofactors are the same, the oxidative decarboxylation of homo-isocitrate to α-oxo-adipic acid, catalysed by homo-isocitrate dehydrogenase, is not stimulated by AMP which activates isocitrate dehydrogenase. This would be expected since the role of the AMP activation of isocitrate dehydrogenase is to enhance the activity of the citrate cycle at a time when increased energy metabolism is required. Such considerations would not be expected to apply to lysine biosynthesis.

The formation of α-amino-adipic semialdehyde appears to be similar to the formation of aspartic semialdehyde from aspartate, in that both ATP and NADPH are required. However, no phosphorylated intermediate has been detected, and ATP is hydrolysed to AMP and pyrophosphate in this reaction. The enzyme catalyses a pyrophosphate exchange, suggesting that the activated intermediate, if any, must be enzyme-bound α-amino-adipyl-δ-AMP, rather than the δ-phosphate.

A side-reaction which can occur spontaneously is the rapid cyclization of α-amino-adipic semialdehyde to Δ^1-piperidine-6-carboxylate in free solution. To prevent this, the semialdehyde must be almost entirely enzyme-bound with very little free in solution. The amination of α-amino-adipic semialdehyde to lysine does not proceed directly, but by the intermediate formation of saccharopine by a reductive condensation between the semialdehyde and glutamate. Saccharopine is then oxidatively hydrolysed to lysine and α-oxo-glutarate.

Lysine catabolism

Two pathways of lysine catabolism found in many bacteria are shown in Figure 5.4. One, which is the reverse of the pathway used for lysine biosynthesis in yeasts, involves the reductive condensation of lysine with α-oxo-glutarate to form saccharopine, followed by oxidative cleavage to glutamate and α-amino-adipic semialdehyde, which is reduced to α-amino-adipic acid. In this pathway, the ε-amino group of the lysine is lost, so that the Δ^1-piperidine-6-carboxylate formed by spontaneous cyclization of α-amino-adipic semialdehyde retains the label from the α-amino group of the initial substrate.

The other pathway for lysine catabolism is by deamination to α-oxo-ε-amino caproic acid, which spontaneously cyclizes to Δ^1-piperidine-2-carboxylate. This can be isomerized to Δ^1-piperidine-6-carboxylate by reduction to the satur-

120

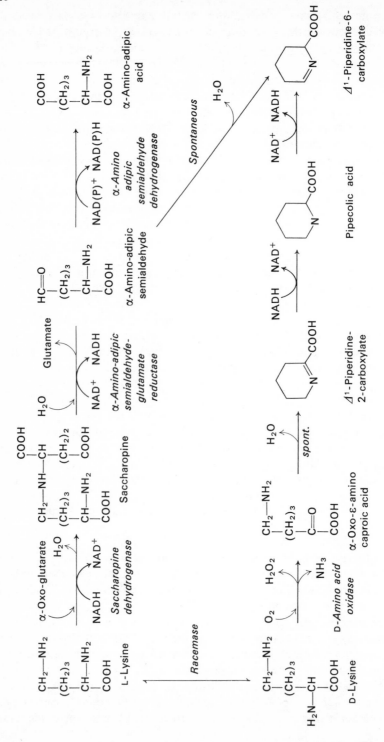

Figure 5.4. Lysine catabolism

ated compound, pipecolic acid, followed by unsaturation. The Δ^1-piperidine-6-carboxylate formed by this route can be distinguished from that produced by way of saccharopine since in this case it is the α-amino group that is lost, so that the final product retains the ε-amino group of lysine.

The immediate precursor of the cyclic pathway of lysine catabolism appears to be D-lysine. Although most bacteria are capable of racemizing lysine, this reaction appears to be little used, and in general it is possible to demonstrate that, as shown in Figure 5.4, L-lysine is mainly catabolized by way of saccharopine, while the D-isomer is normally degraded by way of pipecolic acid.

In pseudomonads, D-lysine catabolism proceeds as in other organisms, by the pipecolate pathway described above, but the Δ^1-piperidine-6-carboxylate formed is hydrolysed to the open chain α-amino-adipic semialdehyde, which is then reduced to α-amino-adipic acid. The pathway of L-lysine catabolism in these organisms is shown in Figure 5.5, formation of acetyl-SCoA by way of glutaric acid.

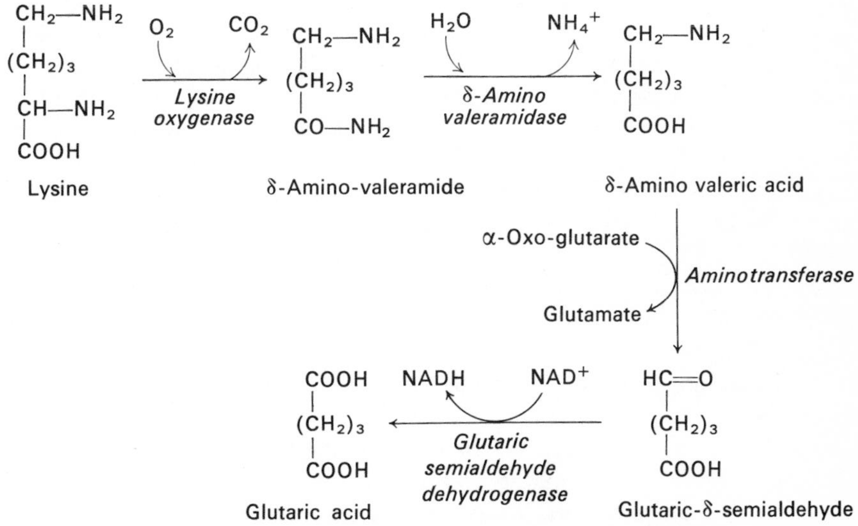

Figure 5.5. L-Lysine catabolism of pseudomonads

The first step is a mixed oxidative decarboxylation and deamination, catalysed by the flavoprotein lysine oxygenase. The reaction is assumed to proceed by way of an initial dehydrogenation of the α-amino group, leading to the formation of the α-imino acid. This is then attacked by oxygen, with decarboxylation and formation of an amide at the former α-carbon, so that the product is δ-amino valeramide. Under anaerobic conditions *in vitro* it has been possible to manipulate lysine oxygenase so that the reaction follows the same pathway as the amino acid oxidases, forming α-oxo-δ-amino caproic acid, but it is unlikely that this activity is seen under physiological conditions.

When it occurs, α-deamination of lysine is probably catalysed by amino acid oxidases rather than lysine oxygenase. However, it has been shown that purified preparations of lysine oxygenase do display a general amino acid oxidase activity, for example converting ornithine to α-oxo-δ-amino-*n*-valerate. This reaction consumes oxygen, and produces ammonia and hydrogen peroxide in stoichiometric amounts. Ornithine acts as a competitive inhibitor of lysine oxygenase activity, suggesting that the two activities are associated with the same catalytic site. D-lysine is not a substrate for this enzyme, although it does act as an inducer. In organisms grown on D- or L-lysine rich media the activity of lysine oxygenase is much increased.

The second enzyme of the pathway, δ-amino-valeramidase, is also induced by either stereoisomer of lysine. Amino-valeramidase catalyses removal of the amide from the carboxyl group of the substrate, forming δ-amino-valeric acid, which then undergoes transamination, using α-oxo-glutarate as the amino acceptor, to form glutaric semialdehyde. This semialdehyde can be oxidized to glutarate, and after formation of glutaryl-SCoA can be degraded to crotonyl-SCoA, and thence to acetyl-SCoA.

In yeasts there is evidence that saccharopine formation is not involved in the catabolism of lysine; indeed it would be surprising if it were. In *Hansenula saturnalis*, a yeast which is able to use the nitrogen of lysine but not the carbon for growth, it has been shown that during growth in the presence of large amounts of lysine there is an accumulation of ε-*N*-acetyl lysine, as well as glutaric acid. It appears that in most yeasts the pathway of lysine catabolism is via *N*-acetylated intermediates, as shown in Figure 5.6. Acetylation of the ε-amino group, by acetyl transfer from acetyl-SCoA, protects the substrate against cyclization when the α-amino group is removed by amino transfer.

Before deacetylation, the resultant oxo-acid is reduced to the hydroxy-derivative, ε-acetamido-α-hydroxycaproic acid. The deacetylated ε-amino-α-hydroxy-caproic acid undergoes amino transfer with α-oxo-glutarate to yield glutaric semialdehyde. In most yeasts this can be metabolized as described above, eventually yielding acetyl-SCoA, but in *H. saturnalis* it appears that there is a defect in glutarate utilization, and therefore when the organism is grown in the presence of large amounts of lysine, glutarate accumulates.

A number of anaerobic organisms, notably the *Clostridia*, can be shown to ferment lysine anaerobically. The ultimate yield per mole of lysine fermented is 1 mol each of acetate and butyrate and 2 mol of ammonia. One mole of ADP is phosphorylated to ATP in the process (see Figure 5.7).

Although the ultimate products from both stereoisomers are the same, the distribution of label from radioactive lysine is different. In D-lysine fermentation, C-6 of lysine becomes the methyl group of acetate, and C-1 of lysine becomes the carboxyl group of butyrate. In the fermentation of L-lysine, the carboxyl group of butyrate is formed from C-6 of lysine, and the acetate incorporates C-1 and C-2 of the initial substrate.

Three enzymes are involved in the initial stages of the reactions of D- and L-lysine; they have been discussed in detail by Stadtman (1963). All three activities are very similar, in that they involve migration of an amino group to an adjacent carbon atom, and all three reactions require coenzyme B_{12} and pyridoxal-*P*.

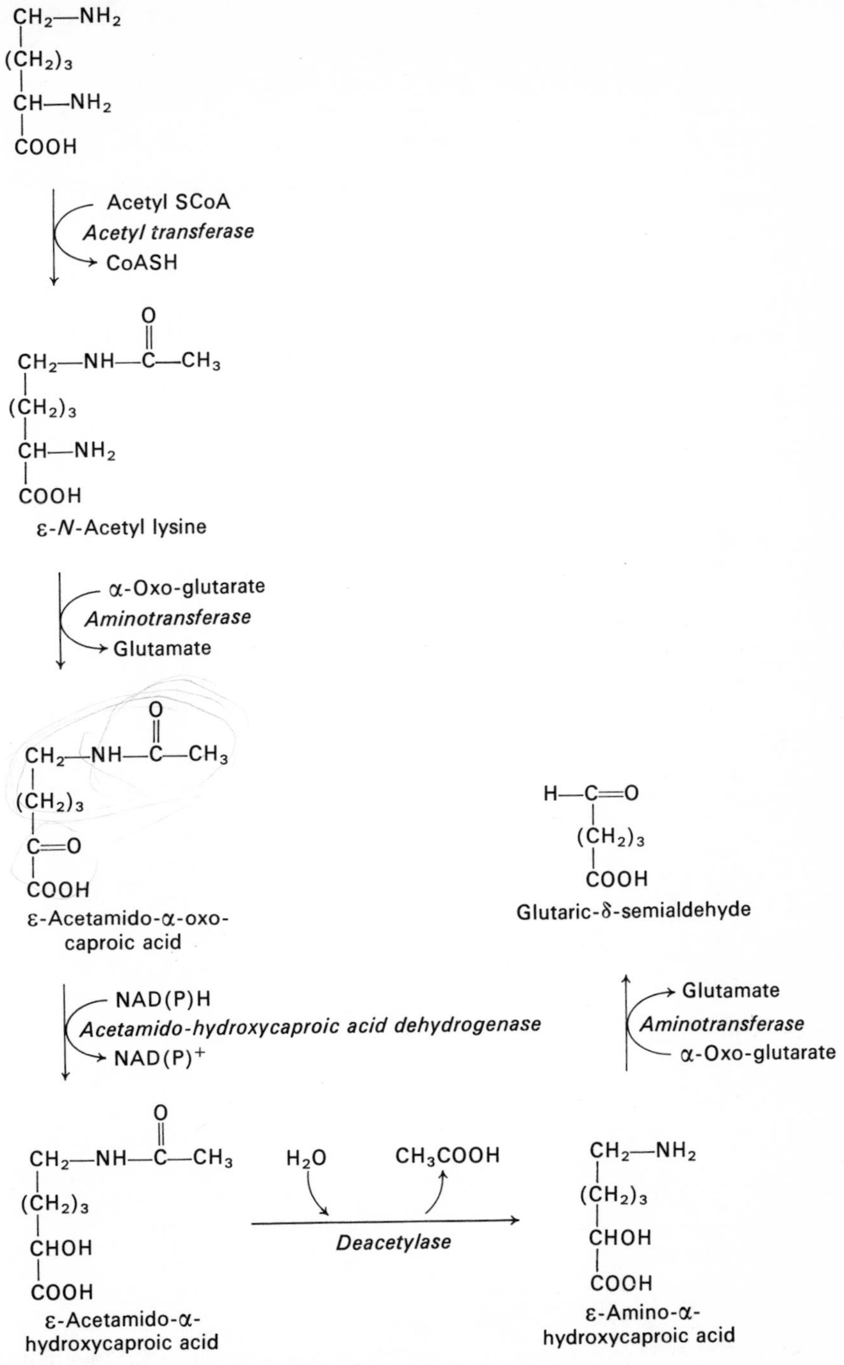

Figure 5.6. The *N*-acetylated pathway of lysine catabolism in yeasts

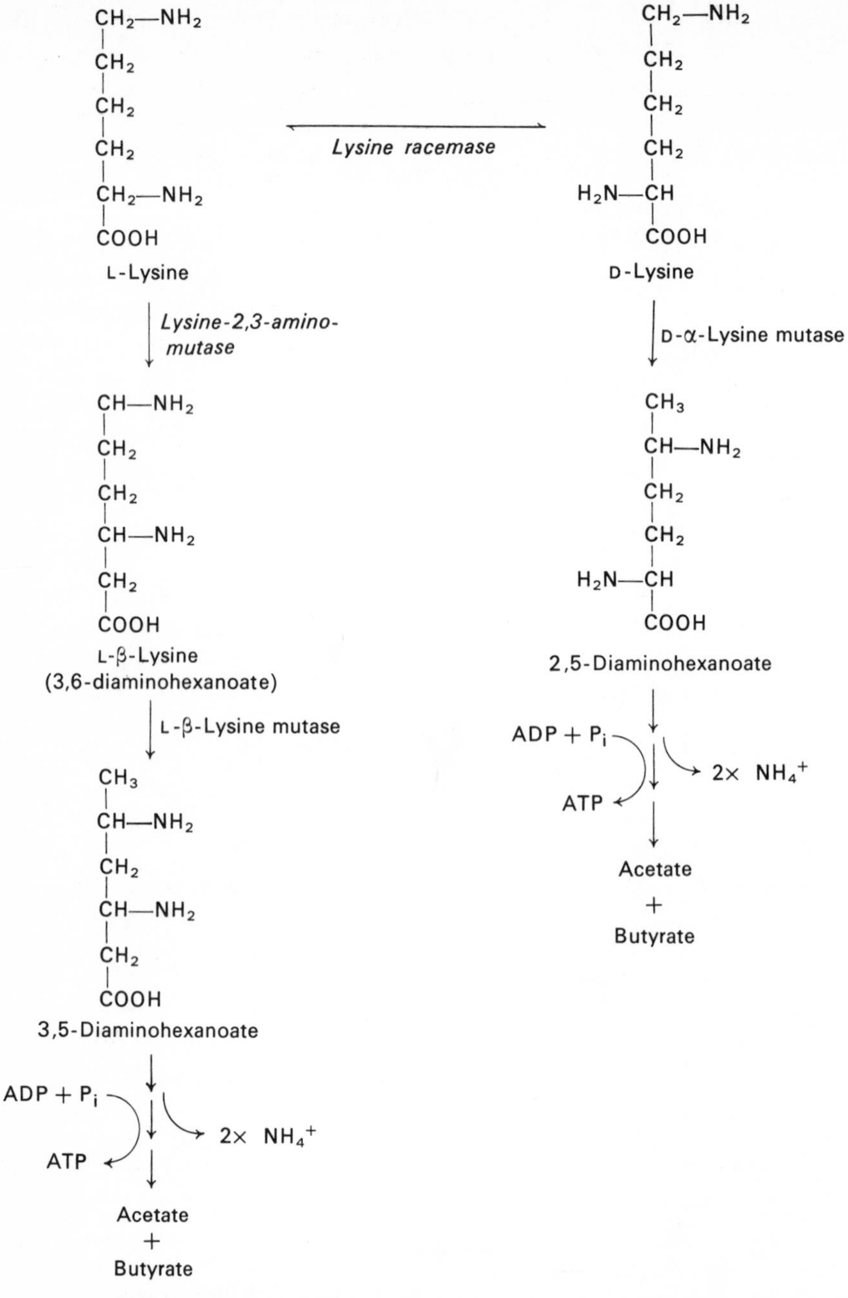

Figure 5.7. Anaerobic fermentation of lysine in *Cl. sticklandii*

There is no exchange of the amino groups with ammonium ions in the incubation medium *in vitro*, so it appears that the amino migration proceeds by way of tightly enzyme-bound amino intermediates, probably as pyridoxamine-*P*.

D-Lysine undergoes a single amino migration, from C-6 to C-5, to form 2,5-diamino hexanoate, which is then deaminated, presumably oxidatively, and cleaved to acetate and butyrate. L-Lysine undergoes two successive amino migrations, initially from C-2 to C-3, forming 3,6-diamino hexanoate (β-lysine), and then from C-6 to C-5, to form 3,5-diamino hexanoate, which is then deaminated and cleaved to acetate and butyrate. The lysine mutase complexes are activated by ATP, which reduces the K_m of the enzyme for its substrate about 10-fold, without being hydrolysed. *Clostridium sticklandii* also has an ornithine mutase, which catalyses the migration of the δ-amino group of D-ornithine to C-4, yielding 2,4-diamino pentanoate. Although it has not been studied in detail, this enzyme appears to be very similar to the three lysine mutases, although it can be separated from them. The reactions involved in the cleavage of 3,6- and 2,5-diamino hexanoates to acetate and butyrate have not yet been elucidated.

In mammals, L-lysine is degraded to α-amino-adipic acid, by way of saccharopine; the pathway is the same as that shown in Figure 5.4. Administered D-lysine is converted to pipecolic acid. This was demonstrated by Grove and coworkers (1969), in a series of experiments using ^{14}C- and ^{15}N-labelled lysine. The work was somewhat inconclusive, in that the recovery of α-amino adipic acid was not sufficient to allow determination of the ^{14}C/^{15}N ratio, to decide whether the amino-adipate formed from L-lysine arose by way of saccharopine or pipecolic acid. However, the poor formation of pipecolate from L-lysine, compared with its ready formation from D-lysine, was considered good evidence that L-lysine catabolism in mammals does not proceed by way of cyclic intermediates.

Other workers have demonstrated the presence in mammalian tissues of an active lysine–α-oxo-glutarate reductase (saccharopine dehydrogenase), forming saccharopine from lysine. Dancis and coworkers (1969) showed that in three hyperlysinaemic siblings there was a deficit of saccharopine dehydrogenase in cultured fibroblasts compared with fibroblasts from normal controls. These patients had a poor overall capacity to catabolize lysine and a very low capacity to synthesize saccharopine.

Fellows (1973) has demonstrated that under conditions of total inhibition of saccharopine synthesis, mammalian liver preparations *in vitro* will oxidatively cleave saccharopine to lysine and α-oxo-glutarate. The enzyme catalysing this reaction has been named lysine-oxo-glutarate oxidoreductase, and has been purified and shown to be distinct from the lysine–oxo-glutarate reductase responsible for saccharopine formation. The physiological significance of saccharopine cleavage to lysine in mammals in unclear, but it may represent a mechanism for short-term storage of the amino acid as saccharopine prior to final catabolism. Simell and coworkers (1972) reported one case, and cited another, of hyperlysinaemia with simultaneous saccharopinuria, indicating that if saccharopine is indeed an intermediate in human lysine catabolism then the defect in these two patients must lie not, as in the cases described above, in the synthesis of saccharopine, but in some later stage of its metabolism. In these two patients, as well as in some of the other cases described, there was considerably more ε-*N*-acetyl lysine present in both blood and urine than the small amounts previously reported in normal subjects. It appears probable that ε-N-acetyl lysine is an intermediate in the mammalian catabolism of D-lysine via pipecolic acid. Mammalian D-amino acid oxidase does not act readily on lysine, but the ε-amino substituted derivatives are good substrates. The increased levels of ε-N-acetyl lysine in blood of hyperlysinaemic patients suggests that it is also possible for some L-lysine to be catabolized by this route, although it has not been established whether the N-acetyl derivatives arise from intestinal bacteria in normal subjects or not.

The catabolism of δ-hydroxylysine from the degradation of collagen and elastin appears to be by way of formation of 5-hydroxypipecolic acid in mammals. This can be metabolized slowly to α-amino-δ-hydroxycaproic acid, in a reaction sequence similar to that described above for D-lysine catabolism in pseudomonads.

METHIONINE

Biosynthesis in plants and micro-organisms

Homoserine-O-phosphate, the last intermediate of the aspartate pathway common to methionine and threonine biosynthesis, can either be methylated to threonine, a reaction catalysed by threonine synthetase, or undergo displacement of the phosphate by a succinyl group catalysed by homoserine succinyl transferase. Threonine synthetase is inhibited by accumulation of isoleucine (and to a lesser extent by threonine), while the succinyl transferase is strongly inhibited by excess methionine and S-adenosyl methionine together, although either of these end-products alone is a poor inhibitor. Thus, the pathway followed by homoserine-O-phosphate is determined by the relative concentrations of the two end-products of the two pathways for which it is the precursor.

As shown in Figure 5.8, succinyl homoserine is attacked by cysteine, in a reaction catalysed by cystathionine-γ-synthetase displacing succinate and forming cystathionine, which is then cleaved by β-cystathionase to yield homocysteine, pyruvate and ammonia.

In bacteria and plants, cysteine is synthesized by a two-step reaction from serine. Serine is O-acetylated by acetyl transfer from acetyl-SCoA, and this intermediate reacts with inorganic sulphide to yield cysteine and acetate. Serine acetyl transferase is a pyridoxal-P-dependent enzyme. Its synthesis is repressed in bacteria grown on cysteine-rich media, although the formed enzyme is not inhibited by cysteine. In some organisms, including chick embryos but not the adult bird, there is an alternative pathway of cysteine synthesis. Inorganic sulphide displaces the hydroxyl group of serine directly, without O-acylation. The same enzyme catalyses an exchange between inorganic sulphite and the sulphydryl group of cysteine, forming cysteic acid, and liberating hydrogen sulphide.

In some bacteria. there is an alternative pathway of homocysteine synthesis, also shown in Figure 5.8, whereby O-acyl homoserine (normally the acetyl rather than the succinyl derivative) is attacked by inorganic sulphide, displacing the acyl group, and forming homocysteine directly. The reaction is apparently

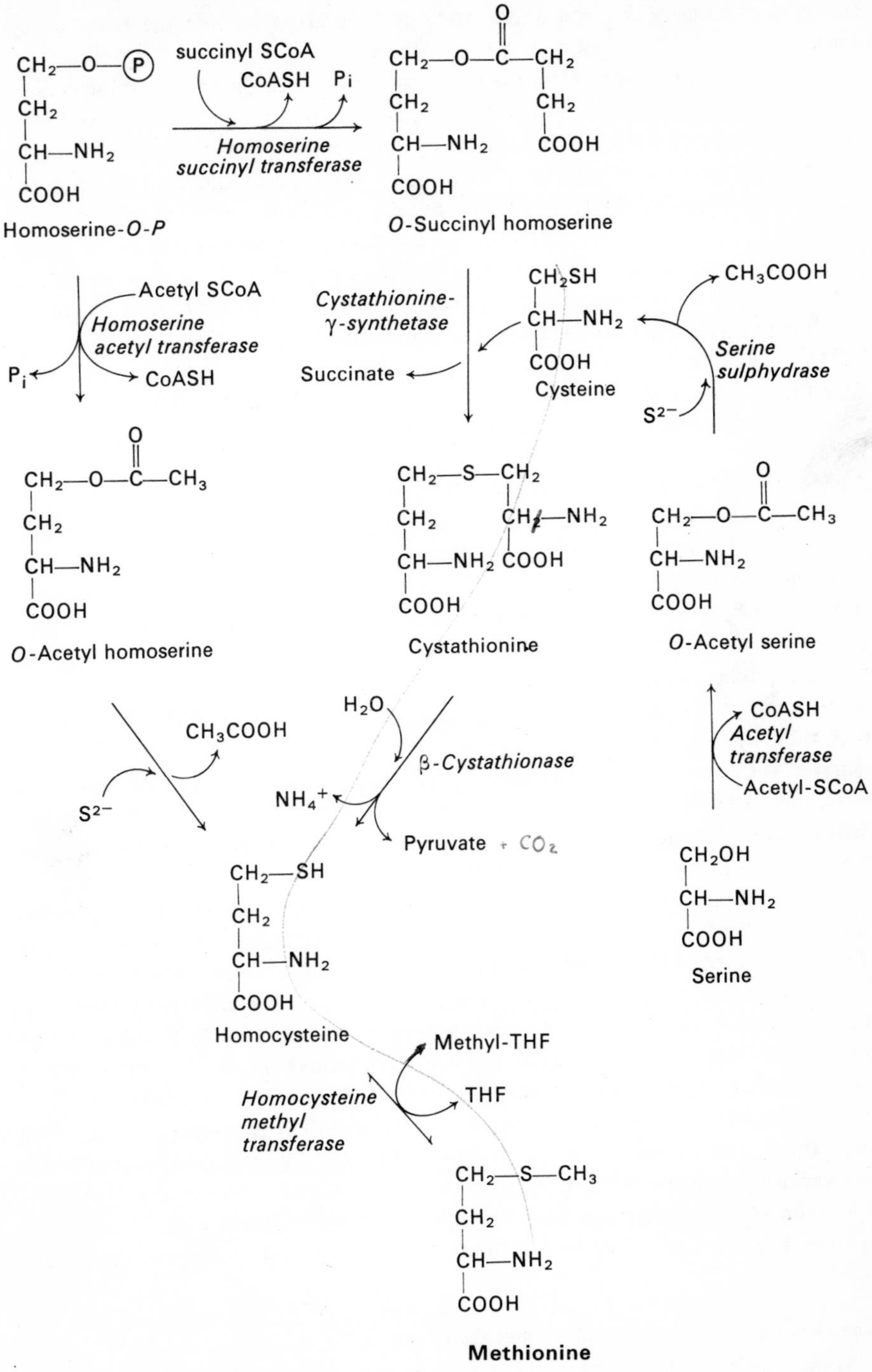

Figure 5.8. Methionine biosynthesis in micro-organisms and plants

the same as that described above for the formation of cysteine from acetyl serine.

It is uncertain to what extent the formation of cystathionine is an intermediate step in the formation of homocysteine, and hence methionine, in bacteria. Incorporation of label from radioactive cystathionine into methionine in bacteria is generally poor, although the label from homoserine-O-phosphate is incorporated in good yield. Whether this represents merely the dilution of the added material by a large intracellular pool of cystathionine, or whether most homocysteine synthesis is by the more direct pathway, is unclear. It is possible that the formation of cystathionine mainly represents a mechanism for storage of organic sulphur in a readily usable and relatively non-toxic form.

Homocysteine is methylated to methionine in a coenzyme B_{12}-dependent reaction, in which the methyl donor is normally N^5-methyl tetrahydrofolate, although betaine and occasionally other methyl donors can also be involved.

The formation of cysteine from methionine in animal tissues

As was shown in Figure 3.10, S-adenosyl methionine transfers its methyl group to a variety of methyl acceptors, and the resultant S-adenosyl homocysteine is deadenylated, and can then undergo one of two fates. In times of poor methionine supply, homocysteine can be remethylated to methionine, and then converted to S-adenosyl methionine by methionine S-adenosyl transferase. However, when there is less need for the remethylation of homocysteine to methionine, it can be condensed with serine to form cystathionine. By analogy with the β-cleavage of cystathionine in bacteria, which yields homocysteine, this reaction is known as the β-synthesis of cystathionine, and the enzyme catalysing it is therefore cystathionine-β-synthetase. In animals, cystathionine is then cleaved by γ-cystathionase to yield cysteine and α-oxo-butyrate (the deaminated derivative of homoserine) as shown in Figure 5.9.

Cystathionine can be cleaved in two modes, the γ-cleavage yielding cysteine, and the β-cleavage found in bacteria and plants, yielding homocysteine and involved in methionine synthesis. Bacteria and plants do not appear to have a γ-cystathionase, but in N. crassa, both β- and γ-cystathionases are found. Just as cystathionine can be cleaved in two separate reactions, so its synthesis can be either from homoserine and cysteine, the γ-synthetase reaction of bacteria and plants, or from homocysteine and serine, the β-synthetase of animals.

Cystathionine synthetases are pyridoxal-P-dependent enzymes, and for some time there was confusion in the literature because cystathionine β-synthetase and serine and threonine deaminases appeared to be the same enzyme. However, the activities have been separated, and it has been conclusively established that purified preparations of serine deaminase are without cystathionine-β-synthetase activity.

The catabolism of cysteine in mammalian tissues

Mammalian γ-cystathionase can also catalyse the desulphydration of cysteine, shown in Figure 5.11. The reaction is an α-β elimination, forming thiocysteine

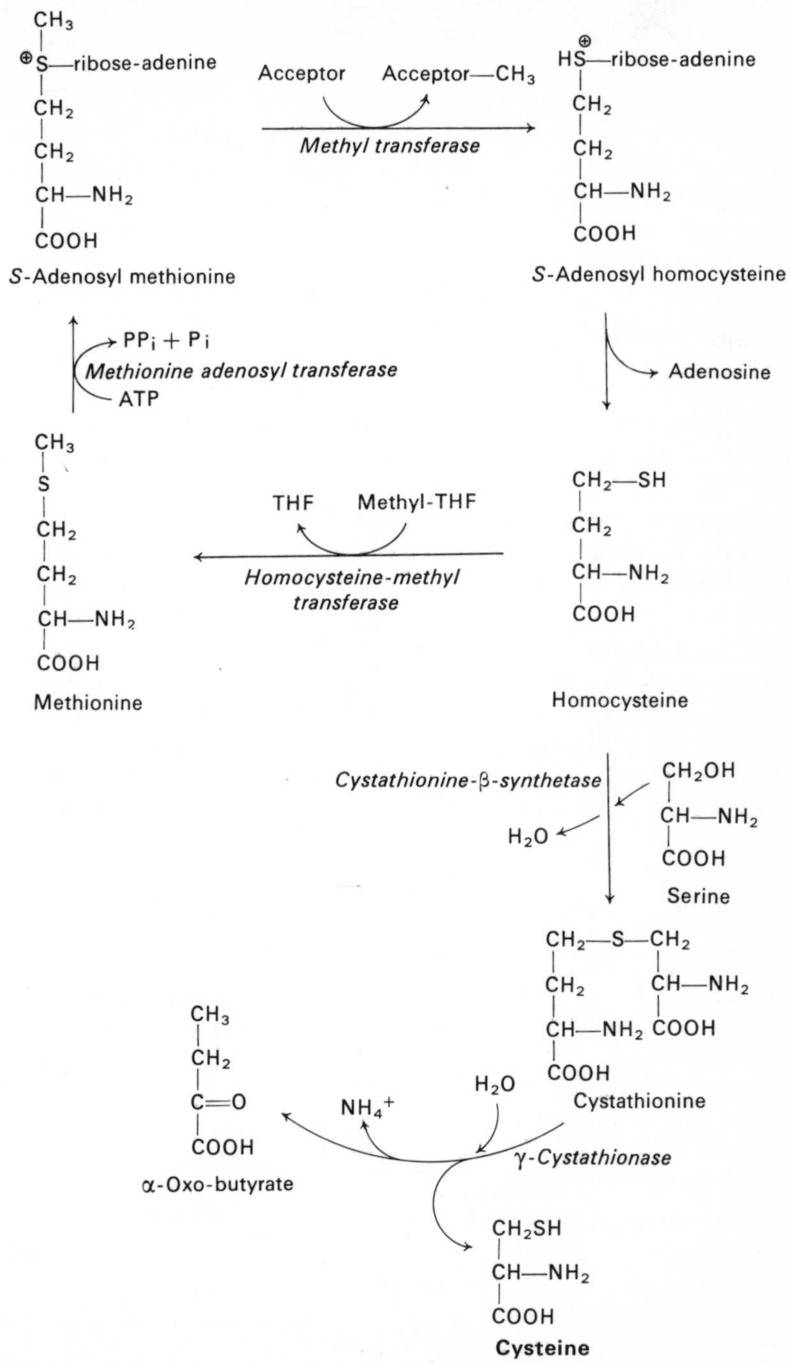

CH$_3$
|
$\oplus$S—ribose-adenine
|
CH$_2$
|
CH$_2$
|
CH—NH$_2$
|
COOH

S-Adenosyl methionine

Acceptor   Acceptor—CH$_3$

$\xrightarrow{\textit{Methyl transferase}}$

HS$\oplus$—ribose-adenine
|
CH$_2$
|
CH$_2$
|
CH—NH$_2$
|
COOH

S-Adenosyl homocysteine

→ PP$_i$ + P$_i$

Methionine adenosyl transferase

ATP

→ Adenosine

CH$_3$
|
S
|
CH$_2$
|
CH$_2$
|
CH—NH$_2$
|
COOH

Methionine

THF   Methyl-THF

Homocysteine-methyl transferase

CH$_2$—SH
|
CH$_2$
|
CH—NH$_2$
|
COOH

Homocysteine

Cystathionine-β-synthetase

CH$_2$OH
|
CH—NH$_2$
|
COOH

Serine

H$_2$O ←

CH$_2$—S—CH$_2$
| |
CH$_2$ CH—NH$_2$
| |
CH—NH$_2$ COOH
|
COOH

Cystathionine

CH$_3$
|
CH$_2$
|
C=O
|
COOH

α-Oxo-butyrate

NH$_4$$^+$ H$_2$O

γ-Cystathionase

CH$_2$SH
|
CH—NH$_2$
|
COOH

Cysteine

Figure 5.9. The formation of cysteine from methionine in animals

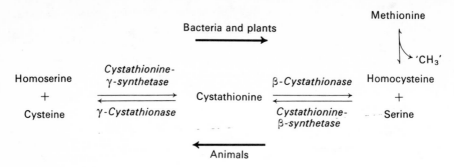

Figure 5.10. The central role of cystathionine in cysteine and methionine metabolism

(the persulphide of cysteine), pyruvate and ammonia. Thiocysteine then spontaneously loses sulphur to yield cysteine. However, when cysteine is present in the incubation medium in moderate amounts, the elemental sulphur is reduced to hydrogen sulphide, and cysteine is oxidized to cystine. In the initial absence of any cysteine in the reaction mixture, the eliminated sulphur remains as elemental sulphur until there is a sufficient accumulation of cysteine as product to catalyse its reduction. When cysteine alone is the substrate, it is necessary to postulate that enough cysteine is produced by atmospheric oxidation to allow the initiation of the reaction. The inhibition of mammalian cystathionase by cysteine may thus represent competition between two alternative substrates for the catalytic site of the enzyme, rather than product inhibition *per se*.

There are two further reactions by which the carbon skeleton of cysteine can be metabolized to pyruvate. Simple transamination of cysteine yields thio-

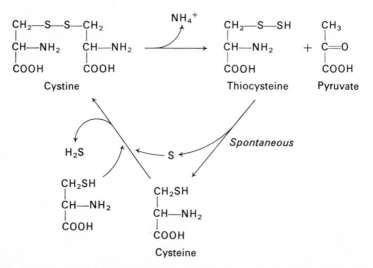

Figure 5.11. Cystine desulphydrase activity of mammalian γ-cystathionase

pyruvate, which then undergoes desulphuration to pyruvate and hydrogen sulphide. Alternatively, the oxidation product of cysteine, cysteine sulphinic acid, can undergo deamination and removal of the sulphinate group as either inorganic or organic sulphate, again yielding pyruvate.

Cysteine sulphinic acid is produced by the action of cysteine oxidase, which is induced by cysteine loading, while the other enzymes involved in cysteine catabolism are not altered by changes in the cysteine intake (Yamaguchi *et al.*, 1973). Therefore, it appears likely that in response to large loads of cysteine, the main metabolic pathway is that initiated by oxidation to the sulphinic acid. As well as degradation to pyruvate, as noted above, cysteine sulphinic acid can undergo either decarboxylation to hypotaurine followed by oxidation to taurine, or oxidation to cysteic acid followed by decarboxylation to taurine, as shown in Figure 5.12. The decarboxylation of cysteine sulphinate and cysteic acid are both believed to be catalysed by the same enzyme.

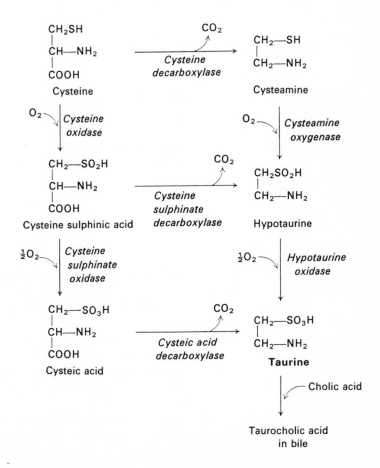

Figure 5.12. The biosynthesis of taurine from cysteine

Taurine can also be produced by decarboxylation of cysteine to cysteamine, followed by oxidation of this amine to hypotaurine. The relative activities of the enzymes involved in different tissues suggests that decarboxylation to cysteamine is mainly of importance in the synthesis of taurine in the central nervous system, but of little significance in the catabolism of cysteine in peripheral tissues. Taurine has been suggested as a possible neurotransmitter in some neurons in the central nervous system. In the liver, taurine is further metabolized by conjugation with cholic acid, a product of steroid catabolism, to form taurocholic acid, which is excreted in the bile, and has an important role in the emulsification of fats in the intestine.

Yamaguchi and coworkers (1973) estimated, by distribution of label in various products after administration of radioactive cysteine, that almost 70% of cysteine catabolism was by way of taurine formation, and less than 30% by way of pyruvate formation. They were unable to determine what proportion of each product was formed by each of the individual pathways.

THE BRANCHED-CHAIN AMINO ACIDS

Biosynthesis of isoleucine and valine

The pathway for the biosynthesis of the two branched chain amino acids, isoleucine and valine, is shown in Figure 5.13. The two amino acids are synthesized by parallel pathways, and there is a considerable amount of evidence that in all systems which have been examined to date the same enzymes are responsible for the synthesis of both. Wagner and coworkers (1965) showed that mitochondrial fractions from *N. crassa* will catalyse simultaneous synthesis of isoleucine and valine, and that pyruvate and α-oxo-butyrate, as well as α-acetolactate and α-aceto-α-hydroxybutyrate, are mutually competitive. To avoid competition between intermediates of the two pathways, it is obviously essential to postulate regulation of the entry of precursors into the pathways. Since pyruvate is a ubiquitous cell constituent, its production cannot be regulated to meet the demands of valine synthesis. Furthermore, both pyruvate metabolism and the synthesis of isoleucine and valine are intra-mitochondrial. The obvious point of regulation is therefore the entry of α-oxo-butyrate, formed from threonine. It was noted on page 70 that organisms which are capable of *de novo* synthesis of isoleucine have two distinct enzymes catalysing the deamination and dehydration of threonine: the so-called catabolic threonine deaminase, which is induced by growth on threonine-rich media, and acts on both serine and threonine; and a separate biosynthetic threonine deaminase, which does not generally act on serine, and is repressed by growth on media rich in isoleucine. Thus while pyruvate will be available for entry into the pathway of branched-chain amino acid biosynthesis at a relatively constant rate, the proportion of isoleucine produced can be controlled by the activity of the biosynthetic threonine deaminase.

In moulds, the enzymes of isoleucine and valine biosynthesis are mitochondrial; in bacteria, which do not have mitochondria, the enzymes have been shown to

133

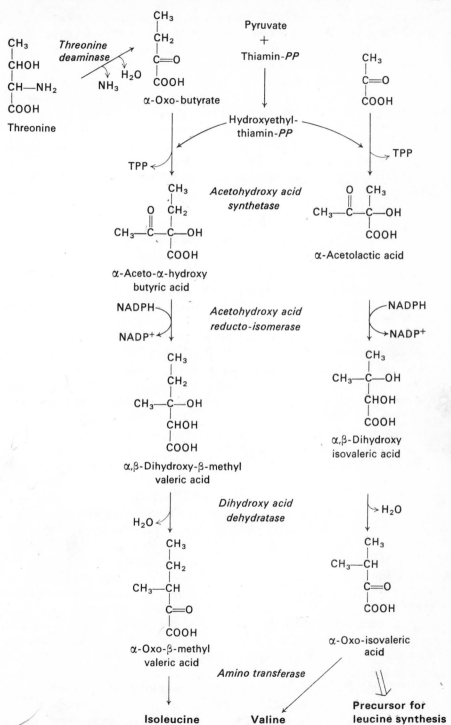

Figure 5.13. The biosynthesis of isoleucine and valine

be tightly membrane-associated. Although all four individual activities can be demonstrated in a membrane-free soluble system, the overall synthesis of valine from pyruvate, or isoleucine from α-oxo-butyrate requires a native, membrane-bound multi-enzyme complex. Vigorously homogenized and diluted preparations show a much reduced activity of the overall pathway, although the individual activities can be demonstrated to be present. In some isoleucine- and valine-requiring mutants of *N. crassa*, it has been shown that all four enzymes are present, and all can be individually demonstrated to be active. It has been suggested that in these mutants the defect lies in the assembly of the multi-enzyme complex rather than a failure of enzyme production.

Free acetaldehyde is not incorporated into any of the branched-chain amino acids, and therefore the substrate for acetohydroxy acid synthetase must be hydroxy-ethyl thiamin pyrophosphate ('active acetaldehyde'). A distinct pyruvate oxidase has been isolated from *E. coli* which catalyses the oxidation of pyruvate to hydroxyethyl thiamin pyrophosphate, which is then transferred to aceto-hydroxy acid synthetase. Unlike the pyruvate oxidase component of the pyruvate decarboxylase complex, which forms acetyl-SCoA, this enzyme is inhibited by valine, one of the end-products of the pathway.

Acetohydroxy acid synthetase in bacterial preparations is both inhibited and repressed by valine, but the enzyme from plants is insensitive to end-product regulation. Preparations of mitochondrial membrane from *N. crassa* which have acetohydroxy acid synthetase activity are sensitive to inhibition by both valine, and to a lesser extent, isoleucine. However, a membrane-free preparation of the enzyme is insensitive to end-product inhibition. The membrane-associated enzyme is also activated by ATP and ADP, which also reverse the end-product inhibition. The solubilized enzyme is insensitive to this nucleotide activation. These findings suggest that inhibitor sensitivity is not a property of the enzyme *per se*, but of the complete multi-enzyme complex.

The activation of acetohydroxy acid synthetase in crude mitochondrial preparations by ATP is of interest in view of the inhibition of pyruvate entry into the citrate cycle by ATP. When excess ATP inhibits conversion of pyruvate to acetyl-SCoA, not only is more pyruvate available for branched-chain amino acid synthesis, but the activity of the enzyme controlling the pathway is also enhanced.

The mechanism of the reductive isomerization of the acetohydroxy acid to the α-β-dihydroxy acid is unclear. No intermediates have yet been isolated, so presumably the reaction proceeds with tightly enzyme-bound intermediates. The reductant for this reaction is specifically NADPH. In bacteria, Mg^{2+} ions are required for the reaction, but no metal requirement has been demonstrated for the plant enzyme. The dehydration of the dihydroxy acids to the oxo-acid precursors of valine and isoleucine is also dependent on Mg^{2+} or Mn^{2+} ions in bacteria.

Two distinct branched-chain amino acid aminotransferases have been isolated from *N. crassa*. Both are active towards valine, leucine and isoleucine. One enzyme is mitochondrial, and will utilize only glutamate as an amino donor, while the other is cytoplasmic, and will utilize phenylalanine, tyrosine or methionine to aminate the branched-chain oxo-acids. Growth of the organism on media rich in the branched-chain amino acids leads to induction of the cytoplasmic aminotransferase, but has no effect on the activity of the mitochondrial enzyme. Since biosynthesis of the branched-chain amino acids is wholly mitochondrial in *Neurospora*, it is probable that the cytoplasmic aminotransferase is mainly concerned with catabolism rather than biosynthesis.

Biosynthesis of leucine

The pathway of leucine biosynthesis is shown in Figure 5.14. Carbons 1 and 2 of leucine are derived from acetate, and the first step unique to the formation of leucine is the condensation of α-oxo-valeric acid, the oxo-acid corresponding to valine, with acetyl-SCoA, forming α-isopropyl malate and releasing CoASH. Isopropyl malate synthetase is, as would be expected from the first enzyme unique to a pathway, sensitive to feed-back inhibition by leucine.

The isomerization of α-isopropyl malate to α-hydroxy-β-carboxy isocaproic acid (β-isopropyl malate) proceeds by way of an α-β unsaturation produced by dehydration of α-isopropyl malate, and subsequent rehydration in the opposite direction across the double bond, a reaction parallel to that of aconitase. However, there is no evidence that the proposed unsaturated intermediate (dimethyl citraconate) does in fact participate in the enzyme-catalysed reaction. Oxidative decarboxylation of β-isopropyl malate (an NAD-dependent reaction) yields α-oxo-isocaproate, the oxo-acid precursor of leucine. Oxo-isocaproate is a substrate for the same aminotransferases as the oxo-acid precursors of valine and isoleucine.

Catabolism of the branched-chain amino acids

So far as is known, the catabolism of the branched-chain amino acids follows the same pathway in all organisms, including mammals. As was noted above, a single aminotransferase appears to catalyse the transamination of all three amino acids, and it is assumed that where there are two branched-chain aminotransferases present in a cell, it is the cytoplasmic isoenzyme that is responsible for the initiation of catabolism.

Two further steps in the catabolism of the branched-chain amino acids are also catalysed by enzymes common to all three, as shown in Figure 5.15. The α-oxo-acid produced by aminotransfer is oxidatively decarboxylated, and condensed with coenzyme A, to form an acyl-SCoA. This is then dehydrogenated to give an unsaturated acyl-SCoA. In cases of maple syrup urine disease (branched-chain ketonuria), the inborn error of metabolism where branched-chain amino acid metabolism is defective, all three branched-chain ketones accumulate in the urine, indicating that if the enzymes for their onward metabolism are not the same, they are at least synthesized from genes under common regulation. Cases of maple syrup urine disease have been investigated in which either the decarboxylation of the branched-chain ketones to acyl-SCoA, or the dehydrogenation of the acyl-SCoA to the unsaturated derivative was defective.

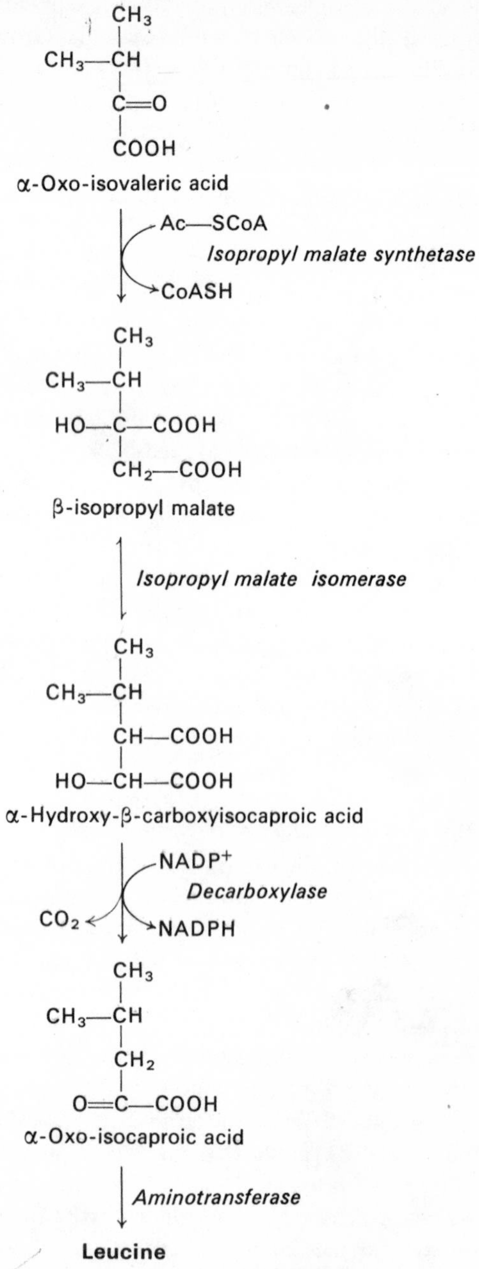

$$CH_3$$
$$CH_3-CH$$
$$C=O$$
$$COOH$$

α-Oxo-isovaleric acid

Ac—SCoA

Isopropyl malate synthetase

CoASH

$$CH_3$$
$$CH_3-CH$$
$$HO-C-COOH$$
$$CH_2-COOH$$

β-isopropyl malate

Isopropyl malate isomerase

$$CH_3$$
$$CH_3-CH$$
$$CH-COOH$$
$$HO-CH-COOH$$

α-Hydroxy-β-carboxyisocaproic acid

NADP$^+$

Decarboxylase

CO_2

NADPH

$$CH_3$$
$$CH_3-CH$$
$$CH_2$$
$$O=C-COOH$$

α-Oxo-isocaproic acid

Aminotransferase

Leucine

Figure 5.14. The biosynthesis of leucine

The disease has its somewhat exotic name because the presence of the branched-chain ketones and other derivatives in the urine gives it an aroma similar to that of maple syrup.

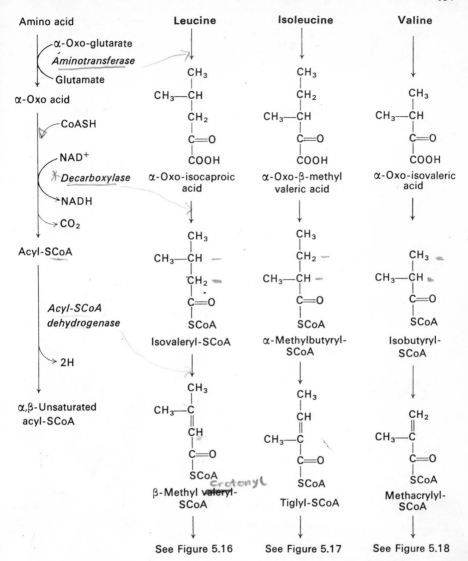

Figure 5.15. Common catabolism of the branched chain amino acids

The onward metabolic pathways of the unsaturated acyl-SCoA derivatives of each of the three amino acids are different, as shown in Figures 5.16, 5.17 and 5.18. Leucine is wholly ketogenic in its metabolism; it yields only acetyl-SCoA and acetoacetate, and no intermediates that can be used in the synthesis of carbohydrate. β-Methyl-crotonyl-SCoA, the unsaturated acyl-SCoA formed from leucine, is carboxylated in a biotin-dependent, ATP-utilizing reaction to β-methyl-glutaconyl-SCoA, which is then hydrated by crotonase (hydroxy-acyl-SCoA hydro-lyase) to β-hydroxy-β-methyl glutaryl-SCoA. This can be used in the synthesis of mevalonic acid, and hence in steroid synthesis, but the major

138

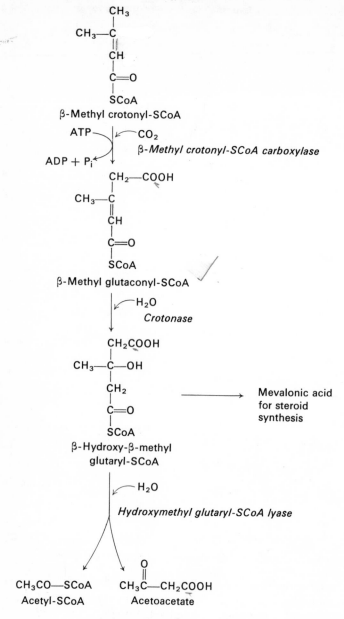

Figure 5.16. Leucine catabolism

fate of the hydroxy-methyl glutaryl-SCoA formed from leucine is hydrolysis to acetyl-SCoA and acetoacetate. The carboxyl group of acetoacetate retains the label of radioactive bicarbonate incorporated at the carboxylation reaction. In experimentally-induced biotin deficiency in laboratory animals, oral loading with leucine leads to excretion of β-hydroxy-isovalerate arising from crotonase action on β-methyl-crotonyl-SCoA, which does not normally accumulate in sufficient quantity to be hydrated. To some extent, isovaleric and β-methyl-crotonic acids also accumulate in the blood, due to the failure of β-methyl-crotonyl-SCoA carboxylase in the absence of its cofactor. In man, β-hydroxy-

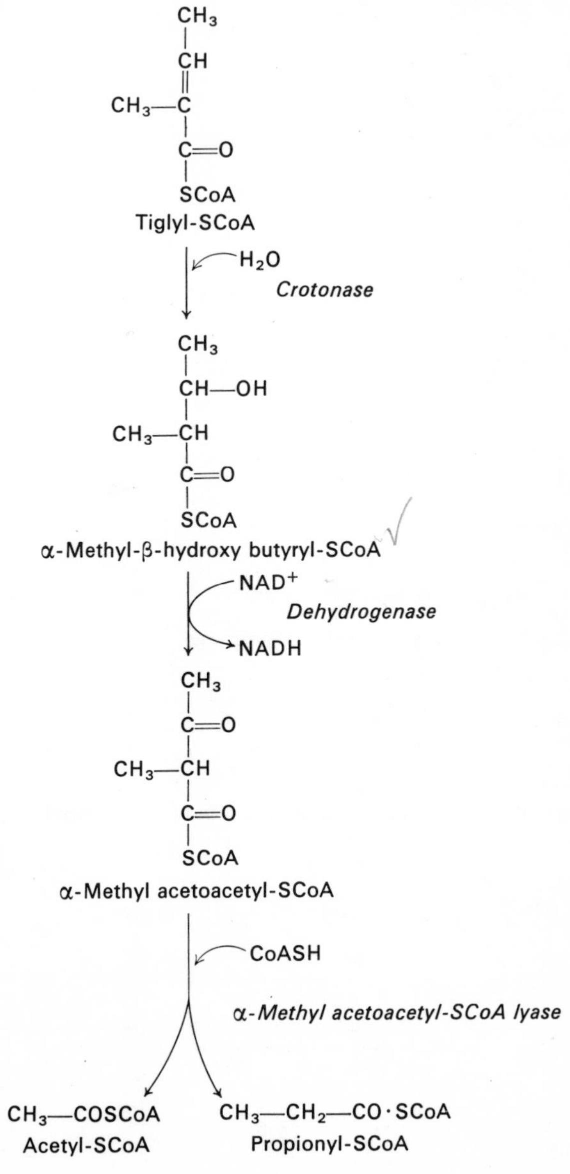

Figure 5.17. Isoleucine catabolism

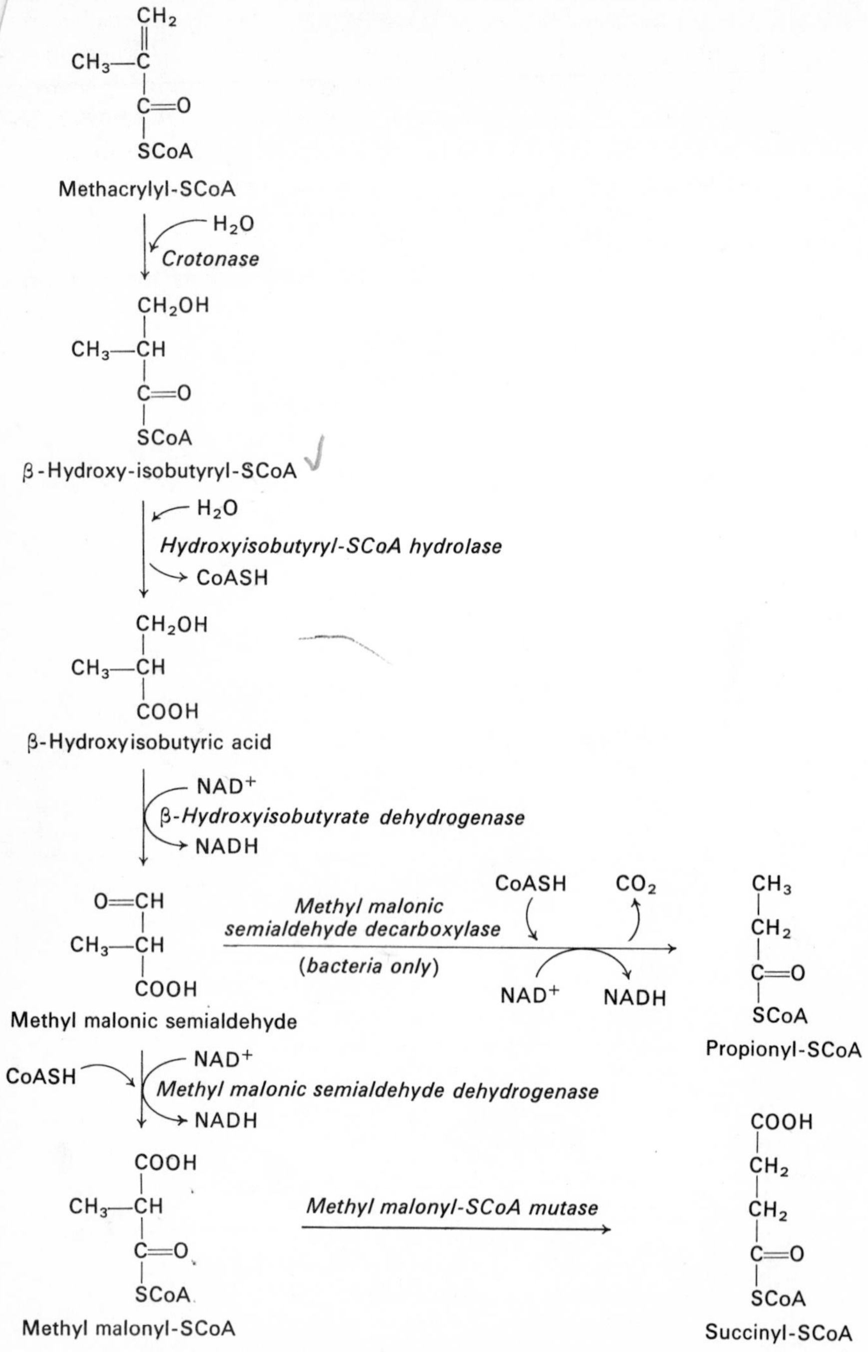

$$CH_2$$
$$\|$$
$$CH_3\!-\!C$$
$$|$$
$$C\!=\!O$$
$$|$$
$$SCoA$$

Methacrylyl-SCoA

$\curvearrowright$ H$_2$O
Crotonase

$$CH_2OH$$
$$|$$
$$CH_3\!-\!CH$$
$$|$$
$$C\!=\!O$$
$$|$$
$$SCoA$$

β-Hydroxy-isobutyryl-SCoA ✓

$\curvearrowleft$ H$_2$O
Hydroxyisobutyryl-SCoA hydrolase
$\searrow$ CoASH

$$CH_2OH$$
$$|$$
$$CH_3\!-\!CH$$
$$|$$
$$COOH$$

β-Hydroxyisobutyric acid

$\curvearrowright$ NAD$^+$
β-Hydroxyisobutyrate dehydrogenase
$\rightarrow$ NADH

$$O\!=\!CH$$
$$|$$
$$CH_3\!-\!CH$$
$$|$$
$$COOH$$

Methyl malonic semialdehyde

Methyl malonic semialdehyde decarboxylase
(*bacteria only*)

CoASH   CO$_2$
NAD$^+$ NADH

$$CH_3$$
$$|$$
$$CH_2$$
$$|$$
$$C\!=\!O$$
$$|$$
$$SCoA$$

Propionyl-SCoA

CoASH $\curvearrowright$ NAD$^+$
Methyl malonic semialdehyde dehydrogenase
$\rightarrow$ NADH

$$COOH$$
$$|$$
$$CH_3\!-\!CH$$
$$|$$
$$C\!=\!O$$
$$|$$
$$SCoA$$

Methyl malonyl-SCoA

Methyl malonyl-SCoA mutase

$$COOH$$
$$|$$
$$CH_2$$
$$|$$
$$CH_2$$
$$|$$
$$C\!=\!O$$
$$|$$
$$SCoA$$

Succinyl-SCoA

Figure 5.18. Valine catabolism

isovaleric aciduria (and possibly also β-methyl-crotonic aciduria) may occur as a result of an inherited defect of the carboxylase.

The unsaturated acyl-SCoA from isoleucine catabolism is tiglyl-SCoA. This is hydrated by crotonase, and the resultant hydroxy-acid is oxidized by a specific NAD-dependent dehydrogenase to yield α-methyl-acetoacetyl-SCoA. This is then lysed by coenzyme A to yield acetyl-SCoA and propionyl-SCoA. Since propionyl-SCoA can be readily converted to succinyl-SCoA and, via the citrate cycle, to oxaloacetate, isoleucine yields both glucogenic and ketogenic fragments on catabolism, as shown in Figure 5.17.

The unsaturated acyl-SCoA in valine catabolism, is methacrylyl-SCoA, which, like tiglyl-SCoA, is hydrated by crotonase, although it can also undergo a parallel spontaneous hydration. The resultant β-hydroxy-isobutyryl-SCoA is believed to undergo removal of the coenzyme A moiety to yield β-hydroxy-isobutyric acid. This is then oxidized to methylmalonic semialdehyde by β-hydroxy-isobutyrate dehydrogenase, which will only act on the free acid; the acyl-SCoA is not a substrate. In some bacteria grown on valine as the sole source of carbon, methylmalonic semialdehyde can be oxidatively decarboxylated to propionyl-SCoA. However, in mammals it is dehydrogenated and condensed with coenzyme A to form methylmalonyl-SCoA, which then undergoes isomerization, catalysed by a coenzyme B_{12}-dependent enzyme, methylmalonyl-SCoA mutase, to succinyl-SCoA. Thus, valine catabolism yields a purely glucogenic fragment in mammals.

Methylmalonic acid also arises in the catabolism of isoleucine, and, quantitatively most important in mammalian metabolism, in the oxidation of odd-chain fatty acids by carboxylation of propionyl-SCoA. In vitamin B_{12} deficiency, methylmalonic acid appears in the urine because of the failure of the mutase in the absence of its cofactor. Methylmalonic aciduria is a purely biochemical lesion with no associated clinical signs, and is therefore diagnostically useful for detection of avitaminosis B_{12} before pernicious anaemia has developed. The occurrence of methylmalonic aciduria is also clinically useful in allowing differentiation between the haematologically very similar anaemias due to defective red cell maturation in avitaminosis B_{12} and folic acid deficiency. Methylmalonic aciduria can also occur, in a few patients, with normal levels of vitamin B_{12}, due to a genetic defect of the mutase.

In a number of insect-pollinated plants, including the arum lily (*Arum maculatum*), the rowan (*Sorbus aucuparia*) and the hawthorn (*Crataegus monogyna*), valine and leucine are decarboxylated in newly opened flower buds, and the volatile amines so produced act as insect attractants.

Further reading

Cronenwett, C. S. and Wagner, R. P. (1965). Overall synthesis of isoleucine by membrane fragments of *S. typhimurium. Proc. Nat. Acad. Sci. U.S.A.*, **54**, 1643–1650.

Flavin, M. and Slaughter, C. (1967). Enzymic synthesis of homocysteine or methionine directly from *O*-succinyl homoserine. *Biochim. Biophys. Acta*, **132**, 400–405.

Grove. J. A., Young, F., Roghair, H. G. and Schimke, P. (1972). Lysine metabolism in rabbits. *Arch. Biochem. Biophys.*, **151**, 464–467.

Lombardini, J. B. and Talalay, P. (1971). Formation, functions and regulatory importance of *S*-adenosyl methionine. *Adv. Enz. Reg.*, **9**, 349–384.

Miller, D. L. and Rodwell, V. W. (1971). Metabolism of basic amino acids in *Ps. putida:*
catabolism of lysine by cyclic and acyclic intermediates. *J. Biol. Chem.*, **246**, 2758–
2764.

Patte, J-C., LeBras, G. and Cohen, G. N. (1967). Regulation by methionine of a third
aspartokinase and of a second homoserine dehydrogenase in *E. coli* K_{12}. *Biochim.
Biophys. Acta*, **136**, 245–257.

Radhakrishnan, A. N. and Snell, E. E. (1960). Biosynthesis of valine and isoleucine:
(ii) formation of α-acetolactate and α-aceto-α-hydroxybutyrate in *N. crassa* and *E. coli*.
J. Biol. Chem., **235**, 2316–2321.

Radhakrishnan, A. N., Wagner, R. P. and Snell, E. E. (1960). Biosynthesis of valine
and isoleucine: (iii) α-keto-β-hydroxy-acid reductase and α-hydroxy-β-keto acid
reducto-isomerase. *J. Biol. Chem.*, **235**, 2322–2331.

Sturani, E., Datta, P., Hughes, M. and Gest, H. (1963). Regulation of enzyme inhibition
by specific reversal of feed-back inhibition. *Science*, **141**, 1053–1054.

Truffa-Bachi, P. and Cohen, G. N. (1968). Some aspects of amino acid biosynthesis
in micro-organisms. *Ann. Rev. Biochem.*, **37**, 79–108.

Tucci, A. F. and Ceci, L. N. (1972). Control of lysine biosynthesis in yeast. *Arch.
Biochem. Biophys.*, **153**, 751–754.

Umbarger, H. E. (1973). Threonine deaminases. *Adv. Enzymol.*, **37**, 349–395.

Veron, M., Saari, J. C., Villar-Palasi, C. and Cohen, G. N. (1973). The threonine-
sensitive homoserine dehydrogenase and aspartokinase of *E.coli* K_{12}. *Eur. J. Biochem.*,
38, 325–335.

Wagner, R. P., Bergquist, A. and Barbee, T. (1965). The synthesis *in vitro* of valine and
isoleucine from pyruvate and α-oxo-butyrate in *Neurospora*. *Biochim. Biophys. Acta*,
100, 444–450.

Wixom, R. L., Heinemann, M. A. and Semeraro, R. J. (1971). Studies on valine biosynthesis: (ii) the enzymes in photosynthetic and auxotrophic bacteria. *Biochim.
Biophys. Acta*, **244**, 532–546.

References cited in the text are listed in the bibliography

CHAPTER 6

HISTIDINE AND THE AROMATIC AMINO ACIDS, PHENYLALANINE, TYROSINE AND TRYPTOPHAN

The three aromatic amino acids are essential to mammals. However, since tyrosine can readily be formed from phenylalanine, it is not strictly an essential amino acid as long as adequate phenylalanine is available.

Histidine can be readily synthesized by most mammals, and is therefore not a dietary essential under normal conditions. In children and in young rats and mice the rate of histidine synthesis, like that of arginine, is not adequate to meet the demands of growth, and therefore under these conditions histidine is an essential amino acid.

Apart from its role in protein synthesis, and especially in the catalytic site of many enzymes, histidine is needed for synthesis of the pharmacologically active amine, histamine, discussed below, and the dipeptide carnosine (β-alanyl-histidine), found in muscle. In some species, carnosine is replaced wholly or in part by the *N*-methyl histidine derivative, anserine.

HISTIDINE

Biosynthesis

Histidine is synthesized by a simple pathway which does not involve any branch points, and does not lead to any other metabolically important intermediates. The pathway appears to be the same in all organisms, including mammals.

The first step is the condensation of phosphoribosyl pyrophosphate with ATP, to form phosphoribosyl-ATP. This reaction is catalysed by ATP phosphoribosyl transferase, which is freely reversible *in vitro*. *In vivo*, the equilibrium is maintained in the direction of phosphoribosyl-ATP synthesis by the action of pyrophosphatase which hydrolyses the pyrophosphate released in the condensation reaction, and thus effectively prevents reversal by removal of one of the products. As would be expected, the phosphoribosyl transferase is strongly inhibited by histidine. This inhibition is non-competitive with respect to either substrate, and involves a conformational change in the enzyme. In some bacterial mutants, in which this enzyme is not inhibited by histidine, although it can be shown that the amino acid binds to the enzyme, there is no conformational change on binding. It therefore appears probable that it is the conformational change in the wild-type enzyme which is responsible for the inhibition. The normal enzyme appears to be a hexamer of identical subunits.

143

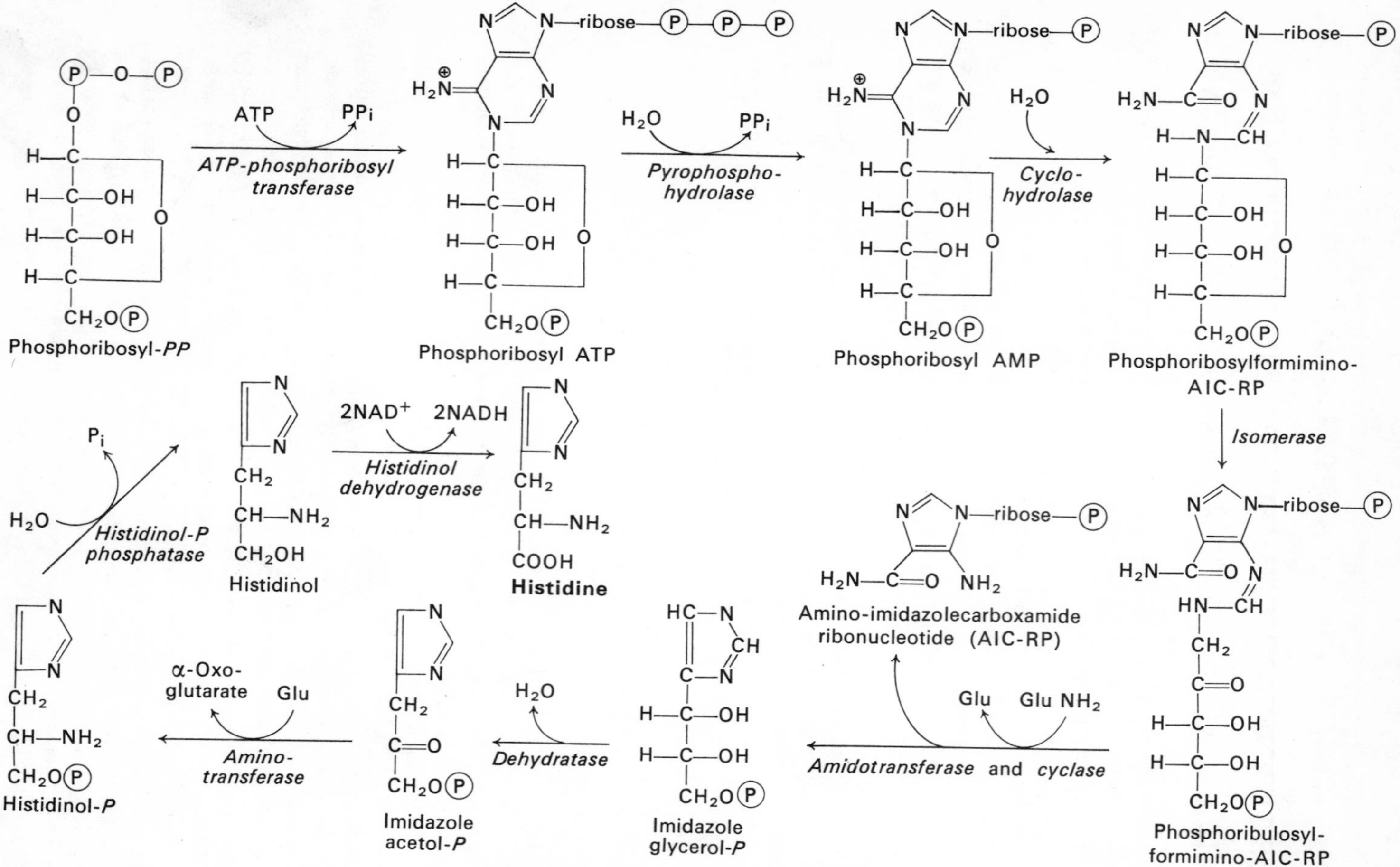

Figure 6.1. The biosynthesis of histidine

As shown in Figure 6.1, phosphoribosyl-ATP is then hydrolysed to phosphoribosyl-AMP by a pyrophosphohydrolase, which, like the first enzyme of the pathway, releases pyrophosphate. The adenine ring of phosphoribosyl-AMP is hydrolytically cleaved between C-6 and N-1, to yield phosphoribosylformimino aminoimidazole-carboxamide ribonucleotide (PR-formimino-AIC-RP). The enzyme catalysing this reaction is phosphoribosyl-AMP cyclohydrolase.

PR-formimino-AIC-RP undergoes isomerization to the ribulosyl derivative, which is aminated by transfer of the amide group of glutamine. This intermediate undergoes cyclization and cleavage to yield amino-imidazole-carboxamide ribonucleotide from the ATP moiety, and imidazole glycerol phosphate from the ribulosyl moiety and C-2 and N-1 of the adenine ring. Thus, while the synthesis of histidine incorporates C-2 and N-1 of the imidazole ring of adenine into the equivalent positions of the ring of the amino acid, it does not incorporate the formed imidazole ring of the purine *per se*. Although two separate enzymes, an amidotransferase and a cyclase, are known to catalyse these two reactions, no intermediate has been isolated to date, so it appears that the two enzymes act in close concert, and the intermediate must be transferred from one enzyme to the other without appearing in free solution.

Imidazole glycerol phosphate is dehydrated to the 2-oxo derivative, imidazole acetol phosphate, which is a substrate for aminotransfer from glutamate to form histidinol phosphate. This product is hydrolysed to the free amino alcohol, histidinol.

Although in *Neurospora* it can be shown that there is a specific histidinol phosphate phosphatase, in *Salmonella* it appears that the reaction is catalysed by the same enzyme as catalyses the dehydration of imidazole glycerol phosphate. Such catalysis of two non-adjacent steps in a pathway by the same enzyme is very unusual.

Histidinol is oxidized to histidine in a two-step reaction. A single enzyme appears to be responsible for both oxidations, and although the postulated intermediate aldehyde, histidinal, is a substrate *in vitro*, it is not normally detected *in vivo*, so it must remain firmly enzyme-bound, and be rapidly oxidized.

Genetic control of histidine biosynthesis in Salmonella typhimurium

Salmonella is typical of a group of micro-organisms in which all ten enzymes required for histidine biosynthesis are coordinately derepressed when the organism is grown in the absence of histidine. When histidine is present in the culture medium, none of the enzymes is synthesized, all are repressed by the end-product of the pathway. However, when there is a need for histidine biosynthesis, all ten enzymes are synthesized simultaneously.

It has been established that in *Salmonella* a single length of DNA codes for all ten enzyme activities, i.e. the entire pathway of histidine biosynthesis is coded for by a single polycistronic operon containing eight separate genes. Two of the genes code for two enzyme activities each. The *E* gene is bicistronic, coding for both ATP-phosphoribosyl transferase and phosphoribosyl-AMP cyclohydrolase. The other apparently bicistronic gene is the *B* gene, which codes for imidazole glycerol phosphate dehydratase and histidinol phosphate phosphatase activities. However, as was noted above, in *Salmonella* these two activities are associated with the same protein and cannot be separated, suggesting that gene fusion has occurred during the evolution of the organism. The assignment of names to the genes of the histidine (*his*) operon in Salmonella is shown in Table 6.1.

Table 6.1. The genes of the histidine operon of *Salmonella typhimurium*

Gene	Enzyme
Regulator	—
E	⌠ATP-phosphoribosyl transferase
	⌡Phosphoribosyl-AMP cyclohydrolase
F	Phosphoribulosyl-formimino-AIC-RP cyclase
A	Phosphoribosyl-formimino-AIC-RP isomerase
H	Phosphoribulosyl-formimino-AIC-RP amidotransferase
B	⌠Imidazole glycerol phosphate dehydratase
	⌡Histidinol phosphate phosphatase
C	Imidazole acetol phosphate aminotransferase
D	Histidinol dehydrogenase
G	PRPP-ATP pyrophosphorylase

Note: the genes are listed here in the order in which they have been mapped in the *his* operon of *S. typhimurium*.

About half the point mutations of the *his* operon that have been investigated have a dual effect. Not only is there a single defective enzyme, as would be expected, but the activity of all enzymes that are coded for by genes that map distal to the enzyme affected are produced in much reduced amounts. This has been interpreted as indicating that the *his* operon is transcribed as a single poly-cistronic messenger, which is then translated on the ribosome in the same way. It is postulated that a large number of ribosomes would be associated with any such messenger, each reading sequentially along the messenger from the end distal to the regulator gene (i.e. upwards through the genes as they are listed in Table 6.1). Such an arrangement would account for the observation that enzymes coded for by genes mapped as distal to the regulator are produced in greater amounts than those coded for by genes nearer to the regulator. It is assumed that not all ribosomes succeed in translating the whole messenger. This means that ATP-phosphoribosyl transferase, the first enzyme of the pathway, which is subject to feedback inhibition by histidine, will also be the enzyme present in least amount.

Histidinyl-tRNA synthetase is also apparently coded for by a gene of the *his* operon, and it is noteworthy that while the enzymes of the histidine bio-synthetic pathway are derepressed by growth in a histidine-free medium, it appears that the active repressor is not histidine *per se*, but charged histidinyl-tRNA. Mutations in the gene for the tRNA synthetase will therefore lead to de-repressed organisms, which produce all the enzymes of the pathway even when grown in the presence of the amino acid. Histidinyl-tRNA also binds to ATP phosphoribosyl transferase, at a site distinct from histidine or either substrate.

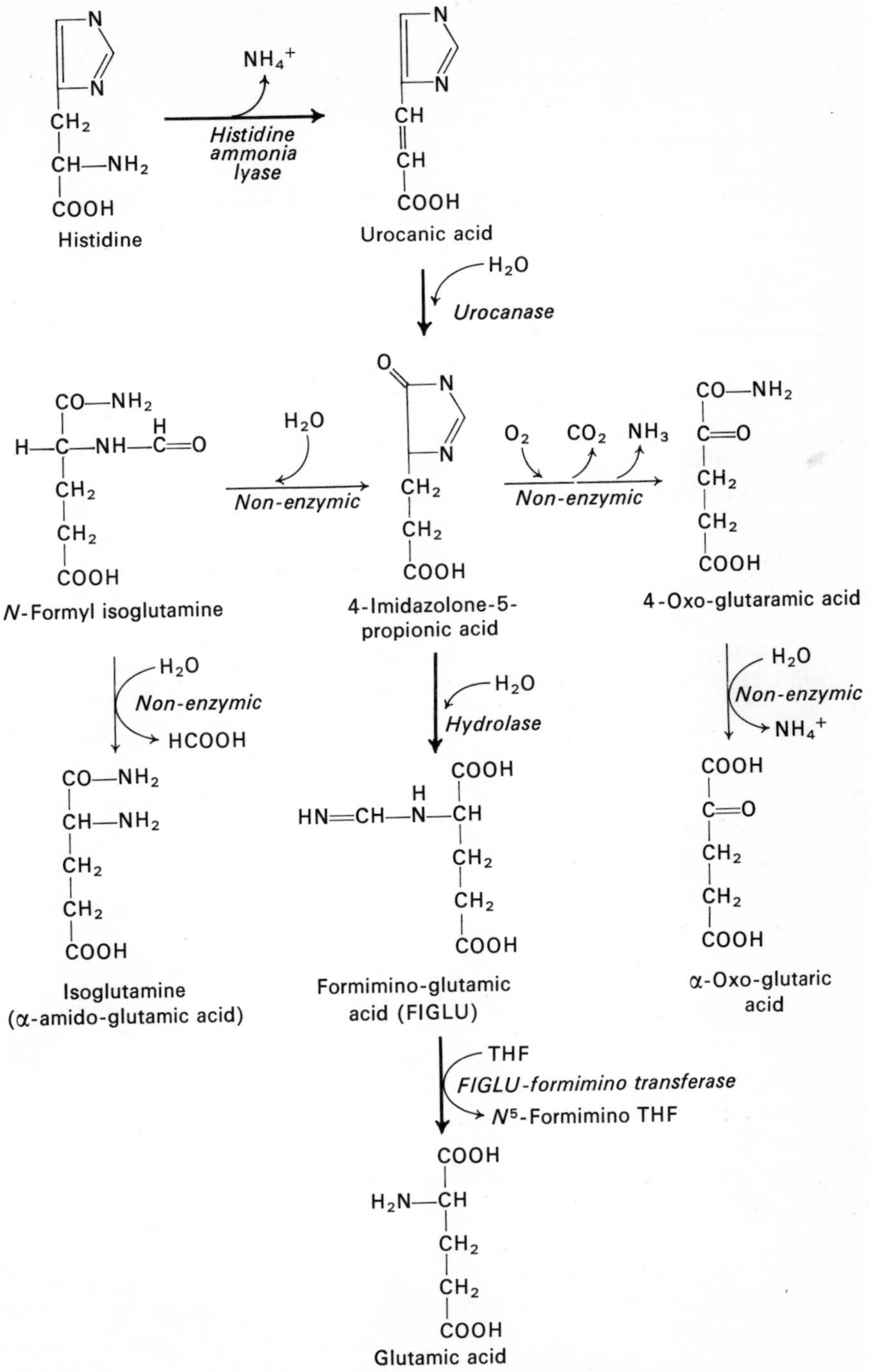

Figure 6.2. The catabolism of histidine

Histidine catabolism

In both bacteria and animals the main pathway of histidine catabolism is that shown in Figure 6.2. It is initiated by the formation of urocanic acid (imidazole acrylic acid) by the non-oxidative deamination of histidine. Urocanic acid has been identified in the urine of dogs and other animals which have been fed with large amounts of histidine, but not in sufficient amount to account for all the excess amino acid fed. Some imidazole propionic acid is formed in mammals by reduction of urocanic acid, and is excreted in the urine. However, this is a minor pathway of urocanate metabolism. It has been shown that when [^{14}C]-histidine is fed to experimental animals, almost all of the radioactivity is recovered as carbon dioxide.

The cells of the *stratum corneum* of the skin contain histidine ammonia lyase (histidase), the first enzyme of the urocanate pathway, but none of the later enzymes. Because of this, sweat normally contains urocanic acid. In patients suffering from histidinaemia, an inborn error of histidine metabolism, histidine ammonia lyase is absent from all cells of the body, including the *stratum corneum*. This is useful in the diagnosis of the cause of elevated blood and urine histidine in patients.

In histidinaemic patients, the blood histidine level is considerably elevated, and large amounts of histidine, and its transamination product imidazole pyruvic acid, are found in the urine. Histidine aminotransferase is found in the liver in large amounts; it is distinct from the glutamate-linked imidazole acetol

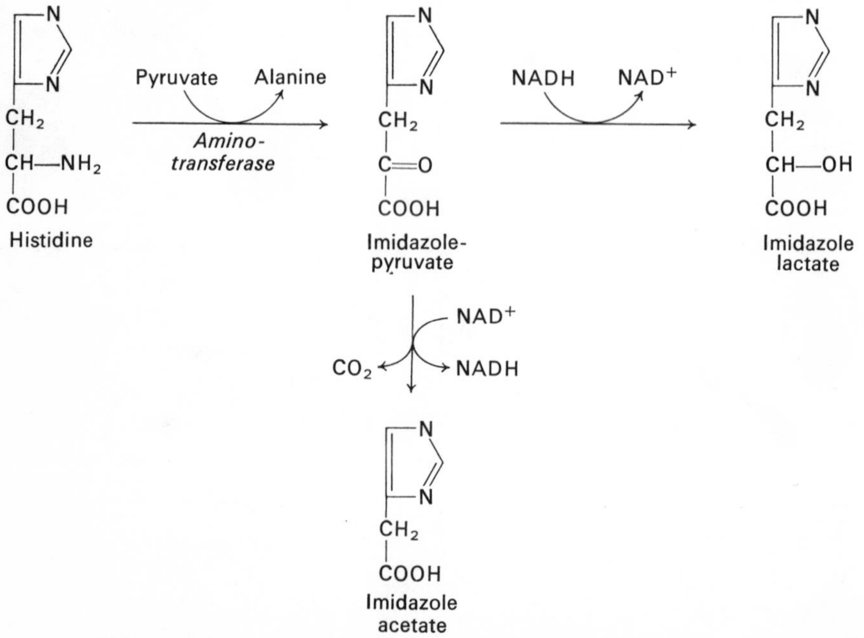

Figure 6.3. Histidine catabolism by aminotransfer

phosphate aminotransferase which is required for histidine synthesis. Histidine aminotransferase is linked to pyruvate as the amino acceptor. The role of this enzyme in normal subjects, who form very little imidazole pyruvate even after a loading dose of histidine, is unclear. Some of the products of further metabolism of imidazole pyruvate are also excreted by histidinaemic patients, including imidazole lactate, formed by reduction, and imidazole acetate, formed by oxidative decarboxylation (see Figure 6.3).

Urocanic acid is degraded by the action of urocanase to yield 4-imidazolone-5-propionic acid. The reaction is an internal oxidation–reduction reaction, with the addition of the elements of water.

Imidazolone propionic acid is chemically unstable, and apart from enzymic degradation, can be shown to undergo two non-enzymic reactions, one to yield isoglutamine (the α-amide of glutamate) by way of formyl-isoglutamine, and the other by an oxidative pathway to 4-oxo-glutamic acid, and thence to α-oxo-glutarate.

In vivo, the main pathway of imidazolone propionate degradation is enzymic cleavage of the imidazolone ring to yield formiminoglutamic acid (FIGLU). FIGLU is then converted to glutamate by transfer of the formimino moiety to tetrahydrofolate.

In cases of megaloblastic anaemia, where it is uncertain whether the primary cause is a deficiency of folate or vitamin B_{12}, patients are tested with an oral load of histidine. When folic acid is deficient, FIGLU cannot be further metabolized, and is excreted in the urine in large amounts. Differential diagnosis is

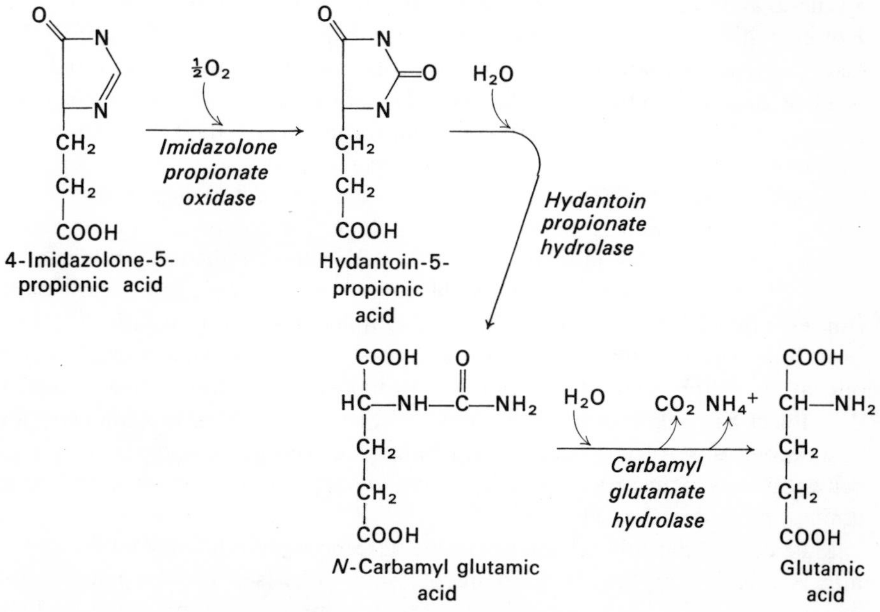

Figure 6.4. The hydantoin propionate pathway of histidine catabolism

of clinical importance because administration of folic acid to patients suffering from pernicious anaemia (avitaminosis B_{12}) may precipitate the neurological degeneration typical of advanced pernicious anaemia.

In the liver of most animals examined to date there is an imidazolone propionate oxidase which catalyses the oxidation of imidazolone propionate to hydantoin propionate. This latter is not further metabolized, but is excreted in the urine. The small amount of hydantoin propionate, excreted by most mammals, suggests that this is normally a minor pathway of histidine catabolism. However, in a number of bacteria, hydantoin propionate can be further metabolized as shown in Figure 6.4, by initial hydrolysis to N-carbamyl glutamate, followed by hydrolysis to give glutamate, and liberating ammonia and carbon dioxide from the carbamyl moiety.

Histamine

Histamine is the primary amine formed by decarboxylation of histidine. It has its main pharmacological effect on smooth muscle, where it causes contraction. In many species, although not in man, it is a potent inducer of uterine contraction.

Histamine also acts on the mucosa of the stomach causing a marked stimulation of acid secretion. It is generally believed that it acts either to maintain gastric secretion in response to stimulation by the vagus nerve, or possibly as a second messenger following gastrin release.

In mammalian tissues, there are believed to be two enzymes responsible for decarboxylation of histidine to histamine, a specific histidine decarboxylase, and a general amino acid decarboxylase, possibly the same as DOPA decarboxylase. However, histidine is not a substrate for partially purified preparations of DOPA decarboxylase. Although most histidine decarboxylases are pyridoxal-P dependent, as noted on page 53 in *Lactobacillus 30a* and some *Micrococcus* species, the enzyme has an attached pyruvate group, which serves the same function as pyridoxal-P in the majority of amino acid decarboxylases.

Histidine decarboxylase in mammalian tissues is found mainly in mast cells; among other factors it is induced by psychological stress, or repeated injection of noradrenaline. Such induction leads to a considerable increase in histamine levels. Mast cells in the lung release histamine in response to physical assault (for example in allergic reactions) and administration of histamine causes bronchospasm. This may explain the respiratory distress which is often the cause of death in anaphylactic shock, caused by administration of an antigen to which the subject has only recently been sensitized, such as over-hasty administration of a second dose of a vaccine. The administered antigen combines with mast cell antibodies to the protein, causing lysis and release of the histamine (and other amines) present in the cells.

Mast cells of the skin release histamine in response to relatively mild trauma; after scratching or heavily stroking the skin there is a characteristic 'triple response'. Initially, after a brief latent period, a thin red line appears in the path of the scratch, due to capillary dilatation. After a further 30 sec, a flare or flash develops on either side of this red line, associated with a rise in the local skin temperature, due to arteriolar dilatation. This persists for some time, then a raised oedematous area develops on either side of the scratch due to increased permeability of the skin capillaries. This change in capillary permeability is due to a morphological change in the endothelial cells of the capillary wall induced by histamine; the cells lose their normal close contact and expose the freely permeable basement membrane. As this weal reaches its maximum size, there is compression of local blood vessels, and the area becomes pale. The same sequence of events can be observed following injection of small amounts of histamine subcutaneously. In subjects with great sensitivity, such an injection of histamine can lead to the development of severe headache, and to increased gastric secretion.

A number of arylalkylamines are used clinically as anti-histamines to antagonize the actions of histamine on smooth muscle and capillary permeability. They are not generally effective in antagonizing the effect of massive mast cell lysis, because of the large amounts of histamine released, and the presence of other pharmacologically active substances in the mast cells, including serotonin and heparin. Anti-histamines are especially effective in controlling such allergic reactions as hayfever (pollen or dust allergy) and skin allergic responses. They do not, however, affect the gastric secretagogue action of histamine. Anti-histamines act by mimicry; they bind at the histamine receptor sites in smooth muscle and capillary walls, have no action themselves, but prevent access by histamine when it is released. Since the anti-histamines do not block the gastric action of histamine, it is possible that the gastric histamine receptors differ from those found in other tissues. Such differences in receptor sensitivity to inhibitors are seen in acetylcholine receptors at neuromuscular junctions and adrenergic receptors. In both of these cases different classes of affector analogues can be used to block the receptors at the two different types of site.

There are three pathways of histamine catabolism in mammals. The formation of N-acetyl histamine by acetyl transfer from acetyl-SCoA to the amino group appears to have been little studied and is of relatively minor importance. Oxidative catabolism of histamine can follow the two pathways shown in Figure 6.5. One pathway involves the direct oxidation of the amine by histaminase, forming imidazole acetaldehyde, followed by oxidation of the aldehyde to imidazole acetic acid. The other pathway involves the same steps, after an initial imidazole-N-methylation, catalysed by N-methyl transferase. Kapeller-Adler (1965) showed that a purified (electrophoretically homogeneous) preparation of histaminase catalysed the oxidation of histamine, or N-methyl histamine, to the corresponding aldehyde, but had no effect on a number of other amines, including amino-N-substituted histamines and the diamines cadaverine and putrescine. This has been interpreted as evidence that histaminase and diamine oxidase are clearly distinct enzymes, but this has been challenged by, for example, Zeller (1965) who argued that, despite the evidence of Kapeller-Adler, the two activities are associated with the same protein. Both pyridoxal-P and FAD are required for histaminase activity. The requirement for pyridoxal-P distinguishes

152

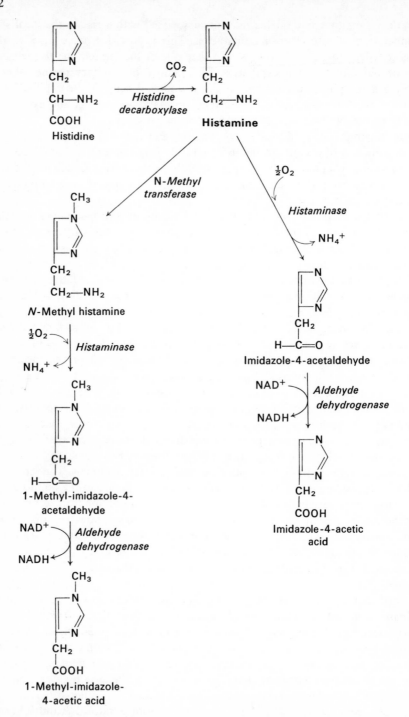

Figure 6.5. Histamine metabolism

this enzyme from the other amino acid and amine oxidases and dehydrogenases. The mechanism of the reaction has not been elucidated in detail, but it is known that excess pyridoxal-P or substrate will inhibit the enzyme, apparently by formation of stable ring-closed adducts between pyridoxal-P and the amine. Imidazole acetaldehyde, formed by histaminase activity, is a substrate for either FAD-linked xanthine oxidase, or NAD-linked aldehyde dehydrogenase.

Oxidation of histamine by histaminase action appears to account for only a relatively small proportion of catabolism *in vivo*. More is catabolized by formation of N-methyl histamine, which is then catabolized by the same route. N-Methyl imidazole acetic acid, formed by the oxidation of N-methyl histamine is generally excreted in the urine unchanged, while imidazole acetic acid, arising from histamine oxidation without prior methylation, is normally excreted as imidazole acetic acid ribonucleotide after conjugation with ribose.

In maternal blood during pregnancy, there is a considerable increase in histaminase activity. Despite this, and the presence in the placenta of an active histaminase, there is also a great deal of unmetabolized histamine excreted during pregnancy. Human foetal liver has an active histidine decarboxylase (the activity is considerably greater than in adult liver), and the foetus produces histamine at a considerable rate. However, there appears to be no foetal mechanism for catabolism of the amine, which is therefore excreted via the umbilical cord to the maternal circulation. The raised maternal histaminase level therefore appears to be a protective mechanism to deal with this constant excretion of a pharmacologically active material by the foetus. The physiological significance of this massive foetal histamine production is unclear.

Alivisatos and coworkers (Alivisatos, 1965) have studied a reaction whereby histamine reacts enzymically with NAD, displacing nicotinamide, and forming histamine adenine dinucleotide (HAD) as shown in Figure 6.6. It was thought at one time that this reaction represented a method of storing histamine in an inactive form in the body, but the great cost to the body in the nicotinamide used and the absence of any detectable enzyme capable of releasing histamine from HAD has led to the abandonment of this hypothesis. No function for this displacement reaction has been proposed, although it may be of importance in inactivating the large amounts of histamine released in allergic reactions. Administration of radioactive histamine to experimental animals leads to the isolation of histamine adenine dinucleotide in small amounts, showing that the reaction can occur *in vivo* as well as *in vitro* with tissue homogenates. However, only small amounts of the dinucleotide can be detected after administration of [^{14}C]histamine-labelled HAD to animals. Radioactive histamine ribonucleotide is found in the urine, suggesting that the dinucleotide can be degraded *in vivo* by cleavage and dephosphorylation. The enzymes most likely to catalyse these two reactions would be nucleotide pyrophosphatase and 5'-nucleotidase. Histamine ribonucleotide is not a substrate for histaminase, or any other oxidase which has been investigated, and cannot be oxidized to imidazole acetic acid ribonucleotide, which, as noted above, arises from conjugation of imidazole acetic acid with ribose.

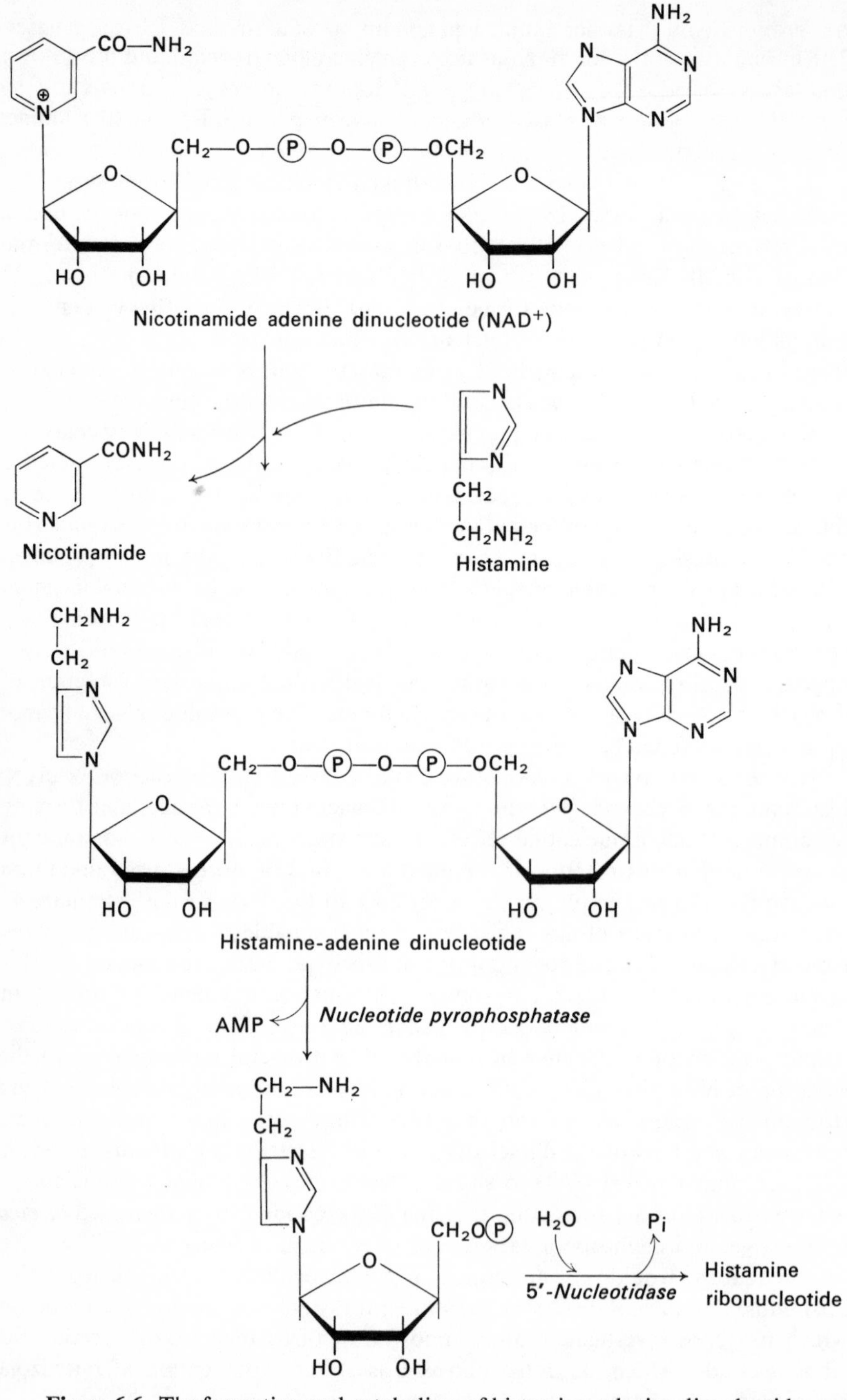

154

Figure 6.6. The formation and catabolism of histamine–adenine dinucleotide

THE AROMATIC AMINO ACIDS

The common pathway of aromatic biosynthesis

The initial stages of synthesis are common to all three aromatic amino acids, phenylalanine, tyrosine and tryptophan; this pathway is shown in Figure 6.7. After the formation of chorismic acid, the pathway of tryptophan synthesis diverges from that of phenylalanine and tyrosine. In most micro-organisms and plants, these two amino acids are synthesized by parallel pathways, which diverge after the formation of prephenic acid. However, in a number of organisms, notably the pseudomonads there is an active phenylalanine hydroxylase, very similar to that found in mammalian liver, which is capable of hydroxylating phenylalanine to tyrosine. Presumably, in these organisms much of the tyrosine is synthesized from phenylalanine rather than directly from prephenic acid.

Early studies with bacterial mutants incapable of synthesizing phenylalanine and tyrosine established the major cyclic intermediates of the pathway. The first to be so identified was shikimic acid, which was shown to be usable by many mutants unable to synthesize aromatic compounds. Other compounds, including 5-dehydroshikimic and 5-dehydroquinic acids, were identified by their accumulation in other mutant strains incapable of forming shikimate. Chorismic acid, the branch point between the phenylalanine/tyrosine and tryptophan pathways is of interest because it can undergo non-enzymic conversion *in vitro* to prephenic acid and even to phenylpyruvate and hydroxyphenylpyruvate when heated in acid.

The first step in the biosynthesis of chorismic acid is the condensation of erythrose-4-P and phospho-enolpyruvate to form 3-deoxyarabinoheptulosonic acid-7-P (DAHP). This synthetase reaction is essentially irreversible, and the enzyme does not catalyse appreciable phosphorolysis of DAHP. Being the first enzyme unique to aromatic biosynthesis, DAHP synthetase is inhibited by the end-products of the pathway; phenylalanine and tyrosine are equally effective as inhibitors, and tryptophan about one quarter as inhibitory. In most organisms, there are three separate isoenzymes of DAHP synthetase, one which is inhibited and repressed by phenylalanine, one which is similarly affected by tyrosine and a third which is repressed, but only slightly inhibited, by tryptophan. Mutants lacking only one of these three isoenzymes have been isolated; it can be shown by genetic mapping that the genes for the three isoenzymes are widely separated in the *E. coli* genome. Any of these mutants will grow adequately on minimal culture medium but, for example, that lacking phenylalanine-sensitive synthetase shows a requirement for phenylalanine when grown in the presence of tyrosine and tryptophan, because these two amino acids repress the formation of the two remaining synthetases, and so cut off completely the supply of DAHP. The two substrates, erythrose-4-P and phospho-enolpyruvate, can be shown to be cooperative allosteric activators of the *E. coli* synthetase although this is not so in most other organisms. The enzyme has a ping-pong mechanism, with phospho-enolpyruvate binding first.

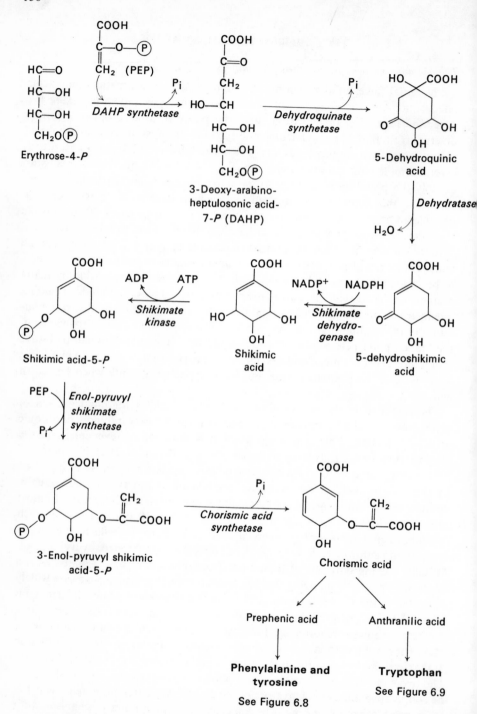

Figure 6.7. The common pathway of aromatic amino acid biosynthesis

The cyclization of DAHP to dehydroquinic acid requires cobalt and catalytic amounts of NAD⁺, which is not reduced in the reaction. No intermediates of the reaction have been isolated, so it is assumed that all are tightly enzyme-bound. To account for the requirement of the enzyme for NAD⁺ in catalytic quantities, it has been proposed that the reaction proceeds by way of an initial dehydrogenation at C-6 to yield the 2,6-di-oxo derivative, which readily loses phosphate at C-7 to yield the 7-deoxy derivative. This is then rehydrogenated by the enzyme-bound NADH, and the product cyclized to 5-dehydroquinic acid. Dehydration of this intermediate, catalysed by 5-dehydroquinate dehydratase, yields dehydroshikimic acid. The dehydratase appears to be absolutely specific for 5-dehydroquinic acid as substrate.

Dehydroshikimic acid is reduced to shikimic acid in an NADPH-dependent reaction catalysed by shikimate dehydrogenase; the enzyme is specific for NADPH and will not use NADH. After phosphorylation, shikimic acid-5-*P* condenses with phospho-enolpyruvate in a reaction similar to that of DAHP synthetase. However, this reaction is readily reversible. *In vitro*, fluoride must be present in the incubation mixture to prevent spontaneous dephosphorylation of the product, 3-enolpyruvylshikimic acid-5-*P* to the next intermediate, chorismic acid. *In vivo*, there is evidence for the existence of a specific enzyme, chorismate synthetase, catalysing this dephosphorylation despite the fact that it will proceed spontaneously.

In *N. crassa*, a single multi-enzyme complex, of molecular weight about 230,000, catalyses the conversion of DAHP to 3-enolpyruvyl-shikimic acid-5-*P*. Encoded by a single gene cluster, the *arom* locus, the multi-enzyme complex can be shown to contain the same five enzyme activities as are found as separate enzymes in *E. coli* and other organisms. However, in Neurospora, there are believed to be only four separate polypeptides in the complex; shikimate dehydrogenase and dehydroquinate dehydratase cannot be separated under conditions which otherwise wholly dissociate the multi-enzyme complex.

Phenylalanine and tyrosine biosynthesis from chorismic acid (IMP)

Two isoenzymes of chorismate mutase, the enzyme catalysing the formation of prephenic acid from chorismic acid, have been isolated from both *K. aerogenes* and *E. coli* preparations. One form is associated with prephenate dehydratase, the first enzyme unique to phenylalanine formation, and is inhibited by phenylalanine, but not by tyrosine; it has therefore been called chorismate mutase P. The other isoenzyme, chorismate mutase T, is sensitive to tyrosine inhibition, but not phenylalanine, and is associated with prephenate dehydrogenase. Prephenate dehydratase is inhibited by phenylalanine, and the dehydrogenase by tyrosine, so that the onward conversion of chorismic acid is doubly regulated. Excess tryptophan activates chorismate mutase, and reverses inhibition by phenylalanine and tyrosine, so aiding removal of chorismate produced in excess.

The synthesis of the two isoenzymes of chorismate mutase appears to be separate. Mutants have been isolated in which mutase P and prephenate dehydratase are inadequately synthesized, but the activities of prephenate dehydro-

158

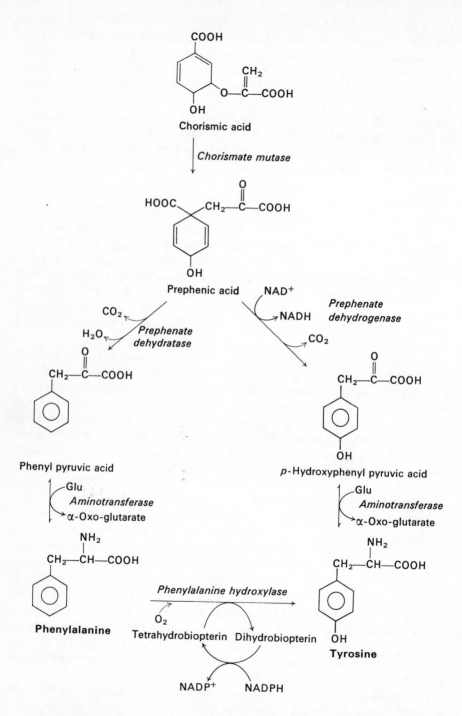

Figure 6.8. The synthesis of phenylalanine and tyrosine from chorismic acid

genase and chorismate mutase T are unaffected. In some organisms, for example *B. subtilis*, there is no evidence of complex formation between chorismate mutase and succeeding enzymes; all three enzymes can be isolated as separate proteins.

In mammals, although phenylalanine is an essential amino acid, tyrosine is not since it can be synthesized readily from phenylalanine by hydroxylation. This, of course, requires that there is adequate phenylalanine present to satisfy the demand for both amino acids. Phenylalanine hydroxylase is an oxygenase, and uses tetrahydrobiopterin (a folic acid derivative) as cosubstrate, forming tyrosine, dihydrobiopterin and water. The dihydrobiopterin is reduced to the active tetrahydro form by an NADPH-dependent enzyme, dihydrofolate reductase, so that the overall reaction of phenylalanine hydroxylation uses NADPH, although the hydroxylase itself does not react with NADPH. In phenylketonuria, an inborn error of metabolism characterized biochemically by a lack of phenylalanine hydroxylase activity, it is the hydroxylase itself, and not the dihydrofolate reductase, which is defective in all cases that have been reported to date.

Tryptophan synthesis from chorismic acid

In *E. coli*, the first two enzymes of tryptophan biosynthesis from chorismic acid, namely anthranilate synthetase and phosphoribosyl transferase, are associated as a multi-enzyme complex, the anthranilate aggregate, containing two subunits of each activity. Both activities of the aggregate are inhibited by tryptophan. Anthranilate synthetase is wholly inhibited by an excess of the amino acid, even in the presence of its two substrates, chorismic acid and glutamine, but the phosphoribosyl transferase is only 70 % inhibited even in the presence of a gross excess of tryptophan.

The reaction of anthranilate synthetase, as shown in Figure 6.9, is the addition of the amide group of glutamine to the ring of chorismate, together with the removal of the enol-pyruvyl side chain. At high concentration *in vitro*, ammonium salts can be shown to substitute for glutamine. It is therefore assumed that the enzyme has a glutaminase activity, and in the *E. coli* system this can be demonstrated to be associated with the phosphoribosyl transferase subunit, rather than the anthranilate synthetase subunit. Anthranilate synthetase separated from the aggregate can use ammonium salts but not glutamine. However, binding of glutamine to the phosphoribosyl transferase subunit requires the presence of chorismate, which has been shown to bind specifically to the anthranilate synthetase subunit. Thus, the subunits in the aggregate exhibit a great deal of cooperation.

Regulation of the aggregate in both *E. coli* and *S. typhimurium* can be shown to involve conformational changes. The *S. typhimurium* system has two competitively related binding sites for tryptophan and chorismate. Since tryptophan will inhibit both activities of the aggregate, it is probable that the tryptophan binding sites on the anthranilate synthetase subunits communicate in some way with the phosphoribosyl transferase subunits. In the same way, chorismate is not only the substrate of the anthranilate synthetase subunit, but relieves the inhibition of both subunits by tryptophan. Pabst and coworkers (1973) have

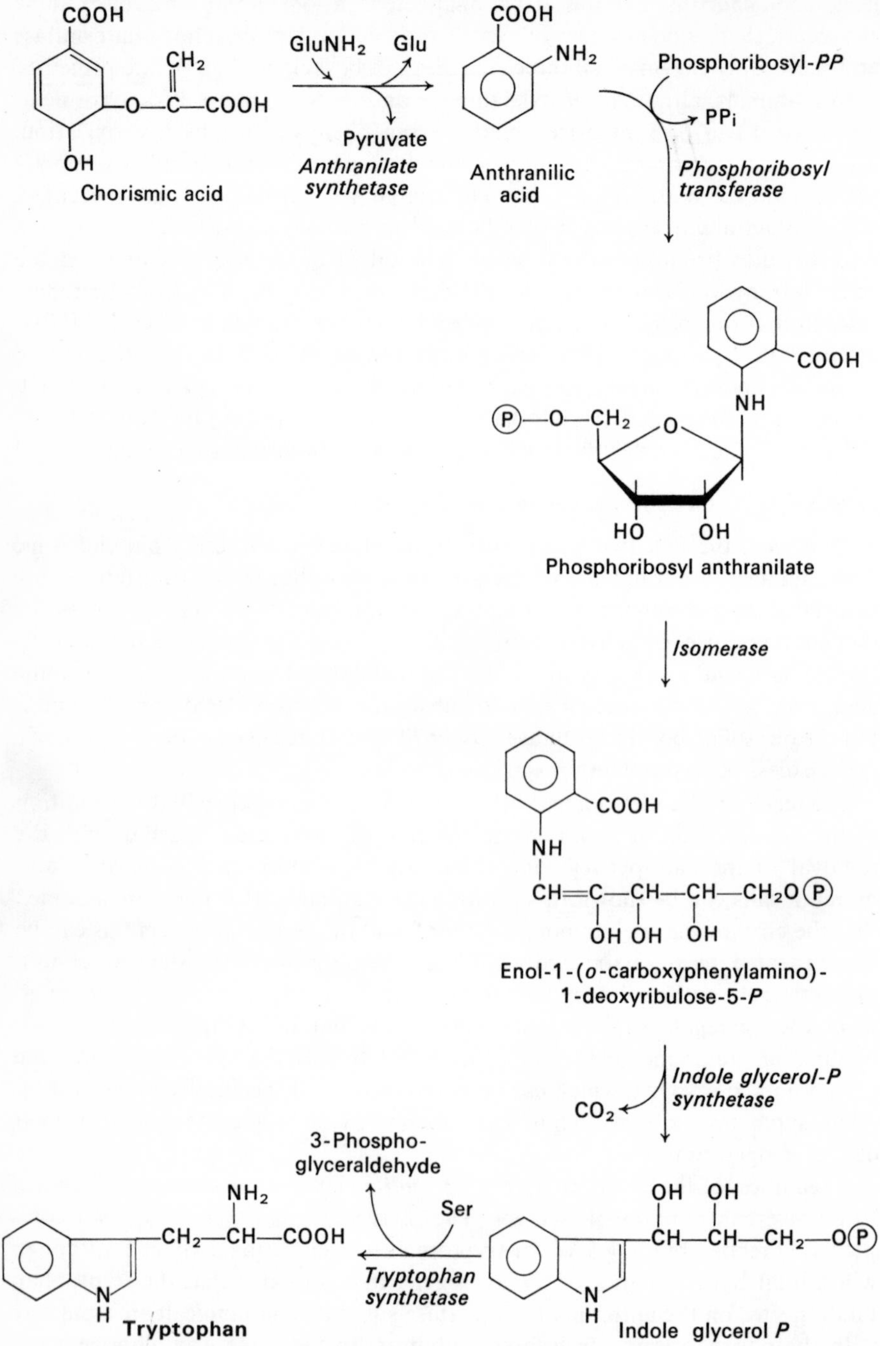

Figure 6.9. The synthesis of tryptophan from chorismic acid

demonstrated that there are indeed conformational changes in the anthranilate aggregate from *E. coli* on binding chorismic acid and tryptophan. They have also shown that although glutamine will bind to the enzyme in the presence or absence of chorismate, it is only when chorismate is also present that there is any detectable glutaminase activity, providing further evidence for conformational changes in the enzyme. Bacterial mutants have been isolated which have normal chorismate binding, and reaction kinetics, but are without tryptophan sensitivity, indicating that the two sites must be separate.

There is considerable evidence that in the *Enterobacteriaciae* the next two activities of tryptophan biosynthesis, phosphoribosyl isomerase and indole glycerol-*P* synthetase, are also associated in a single polypeptide chain. This is presumably a result of gene fusion at some stage in evolution, since in other organisms these two activities are associated with separate proteins, one catalysing the isomerization of phosphoribosyl anthranilate to the enol-deoxyribulosyl derivative, and the other catalysing the decarboxylation of this intermediate to indole glycerol-*P*.

The final stage of tryptophan synthesis is the condensation of indole glycerol-*P* with serine, catalysed by tryptophan synthetase. The mechanism of this reaction was shown in Figure 2.10 (page 48). Enzyme-bound indole is formed from indole glycerol-*P* by the elimination of 3-phosphoglyceraldehyde and this then attacks the Schiff base formed between serine and the pyridoxal-*P* cofactor of the enzyme. In bacteria and plants it has been demonstrated that tryptophan synthetase exists as two separate proteins, a small A-protein, which is essential for the stability and activity of the larger B-protein, which contains pyridoxal-*P*. The active complex catalyses the condensation of serine with indole glycerol-*P* or free indole, and in the absence of serine will catalyse the formation of indole from indole glycerol-*P*. The two proteins of tryptophan synthetase from a wide variety of species have a number of immunologically reactive sites in common, and an active complex has been reconstituted from the purified A-protein isolated from *E. coli*, and the purified B-protein from the flowering plant *Nicotiana tabacum*. In fungi, tryptophan synthetase exists as a single protein which cannot be dissociated by any of the methods which have been tried to date, although there is some evidence that the enzyme consists of two separate polypeptide chains, which are bound by covalent links rather than by the freely dissociable bonds found in bacteria and plants.

In *E. coli* there is coordinate derepression of all the enzymes required for the synthesis of tryptophan from chorismic acid when the organism is grown on a tryptophan-free medium. Strains of the organism with regulator mutations show a constant synthesis of all the enzymes of the pathway, even in the presence of normally repressive levels of the end-product. It therefore appears that not only is anthranilate synthetase, the first enzyme of the pathway, sensitive to tryptophan, but all the other enzymes are repressed by either tryptophan or a metabolite. It is therefore assumed that, as for the enzymes of histidine biosynthesis in *S. typhimurium* discussed above, all the enzymes of tryptophan biosynthesis in *E. coli* must be coded for on a single gene cluster. The repressor role of tryptophan is believed to be in inhibiting the transcription of a polycistronic mRNA, by interaction with the operator gene.

Catabolism of phenylalanine and tyrosine

Under normal circumstances in mammals, phenylalanine is catabolized by hydroxylation to tyrosine, a reaction catalysed by phenylalanine hydroxylase, as noted above. Tyrosine is then transaminated to p-hydroxyphenylpyruvate. This reaction is catalysed by an aminotransferase which appears to be inducible in man, and may be the same as the enzyme which catalyses the transamination of tryptophan. It can also act on phenylalanine, a reaction which becomes important in phenylketonuria, when phenylalanine hydroxylase is congenitally defective.

Although p-hydroxyphenylpyruvate can be reduced to the lactate derivative, this reaction is normally of minor importance. In alcaptonuria, an inborn error of tyrosine metabolism (see below), p-hydroxyphenyllactate can accumulate in the urine in large amounts.

The major pathway of p-hydroxyphenylpyruvate metabolism is through homogentisic acid, as shown in Figure 6.10. Homogentisic acid is formed by a complex series of reactions, involving hydroxylation of the aromatic ring of p-hydroxyphenylpyruvate, migration of the pyruvyl side-chain, and its decarboxylation to an acetyl side-chain. No intermediates of this reaction sequence have been isolated, and it is believed that a single enzyme, p-hydroxyphenylpyruvate hydroxylase, catalyses all three reactions. This hydroxylase is a copper-dependent oxygenase, and it has been demonstrated that in animals rendered deficient in copper there is a considerable reduction in the activity of this enzyme in the liver. It was also thought for some time that the enzyme was ascorbate dependent, and indeed it can be shown that in avitaminosis C there is defective formation of homogentisic acid, and increased urinary excretion of p-hydroxyphenylpyruvate. However, with moderate purification of the enzyme it was shown that the in vitro requirement for ascorbate decreased, and the ability to use a variety of synthetic reducing agents to activate the reaction increased as the purity of the enzyme preparation increased. Hence, while ascorbate may have an effect on the activity of this enzyme in vivo, it is not a specific requirement.

Homogentisic acid is oxidatively cleaved to maleyl acetoacetate, a reaction catalysed by homogentisic acid oxidase. This enzyme is an oxygenase which has several reactive sulphydryl groups in the molecule and requires ferrous ions, presumably bound to the sulphydryl groups as mercaptides, and possibly also in association with histidinyl residues. Maleyl acetoacetate is isomerized to fumaryl acetoacetate. Maleyl acetoacetate isomerase is unusual in that it has an absolute requirement for the reductant tripeptide glutathione (γ-glutamyl-cysteinyl-glycine) for activity. The role of glutathione in this reaction is presumably to maintain the reduced sulphydryl groups of the enzyme; it has been shown that oxidation or reaction of these groups leads to loss of activity. As was noted on page 106, the majority of enzymes which require glutathione in vitro can also

163

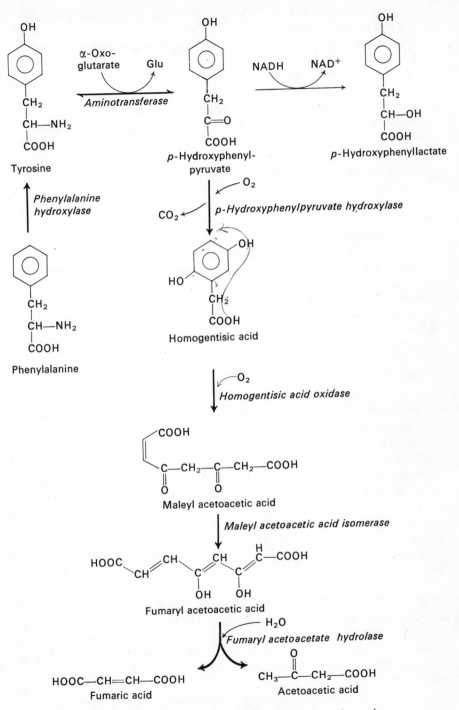

Figure 6.10. The catabolism of phenylalanine and tyrosine

use a variety of other reducing compounds, however this isomerase is unusual in that it does show absolute specificity for glutathione.

The fumaryl acetoacetate is cleaved to yield fumarate and acetoacetate, so that phenylalanine and tyrosine ultimately give rise to both glucogenic and ketogenic fragments. Fumaryl acetoacetate hydrolase appears to be a simple hydrolase, with no cofactor requirements.

In phenylketonuria, there is a defect of phenylalanine hydroxylase, and phenylalanine cannot be converted to tyrosine for catabolism. This means that a number of alternative pathways must be used for catabolism of excess dietary phenylalanine. The major excretory products in this disease are phenylpyruvic acid from transamination of phenylalanine, phenyllactic acid formed by reduction of phenylpyruvate, and phenylacetate formed by oxidative decarboxylation of phenylpyruvate. It is possible that it is these abnormal metabolites, or further products derived from them, which damage the developing nervous system of the phenylketonuric child, so early diagnosis is essential. Diagnosis is by detection of the phenylketones in the urine, confirmed by finding high serum phenyl-alanine and low serum tyrosine concentrations. Phenylketonuria is treated by strict regulation of the dietary intake of phenylalaninine; intake must be adequate to allow normal protein synthesis and growth, but not so great as to allow the blood phenylalanine level to rise above normal. When such treatment is started at a sufficiently early age, there is little damage to the central nervous system, and treated phenylketonuriacs have approximately normal intelligence. Untreated sufferers from the disease have a severely impaired intelligence. The aetiology of this idiocy is uncertain, and while it has been suggested that there is a neuro-toxic metabolite of phenylalanine, such a compound has not been identified.

In tyrosinosis, there is a failure of p-hydroxyphenylpyruvate hydroxylase, so that homogentisic acid is not formed, and p-hydroxyphenylpyruvate, lactate and acetate are excreted in the urine. Blood and urine tyrosine are also raised. The disease appears to be a biochemical lesion with no clinical signs.

In alcaptonuria, homogentisic acid oxidase is defective, and the acid is excreted in the urine. On standing in air this polymerizes to a melanin-like compound, and the urine darkens, although it appears normal at the time of passing. Alcapto-nuriacs suffer no great disability although, for reasons which are unclear, they are more prone to rheumatoid arthritis than normal subjects, and considerable pigmentation of collagen may occur in later life. Their intelligence is unimpaired.

Formation of the catecholamines

Although of great physiological importance because of their role in neuro-transmission and as hormones, the formation of noradrenaline (norepinephrine) and adrenaline (epinephrine) is quantitatively of little significance in the cata-bolism of the aromatic amino acids. Only a minute fraction of the total intake of phenylalanine passes through the catecholamine pathway shown in Figure 6.11.

Tyrosine is hydroxylated to 3,4-dihydroxyphenylalanine (DOPA) in several tissues by a hydroxylase which appears to be very similar to phenylalanine

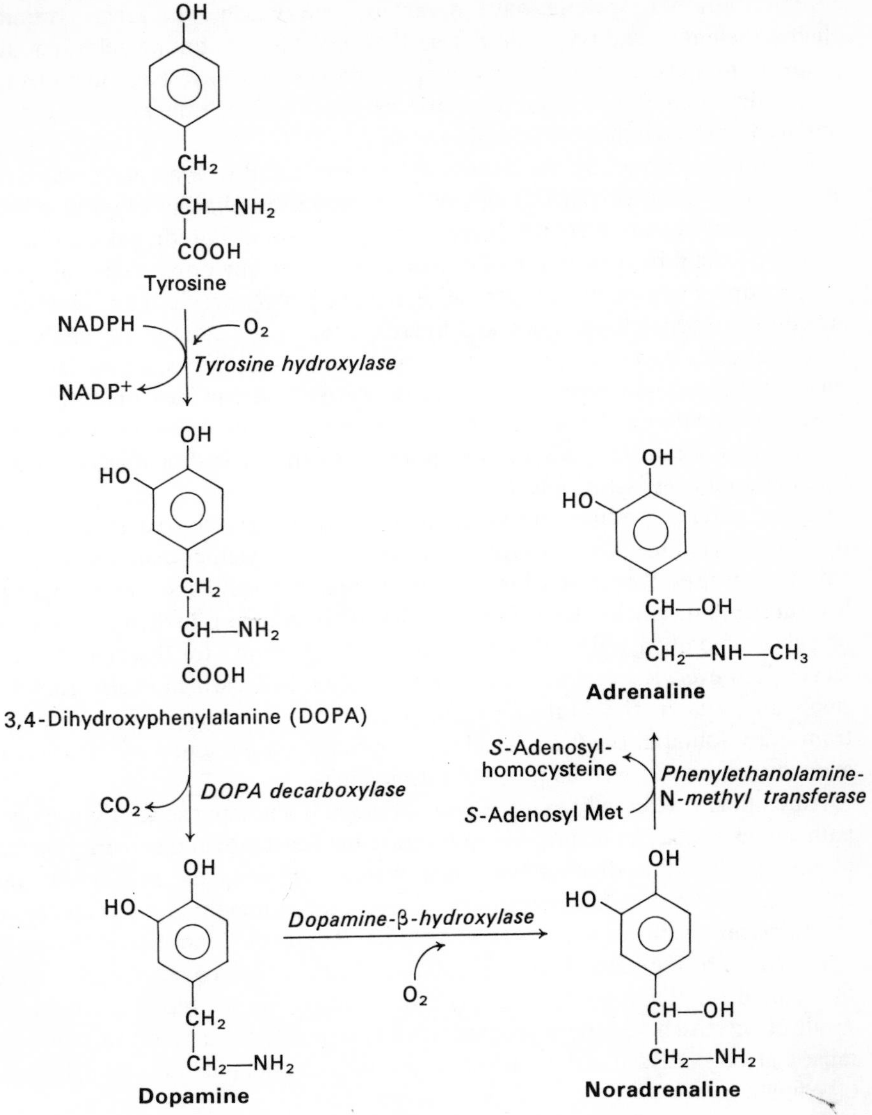

Figure 6.11. The biosynthesis of the catecholamines

hydroxylase, although it can be shown to be a separate protein. DOPA is de-carboxylated to the primary amine dopamine (3,4-dihydroxyphenylethylamine) by DOPA decarboxylase. This enzyme also acts on 5-hydroxytryptophan to yield serotonin, as discussed below. There is some dispute in the literature as to the specificity of this decarboxylase; some workers claim that it also acts on phenylalanine, tyrosine and tryptophan, yielding the corresponding amines, while the majority of workers have been unable to demonstrate any such activity.

Several intestinal bacteria have decarboxylases which will form tyramine, phenylethylamine and tryptamine from the corresponding amino acids, and it is probable that the small amounts of these amines that have been identified in mammalian tissue arise from intestinal bacterial action, rather than by endogenous decarboxylation of the amino acids.

Dopamine, formed by the decarboxylation of DOPA, is a neurotransmitter in its own right (see page 185), and also possesses pharmacological action, being a potent vasoconstrictor. It is also the precursor of noradrenaline, which is formed by the β-hydroxylation of dopamine, catalysed by dopamine-β-hydroxylase, a copper-containing oxygenase of relatively low specificity. A number of substituted phenylethylamines are hydroxylated to noradrenaline analogues. For example, tyramine gives octopamine and α-methyldopamine gives α-methylnoradrenaline, both of which can displace noradrenaline from its receptor sites, and function as 'false' transmitters. These compounds are of some therapeutic use, since they are catabolized more slowly than noradrenaline, and therefore have a longer lasting effect.

In the adrenal medulla, noradrenaline is further metabolized to adrenaline by N-methylation. The enzyme responsible, phenylethanolamine-N-methyl transferase, uses S-adenosyl methionine as methyl donor, and has a relatively low substrate specificity; any of the products of dopamine-β-hydroxylase activity on substituted phenylethanolamines will act as a substrate for the methyl transferase. However, the enzyme from the adrenal medulla, which is also found in small amounts in the brain, is distinct from the lower-specificity N-methyl transferase found in the lung, which acts on indoleamines and a wide variety of aromatic amines as well as phenylethanolamines.

Adrenaline is released from the adrenal medulla in response to fright, anger, pain and asphyxia; its actions are to increase the heart rate and constrict surface blood vessels, while dilating the blood vessels supplying the muscles. It also stimulates respiration, and acts as a bronchodilator; adrenaline and its analogues are therefore useful in treatment of asthma. The main biochemical action of adrenaline is to stimulate the activity of liver and muscle glycogen phosphorylase, thus enhancing the breakdown of glycogen, and raising the blood glucose (as a result of increased hepatic glycogenolysis) and lactate (as a result of increased muscle glycogenolysis). Adrenaline thus prepares the animal either to fight or to take flight.

The regulation of catecholamine biosynthesis is not clear; the first enzyme of the pathway, tyrosine hydroxylase, is present in limiting amounts so any factor that affects the activity of this enzyme will also regulate the production of catecholamines, However, unlike the regulation of serotonin synthesis from tryptophan (see page 183), there is no evidence that the rate of formation of the amines is determined by the availability of the precursor amino acid in the brain. Both phenylalanine and tyrosine hydroxylase activities have been identified in the brain, so that either amino acid can be used as a precursor of the catecholamines. When radioactive phenylalanine is given to animals, the radioactivity of brain tyrosine is very much lower than that of DOPA and the catecholamines, suggesting that brain phenylalanine hydroxylase is closely associated with tyrosine hydroxylase, so that little of the newly formed tyrosine enters the general brain pool of the amino acid; instead it is rapidly metabolized further to catecholamines.

Catabolism of the catecholamines gives rise to a large number of excretory products through the action of two enzymes, monoamine oxidase, and catechol-O-methyl transferase. These two enzymes can act in either order, so that methylated amines and non-methylated acids are excreted as well as methylated acids.

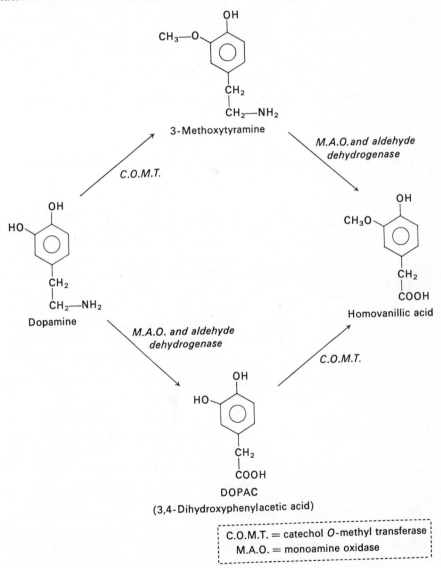

Figure 6.12. The catabolism of dopamine

This is shown for dopamine in Figure 6.12. The immediate product of mono-amine oxidase activity is the aldehyde corresponding to the amine; this is rapidly oxidized to the corresponding acid by aldehyde dehydrogenase. In some cases there may be reduction of the aldehyde to the corresponding alcohol, a reaction catalysed by aldehyde reductase or alcohol dehydrogenase. Monoamine oxidase is a mitochondrial flavoprotein, which has been postulated to exist in a number of different isoenzymes, characterized by their electrophoretic mobility, different substrate specificity and differing sensitivity to inhibitors (Youdim et al., 1969). However, the existence of such isoenzymes has been challenged by Houslay and Tipton (1973) on the grounds that the separable forms merely represent an artefact of the solubilization procedure, different amounts of membrane lipid remaining attached to the enzyme. As well as acting on the catecholamines, monoamine oxidase acts on a variety of primary monoamines, including sero-tonin, tyramine and tryptamine; it does not act on histamine or the diamines and polyamines.

Catechol-O-methyl transferase requires S-adenosyl methionine as methyl donor, and has a broad specificity, methylating the m-hydroxyl groups of a large number of compounds with a catechol (1,2-dihydroxyphenyl) nucleus.

Melanin

The black and brown pigments of most animals are forms of melanin, a com-plex polymer of uncertain structure, which is formed from DOPA by ring closure to a dihydroxyindole derivative. The enzyme responsible for melanin formation is tyrosinase, not the tyrosine hydroxylase which forms DOPA for catecholamine synthesis. To what extent tyrosinase, a copper-containing oxygenase, is respon-sible for the steps which occur after the formation of DOPA is not clear, since, at least *in vitro*, DOPA will readily polymerize to a melanin-like insoluble pigment in the presence of oxygen. DOPA is oxidized to the quinone form, dopaquinone, which then undergoes ring closure to form 2-carboxy-2,3-dihydro-5,6-dihy-droxyindole. This yields 5,6-dihydroxyindole via decarboxylation and reduction, which then forms indole-5,6-quinone, as shown in Figure 6.13. It is the indole-quinone which polymerizes to melanin.

The role of tyrosinase in controlling the initiation of melanin formation is seen in the goldfish, *Carassius auratus*, which exists in three clearly distinguishable forms, a xanthic form (yellow, with almost no melanin, and very low tyrosinase activity in the skin), a black form (the black moor), which has a very high tyro-sinase activity in the skin, and an intermediate form, the grey carp, which has an intermediate level of tyrosinase activity.

Albinism in mammals is due to a deficiency of tyrosinase activity, leading to a failure of melanin formation. In experimental animals, total albinism is common, with no pigmentation of skin, hair or eyes. However, in man, although total albinism has been observed, the commonest form is partial albinism, with unpigmented regions of the skin or hair. Not only the tendency to partial albin-ism, but also the pattern of albinotic patches, is genetically determined; a white forelock is frequently a familial trait.

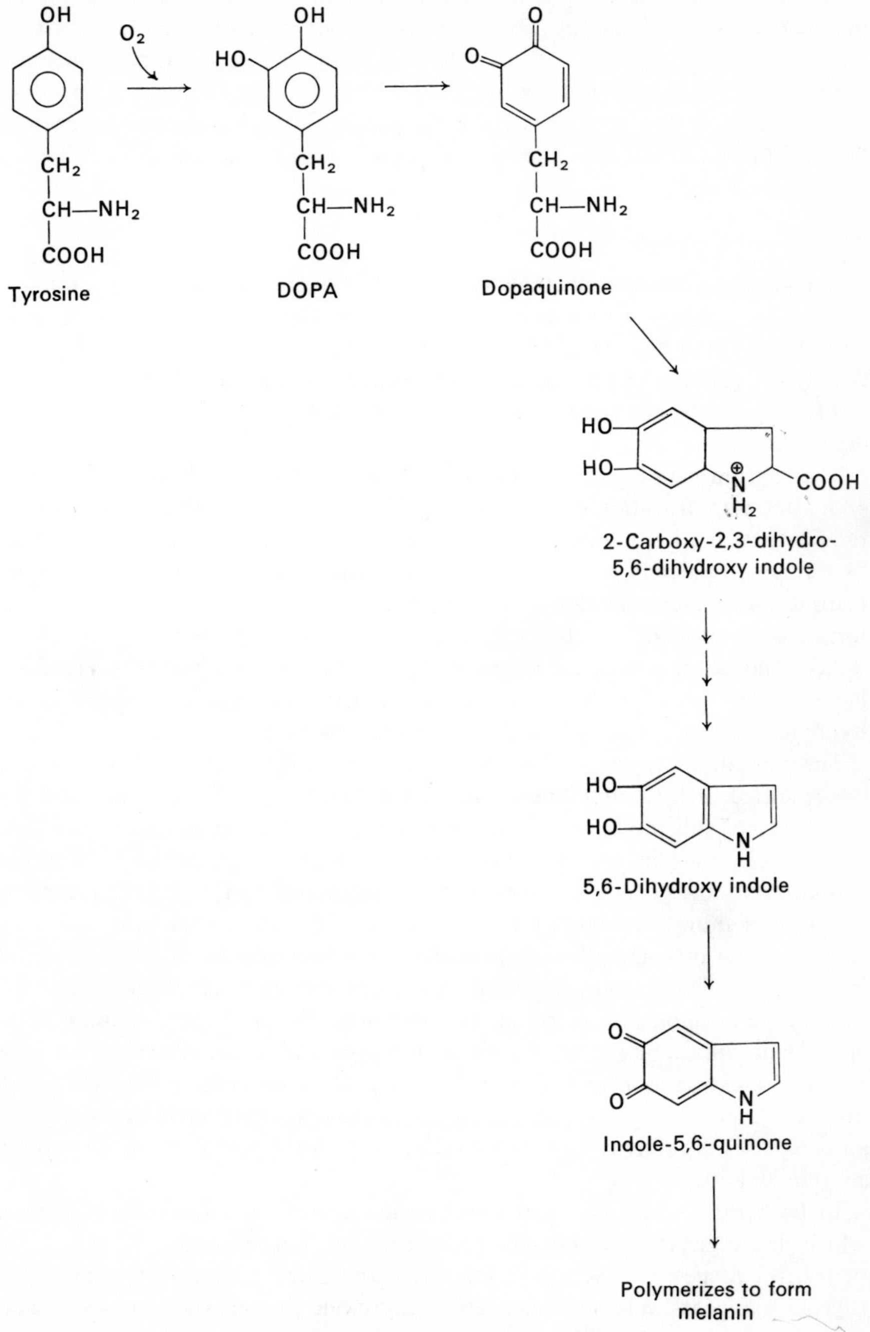

Figure 6.13. Melanin synthesis

In the *substantia nigra* of the brain there is a considerable amount of melanin. This is not DOPA melanin as is found in the skin and hair, but is formed by polymerization of dopamine. Even in wholly albino animals, the *substantia nigra* is normally pigmented. The mechanism of formation of this neuromelanin is unknown. *Post mortem* examination has revealed that there is little or no pigmentation of the *substantia nigra* in patients with Parkinson's disease, a disorder in which there is a deficiency of brain dopamine and considerable motor neuron disability.

Thyroxine and tri-iodothyronine

In common with other phenolic compounds, tyrosine can be readily iodinated *in vitro* by reaction with iodine, to form mono- and di-iodotyrosine by substitution at the *m*-positions of the ring. The same reaction also occurs *in vivo* in the thyroid gland, where it is assumed to be enzyme catalysed. The name iodinase has been given to this enzyme, although its existence has not been conclusively demonstrated.

The thyroid gland accumulates iodine from the blood with great efficiency: 48 h after administration of a test dose of $^{131}I^-$ it can be shown that 80% of the radioactivity has been taken up by the gland. Much of the remainder is taken up by the salivary glands, and is subsequently released into the general circulation. Prior to intestinal absorption, iodine is reduced to the iodide ion, and it is in this form that it circulates in the body and is taken up by the thyroid gland. After uptake, the iodide is oxidized to iodine. The oxidase responsible for this reaction has not been identified, but it is assumed that the reaction is catalysed by the hydrogen peroxide formed by a flavoprotein oxygenase.

The iodination of tyrosine does not occur in free solution *in vivo*, but when it is incorporated into thyroglobulin, one of the thyroid proteins. Mono- and di-iodotyrosine, still incorporated into thyroglobulin, then react in an oxidative reaction catalysed by an enzyme known as 'coupling enzyme' to form either tri-iodothyronine (T_3) or thyroxine (tetra-iodothyronine, T_4). This sequence of reactions is shown in Figure 6.14. Thyroxine and tri-iodothyronine are then released from thyroglobulin by proteolysis and secreted by the thyroid gland into the bloodstream under stimulation from the anterior pituitary thyroid stimulating hormone, thyrotropin. In the blood, T_3 and T_4 are again protein-bound, and clinical measurement of the protein-bound iodine (PBI) is a measure of the circulating levels of T_3 and T_4. As well as stimulating the release of thyroid hormones, thyrotropin also enhances the uptake of iodide by the thyroid and increases the activity of iodide oxidation to iodine, and the rate of coupling enzyme activity.

In both the thyroid and peripheral tissues there are deiodinating enzymes, which dehalogenate free, but not protein-bound, iodotyrosines, T_3 and T_4. In peripheral tissues, this serves to inactivate thyroxine after action, and in the thyroid it appears to regulate the rate of thyroxine production. In cases of congenital lack of the thyroid deiodinase, mono- and di-iodotyrosine are excreted in the urine, suggesting that normally a considerable amount of iodotyrosine is recycled by way of deiodination. Since iodination of tyrosine may well be largely, if not entirely, non-enzymic, such a regulatory mechanism is essential.

Hypothyroidism (underactivity of the thyroid) involves defective production of thyroxine, and consequent abnormally low circulating levels of T_3 and T_4. It is characterized by a very low metabolic rate (the basal metabolic rate may be as much as 40% below normal), and a general mental apathy; exophthalmos (protruding eyes) may also occur. Severe adult hypothyroidism is known as myxoedema; there is subcutaneous oedema, and especially the hands and face have a puffy appearance. Cretinism is the result of infantile hypothyroidism; cretins are considerably stunted in growth, and have a very low mental age.

By contrast, hyperactivity of the thyroid, resulting in abnormally high circulating levels of T_3 and T_4, is characterized by a nervous agitation and a raised basal

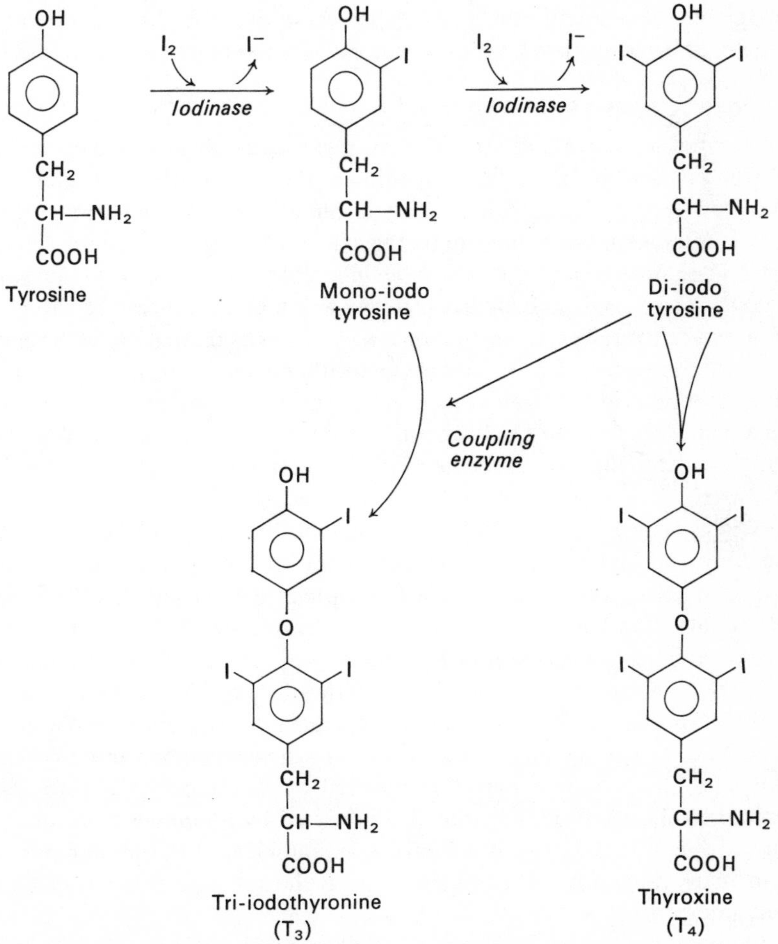

Figure 6.14. Thyroxine and tri-iodothyronine synthesis

metabolic rate. *In vitro*, and presumably also *in vivo*, thyroxine acts as an un-coupler of mitochondrial oxidative phosphorylation, thus allowing increased oxidative metabolism without phosphorylation of ADP to ATP.

Goitre is an enlargement of the thyroid, and is endemic in areas of the world where soil and water iodine levels are low. In Great Britain it has been called Derbyshire neck, because of the former high incidence of endemic goitre in that county. The enlargement is due to hypertrophy of the gland in an attempt to synthesize adequate T_3 and T_4 without adequate supplies of iodine.

A number of compounds interfere with the metabolism of iodine in the thyroid gland, and are termed goitrogens. These include thiocyanate and perchlorate ions, which inhibit the uptake and oxidation of iodide ions, and thio-ureas and some imidazole derivatives, which inhibit the oxidative coupling of iodotyrosine. Many plants, especially members of the genus *Brassica*, contain goitrogens, although in the amounts normally eaten these are not clinically significant. Synthetic goitrogens have been used successfully to control hyperthyroidism.

The kynurenine pathway of tryptophan catabolism

The major oxidative pathway of tryptophan catabolism is shown in Figure 6.15. The first step is the oxidative opening of the heterocyclic ring, catalysed by tryptophan pyrrolase (also known as tryptophan oxygenase), a haem oxygenase. The rate of tryptophan catabolism by this pathway is regulated by the activity of the pyrrolase, which can be shown to be inducible in both micro-organisms and mammals. Oestrogens and hydrocortisone are potent inducers of the enzyme in mammalian liver. Tryptophan loading also increases the activity of the enzyme. This is not, however, a true induction, but rather a stabilization of the pyrrolase in the presence of its substrate. Tryptophan pyrrolase is a very unstable enzyme, and has a half-life *in vivo* of only about 2 h, so that very fine control of the rate of tryptophan catabolism can be achieved by regulation of the amount of pyrrolase synthesized.

As well as protecting the pyrrolase from catabolism *in vivo*, tryptophan appears to enhance the binding of the haem cofactor to the apoenzyme. In animals which have been given large doses of tryptophan, the percentage of the enzyme which is saturated with its cofactor is considerably greater than in liver from untreated animals. This action of tryptophan appears to involve binding to the apoenzyme at a site distinct from the catalytic site, since it has been shown that α-methyl tryptophan, which is neither a substrate nor an inhibitor of the enzyme, enhances haem binding, and reduces the K_m of the enzyme towards oxygen.

Not only is tryptophan pyrrolase induced by a number of hormones, and stabilized by its substrate, but it is also inhibited by a number of nicotinyl de-rivatives. NADPH is especially effective as an inhibitor of tryptophan pyrrolase, and in many ways can be considered to be the ultimate end-product of the kynurenine pathway.

Formylkynurenine, the product of tryptophan pyrrolase action, is deformylated by action of formamidase, an enzyme of low specificity which will release formate from a variety of aryl-formylamines, although its greatest activity is towards

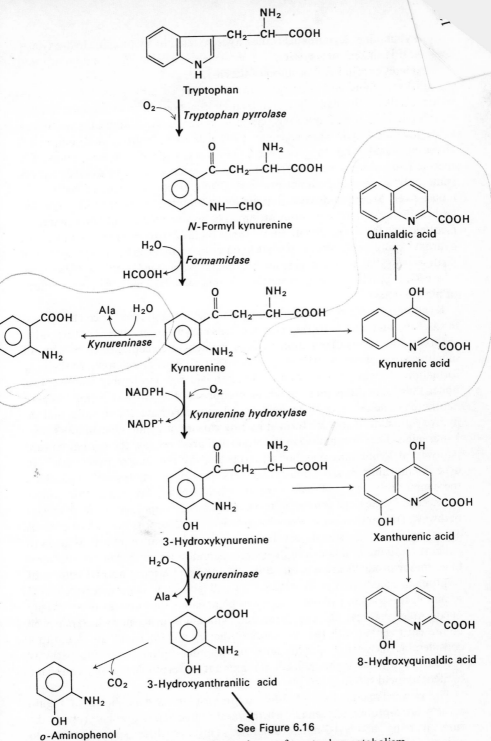

Figure 6.15. The kynurenine pathway of tryptophan catabolism

formylkynurenine. Kynurenine is then hydroxylated by kynurenine hydroxylase, an NADPH-linked oxygenase. The enzyme is specific for kynurenine, and hydroxylates only at the 3-position of the ring.

Both kynurenine and 3-hydroxykynurenine are substrates for kynureninase, which catalyses the hydrolytic removal of the side-chain as alanine, leaving anthranilic acid or its 3-hydroxy derivative. The enzyme is about three times as active towards 3-hydroxykynurenine as towards the unhydroxylated compound. However, McDermot and coworkers (1973) have reported the isolation of a specific hydroxykynureninase from mouse liver which is active towards kynurenine only at very high concentrations. There is no kynureninase activity in mouse liver. Mouse hydroxykynureninase is inhibited by its product, hydroxyanthranilic acid. This inhibition presumably acts to regulate the production of nicotinic acid from tryptophan. In *N. crassa*, there are two enzymes, a constitutive hydroxykynureninase, and a separate kynureninase, induced by growth on tryptophan-rich media, which is presumably mainly concerned with the catabolism of excess tryptophan. The constitutive enzyme is involved mainly in the synthesis of nicotinic acid.

Kynureninase is a pyridoxal-P-dependent enzyme, and it has been shown that in cases of avitaminosis B_6 the activity of this enzyme in the liver is considerably reduced. This means that avitaminosis B_6 is likely to be complicated by signs of nicotinic acid deficiency (pellagra), since in the absence of kynureninase activity formation of nicotinic acid from tryptophan will be considerably reduced. It is under these conditions that the minor products of the pathway, kynurenic and xanthurenic acids, and their dehydroxylated derivatives, quinaldic and 8-hydroxyquinaldic acids, are formed by ring closure of kynurenine and hydroxykynurenine. They accumulate in the blood and urine because the normal onward pathway of kynurenine metabolism is blocked by the lack of pyridoxal-P. In experimental animals and human volunteers given large oral doses of tryptophan, these minor products are found in the urine because the capacity of kynureninase is exceeded by the large amount of tryptophan being catabolized by the pyrrolase pathway. The same effect is also observed when hydrocortisone and oestrogens are taken, and it has been demonstrated that if additional vitamin B_6 is given to patients receiving oral contraceptive steroids and other oestrogen preparations, these minor products are not found in the urine and a more normal pattern of tryptophan metabolites is maintained. In pellagra, there is no excess NADPH to inhibit tryptophan pyrrolase, so tryptophan enters the pathway in a virtually uncontrolled manner. This exaggerates any vitamin B_6 deficiency which may well be present together with the deficiency of dietary nicotinic acid, and leads to a considerable increase in the amounts of the minor products of the pathway excreted. If anything, this reduces the amount of tryptophan being converted to nicotinic acid still further.

The onward metabolism of 3-hydroxyanthranilic acid is shown in Figure 6.16. A ferro-protein oxygenase, hydroxyanthranilic acid oxygenase, opens the ring, forming acroleyl-3-aminofumarate. This recyclizes spontaneously to quinolinic acid, which is converted to quinolinic acid ribonucleotide by the action

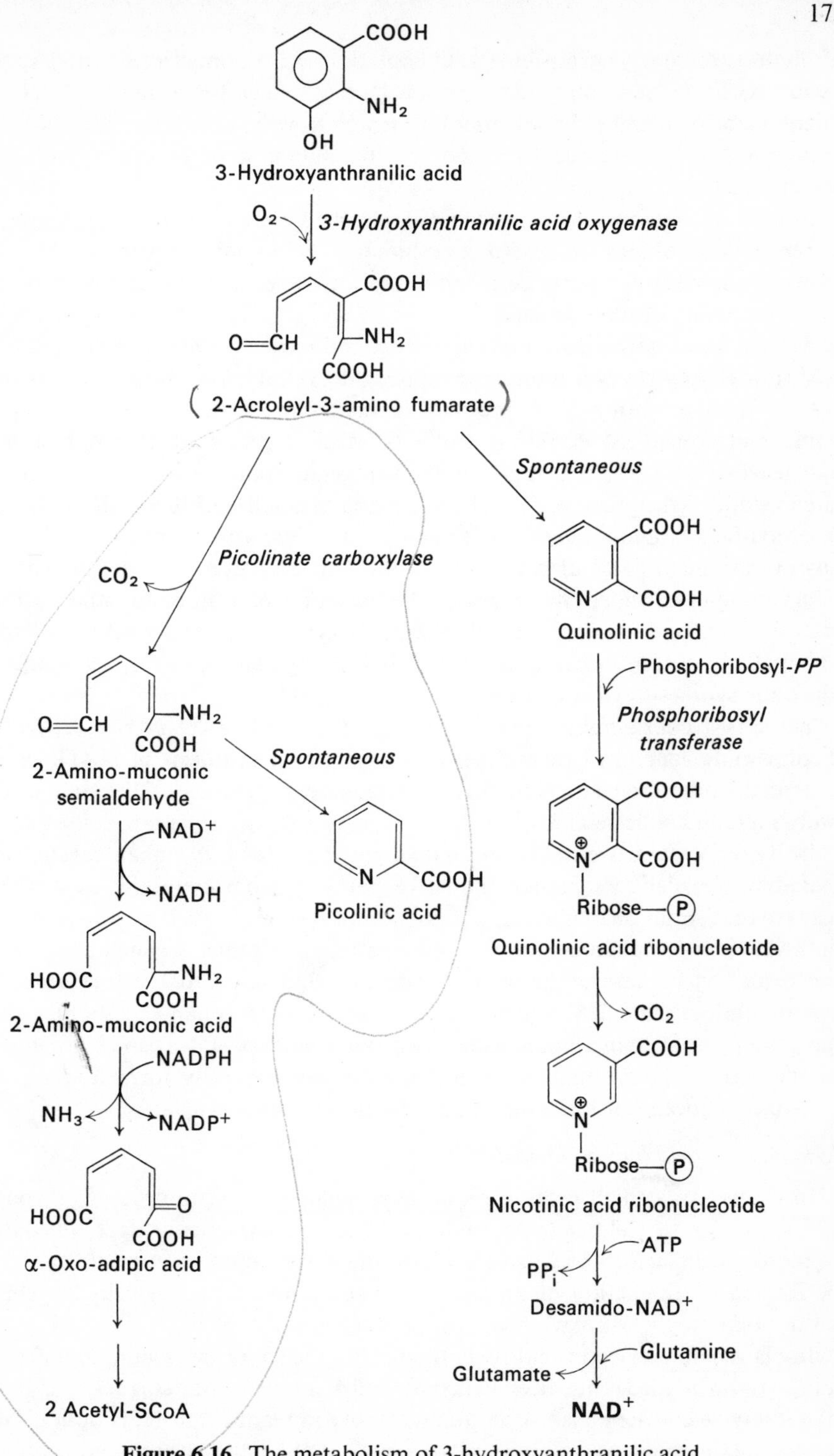

Figure 6.16. The metabolism of 3-hydroxyanthranilic acid

of a phosphoribosyl transferase. Quinolinic acid ribonucleotide undergoes decarboxylation to nicotinic acid ribonucleotide, which forms desamido-NAD (nicotinic acid–adenine dinucleotide) by reaction with ATP. The nicotinic acid moiety is finally amidated by reaction with glutamine in an ATP-dependent amidotransferase reaction.

As well as metabolism to yield NAD, acroleyl aminofumarate can undergo an enzymic decarboxylation to 2-aminomuconic-6-semialdehyde, which can either spontaneously cyclize to picolinic acid, another minor excretion product of tryptophan, or be oxidized to aminomuconic acid. Aminomuconic acid undergoes an oxidative deamination to α-oxo-adipic acid, which can be metabolized further to yield two molecules of acetyl-SCoA. Hence, there is a pathway for the total oxidation of tryptophan in mammals, so that despite the large number of specialized excretion products which it generates, tryptophan can, like leucine, be classified as a wholly ketogenic amino acid. Under normal circumstances, the greatest part of tryptophan catabolized follows this pathway to acetyl-SCoA. Only a very small proportion of daily tryptophan metabolism gives rise to identifiable urinary metabolites. However, even a moderate loading of tryptophan considerably increases the excretion of kynurenine and various intermediates and side-products of the pathway. It is generally estimated that about 60 mg of tryptophan must be metabolized by man and other mammals to allow the synthesis of 1 mg of NAD.

There is a considerable amount of degradation of NAD *in vivo*, releasing nicotinamide which can then either be reutilized for synthesis of NAD, or be degraded, and excreted as *N*-methyl nicotinamide, depending on the state of the body's nicotinamide reserves.

In bacteria, there are many alternative pathways for tryptophan catabolism, including a widely distributed oxidative pathway from kynurenic acid which leads to the formation of glutamate, alanine and acetate. There is also an aromatic pathway of tryptophan catabolism in some micro-organisms which starts with the oxidation of anthranilic acid to catechol, and leads to the formation of acetate and succinate. Many of the more exotic tryptophan metabolites that have been identified in human urine in various abnormal states can be attributed to the action of intestinal bacteria; they are not generally formed when the intestine has been sterilized with an antibiotic such as neomycin.

Indole-acetic acid (auxin) formation

In mammals, a small proportion of tryptophan catabolism proceeds through aminotransfer to yield indolepyruvic acid. This is oxidatively decarboxylated to indole-acetic acid, which is excreted in the urine. Indole-acetic acid can also be formed by the action of monoamine oxidase and aldehyde dehydrogenase on tryptamine, the α-decarboxylation product of tryptophan.

In plants, indole-acetic acid is synthesized in the shoot tip region, and acts as a growth hormone; it has been called auxin. A number of analogues, including naphtholyl acetic acid, also show auxin activity in plants. Since it is biologically active, auxin must be catabolized in plants, unlike the situation in animals where it is an excretory product without any known biological activity. The pathways of auxin synthesis available to plants are shown in Figure 6.17. Little is known of its catabolism, but the main degradation product appears to be indole acetaldehyde, formed by oxidation catalysed by indole-acetic acid oxidase. There are also several biologically inactive conjugates of auxin in plants, which may represent either inactivation products, or storage forms of the hormone. There is some evidence that much of the catabolism of auxin may be by photo-oxidation.

Auxin migrates from the region where it is synthesized to other regions of the plant, where it functions to stimulate growth. Thus, when a plant is subjected to unilateral illumination, it grows towards the source of light because more auxin is formed on the dark side, stimulating growth to a greater extent than on the illuminated side of the stem. Auxin will also stimulate the development of

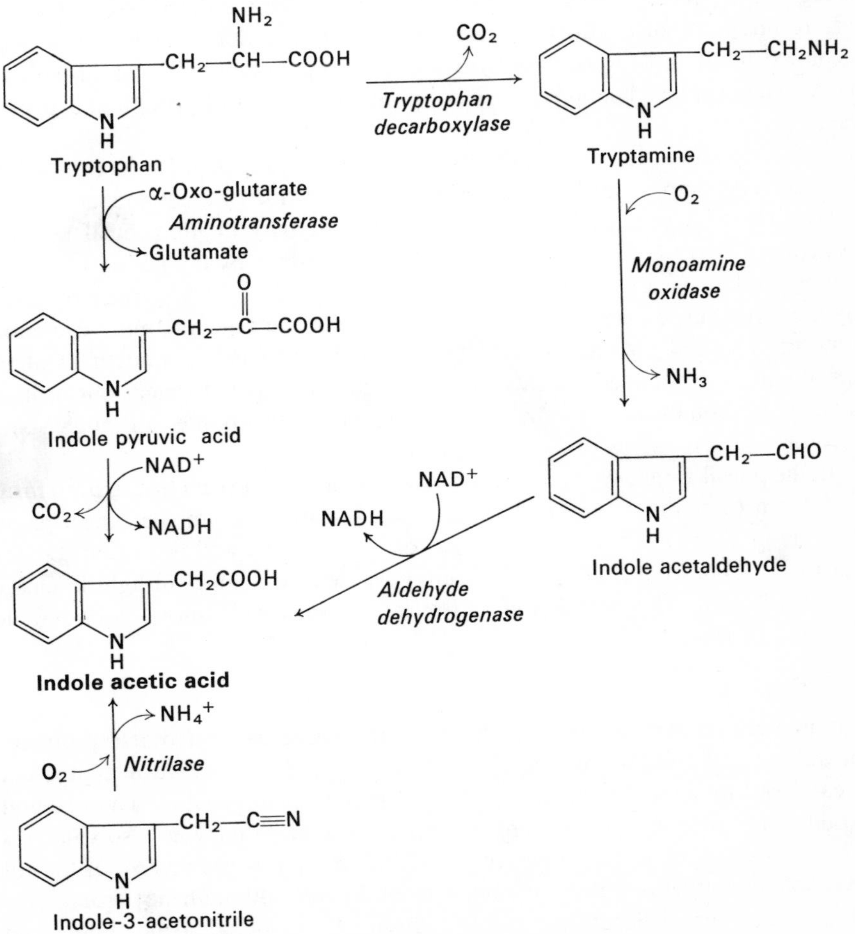

Figure 6.17. Indole-acetic acid (auxin) biosynthesis

roots from stem tissue, and preparations of indole and naphtholyl acetic acids are widely used to aid the rooting of cuttings of plants.

Serotonin (5-hydroxytryptamine)

Serotonin formation is of considerable physiological significance, although only of minor importance as a pathway of tryptophan catabolism.

Tryptophan is hydroxylated to 5-hydroxytryptophan by a specific hydroxylase which appears to be very similar to phenylalanine and tyrosine hydroxylases. Hydroxytryptophan is decarboxylated to serotonin by the same pyridoxal-P-dependent enzyme as acts on DOPA to yield dopamine.

In the brain, serotonin has a neurotransmitter role, as discussed on page 185. It is also important in the gastro-intestinal tract for the maintenance of normal gut motility. Carcinoid tumours of the gut produce large amounts of hydroxy-tryptophan and serotonin, which they release into the blood-stream. It is the serotonin produced which is primarily responsible for the diarrhoea and severe gastro-intestinal discomfort in carcinoid syndrome. Some success has been achieved in attempts to control hydroxyindole production in carcinoid patients using p-chlorophenylalanine, which is a potent inhibitor of tryptophan hydroxy-lase.

Serotonin formation and degradation are shown in Figure 6.18. Its catabolism is relatively simple, since although a number of methylated and acetylated derivatives with considerable pharmacological activity in the central nervous system are formed, the main pathway of metabolism is by the action of mono-amine oxidase yielding 5-hydroxyindole-acetaldehyde, which is then oxidized by aldehyde dehydrogenase to 5-hydroxyindole-acetic acid, the main excretion product. Especially when monoamine oxidase is inhibited, a number of other metabolites are excreted. In rats, serotonin glucuronide is formed, but in man there is no conjugation of the amine to form a glucuronide, although some serotonin-O-sulphate is formed and excreted.

In the pineal gland, serotonin is N-acetylated, and then O-methylated, to form melatonin (5-methoxy-N-acetyl-tryptamine). Melatonin from the pineal gland appears to have an effect on the female gonads, and may well be responsible for seasonal and diurnal rhythms which are governed by changes in light intensity and day length. The production and release of melatonin shows considerable diurnal variation.

Tryptophanase

A number of bacteria are capable of forming free indole from tryptophan, including $E.$ $coli$ and several other $Enterobacteriaciae$. This cleavage of tryptophan is catalysed by tryptophanase, a pyridoxal-P-dependent enzyme. The reaction products are indole, pyruvate and ammonia. The same enzyme also catalyses the deamination of serine, suggesting that the reaction is the reverse of that of tryptophan synthetase. Tryptophanase from $E.$ $coli$, although not from some other organisms, will catalyse the formation of tryptophan from indole and serine.

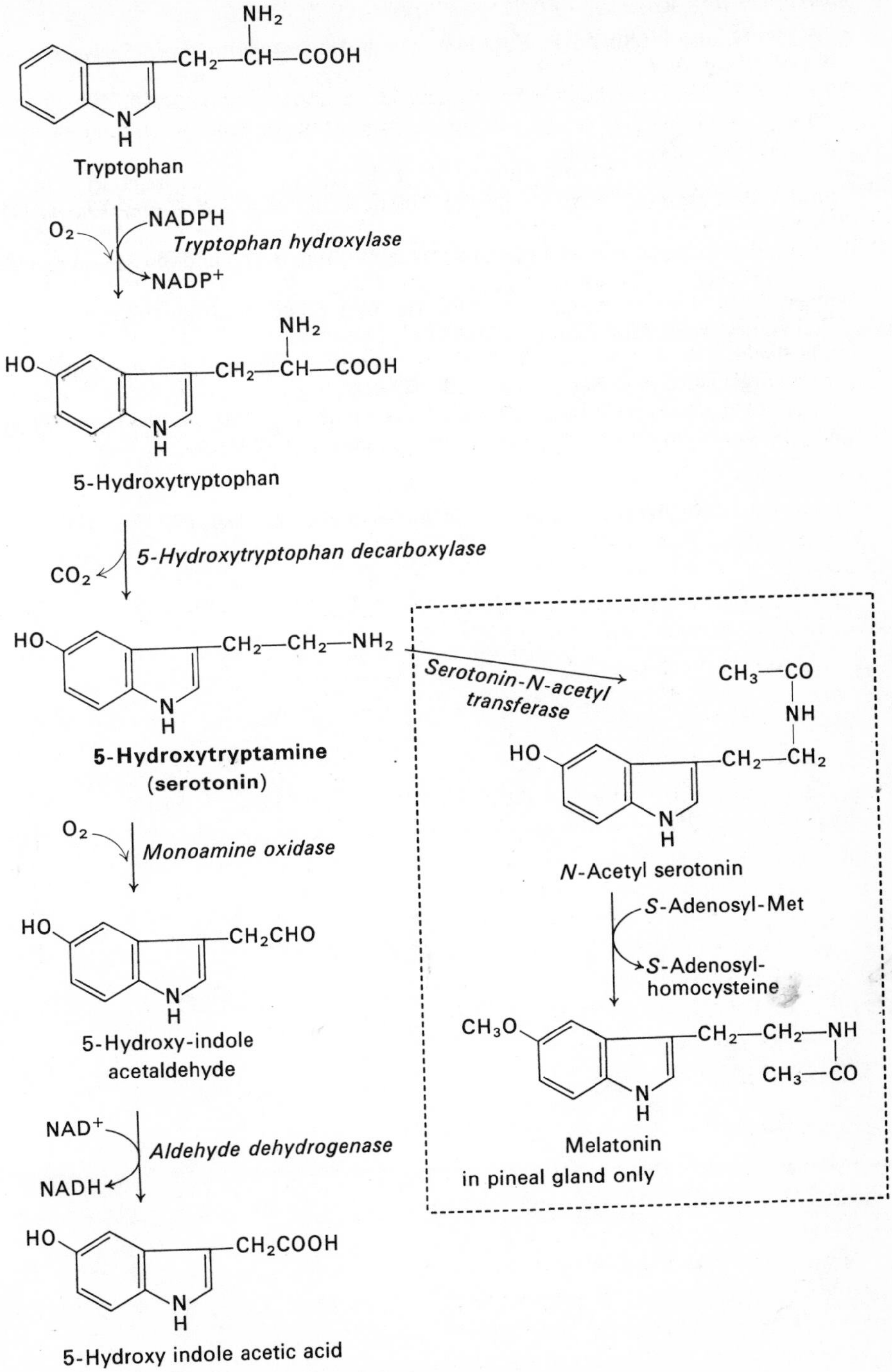

Figure 6.18. The metabolism of serotonin

Further reading

Ames, B. N. and Hartman, P. E. (1963). The histidine operon. *Cold Spring Harbor Symp. Quant. Biol.*, **28**, 349–356.

Gorkin, V. Z. (1966). Monoamine oxidases. *Pharmacol. Rev.*, **18**, 115–120.

Kaufman, S. (1971). The phenylalanine hydroxylating system of mammalian liver. *Adv. Enzymol.*, **35**, 245–320.

Pabst, M. J., Kuhn, J. C. and Somerville, R. L. (1973). Feedback regulation in the anthranilate aggregate of wild-type and mutant strains of *E. coli. J. Biol. Chem.*, **248**, 901–914.

Rose, D. P. (1972). Aspects of tryptophan metabolism in health and disease—a review. *J. Clin. Pathol.*, **25**, 17–25.

Sandler, M. and Ruthven, C. R. (1969). The biosynthesis and metabolism of catecholamines. *Prog. Med. Chem.*, **6**, 200–265.

Truffa-Bachi, P. and Cohen, G. N. (1968). Some aspects of amino acid biosynthesis in micro-organisms. *Ann. Rev. Biochem.*, **37**, 79–108.

Symposium proceedings. (1971.) Biochemistry and pathology of tryptophan metabolism and its regulation by amino acids, vitamin B_6 and steroid hormones. *Amer. J. Clin. Nutr.*, **24**, 655–851.

References cited in the text are listed in the bibliography

CHAPTER 7

AMINO ACIDS IN THE CENTRAL NERVOUS SYSTEM

A number of amino acids have specific roles in the maintenance of normal brain function in animals, and defects in amino-acid metabolism have been associated with a number of psychiatric disturbances in man.

The main specific role of amino acids and derivatives in the central nervous system is as chemical transmitters at synapses. Neuronal transmission is electrical, associated with transient changes in membrane polarization, but between neurons in the central nervous system, and at the junctions between nerves and muscles in the peripheral motor system, there is no electrical conduction. The nerve impulse is carried from one neuron to another by a chemical transmitter, which is synthesized in the presynaptic neuron, and stored in membrane-enclosed vesicles. When there is electrical stimulation of this neuron, the stored transmitter is released into the synaptic cleft. Post-synaptically it interacts with a receptor on the membrane, causing stimulation of electrical transmission in this post-synaptic neuron.

After crossing the synaptic cleft, and activating the post-synaptic neuron, the transmitter can either be taken up by the post-synaptic neuron (or by an adjacent glial cell) and there be catabolized to an inactive form, or can be taken up by the presynaptic neuron, where it is stored in vesicles until required for transmission later. Thus, some of the chemical transmitter can be re-utilized by this pre-synaptic re-uptake mechanism. Post-synaptic catabolism varies according to the chemical transmitter involved. Serotonin and the catecholamines (dopamine and nor-adrenaline) are generally degraded by amine oxidase and methyl transferase action to terminal metabolites, which are then excreted, initially into the cerebro-spinal fluid, and ultimately in the urine. Histamine is similarly degraded to a terminal metabolite. γ-Amino butyrate is catabolized, as noted on page 90, by way of citrate cycle intermediates, and acetylcholine is catabolized by ester hydrolysis to yield acetate, which can be metabolized by common metabolic pathways, and choline which can then be taken up by the presynaptic neuron, and used for further transmitter synthesis. This process of chemical transmission at a synapse is shown diagrammatically in Figure 7.1.

Before a compound can be classified as a neurotransmitter, a number of criteria must be satisfied:

(a) The putative transmitter must be shown to be both synthesized and in-activated or catabolized in the central nervous system, and the rates of synthesis and degradation must be comparable. Much of the evidence for a neurotrans-mitter role for histamine is based on the observation that in the brain the rate of

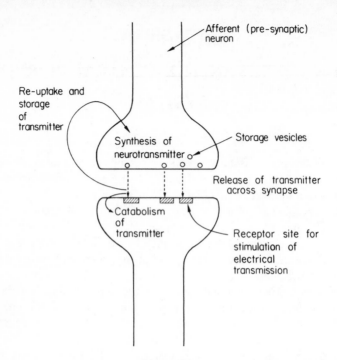

Figure 7.1.
Chemical transmission in the central nervous system

histidine decarboxylation to histamine, and the rate of histamine oxidation (and other catabolic pathways, as shown on page 152) are approximately equal. This contrasts sharply with the situation in other tissues, where there are widely disparate rates of histamine formation and inactivation. This would be expected since in general, histamine acts on a target tissue distant from the mast cell in which it is synthesized and stored, and therefore catabolic mechanisms would not be expected in association with the synthetic system, but only in the target cells. For the catecholamines and serotonin, the rates of synthesis and catabolism in the brain are also very similar, and it was noted on page 90 that γ-amino butyric acid occurs as an intermediate in a pathway which is an important alternative to the citrate cycle in central nervous system energy-yielding metabolism.

(b) The compound must be shown to be located in specific tracts of neurons, rather than distributed diffusely throughout the brain. For dopamine, noradrenaline and serotonin, this has been established by use of fluorescence microscopy. All three amines show characteristic fluorescence in brain sections which have been treated with formaldehyde vapour, and a great many dopaminergic noradrenergic and serotoninergic neuronal pathways have been mapped using this technique. It has been demonstrated that in response to administration of compounds known to inhibit formation of the amines, there is a loss of the amine fluorescence in the neurons in which it is normally seen. Similarly, loss of amine fluorescence has also been observed after surgical transection of neurons. Hence, there is considerable evidence for the role of these three amines as specific neuro-transmitters in the central nervous system.

For other compounds that have been ascribed neurotransmitter function, such localization is less easy, since there are no comparable precise and specific histochemical localization techniques. Some degree of mapping has been achieved by autoradiography following administration of radioactive precursors, but the resolution of autoradiography is not very fine. A further draw-back to such work is that the amino acid precursors are incorporated into proteins throughout the brain, and this confuses the picture considerably.

(c) Application of the putative neurotransmitter to specific groups of neurons (by micro-iontophoretic techniques) should lead to specific initiation or inhibition of neuronal transmission. Evidence of this type has suggested that γ-amino butyric acid, glutamate and glycine are all inhibitory neurotransmitters, func-tioning to inhibit the firing of neurons which would otherwise occur. Such an effect must not be general, but should only occur when the material is applied to specific groups of neurons, i.e. those believed to use the test material as their natural chemical transmitter.

(d) It is generally believed that the pre-synaptic neuron can take up transmitter that has been released, and store it in vesicles together with newly synthesized material. There must therefore be an active uptake mechanism of some kind in the neuronal membrane. Such an amine pump mechanism has been identified for serotonin and the catecholamines, and has been interpreted as further evidence of a neurotransmitter role for these compounds. The clinically-used tricyclic antidepressant drugs, such as imipramine, have been shown to activate these amine pump mechanisms *in vitro*, and it is assumed that they act in the same way *in vivo*. This activation of transmitter re-uptake is possibly the basis of the therapeutic action of these drugs. By activating the re-uptake mechanism, they increase the amount of the transmitter amines available for use, and, as noted below, it is believed that many forms of psychological depression are associated with a deficiency of serotonin or catecholamines.

(e) Specific transmitter-binding proteins must exist in the membrane of the post-synaptic neuron to allow recognition of, and activation by, the amine released by the presynaptic neuron. Such a binding protein has been isolated and partially characterized for serotonin, from the synaptosome fraction of whole brain homogenates. (The synaptosome fraction is generally assumed to represent nerve terminals which are pinched off as discrete membrane-enclosed vesicles when brain tissue is homogenized in isotonic media). Isolation of a specific binding protein, not associated with any of the enzymes known to bind serotonin, is further evidence for its role in chemical transmission at central synapses.

Uptake of amino acids into the brain

Lipid soluble materials can permeate freely into the brain, but the brain membranes form an effective barrier for hydrophilic materials. Therefore all uptake of amino acids into the brain is subject to close regulation by the blood-brain membrane barrier. A number of distinct amino acid carrier mechanisms have been postulated for the brain. As noted on page 106, there is good evidence that the γ-glutamyl cycle, demonstrated in the kidney, may also function in transporting amino acids across the choroid plexus of the brain. If this is so, it is necessary to postulate at least four separate γ-glutamyl transpeptidases, specific for the four groups of amino acids that have been shown to be mutually competitive for transport into the brain. These four groups are: (a) the neutral amino acids (the largest group, consisting of most of those amino acids which have uncharged side chains); (b) the acidic amino acids (glutamate and aspartate) (c) the basic amino acids (including lysine, ornithine, arginine, and possibly also cystine and cysteine); and (d) the two amino acids that do not appear to be substrates for the transpeptidase, namely proline and glycine.

The seeds of *Lathyrus sativus* contain a specific neurotoxin, β-*N*-oxalyl-α,β-diaminopropionate, which causes a paralytic disease, neurolathyrism. It acts by specifically inhibiting the uptake of glutamate and aspartate into cells, and thus inhibits brain protein synthesis. It has no effect on the incorporation of glutamate or aspartate into protein in cell-free systems, nor on their activation to amino acyl-tRNA once they have entered the cell.

As noted on page 164, the specific neurotoxic metabolite in phenylketonuria has not been identified. It has been suggested that the brain damage in this disease is caused in the same way as in neurolathyrism, i.e. a very high circulating level of phenylalanine inhibits the uptake into the brain of other amino acids. Hence the severe mental retardation observed in untreated phenylketonuriacs may be due to defective protein synthesis during the critical post-natal brain growth spurt, rather than to the presence of an endogenously-produced neurotoxic material.

In animal studies of drug-induced phenylketonuria-like conditions, the incorporation into brain protein of radioactive neutral amino acids administered systematically is impaired, although this is not so if the radioactive amino acid is administered by direct injection into the lateral ventricle of the brain. The latter method of administration bypasses the blood–brain barrier, and therefore overcomes any inhibition of uptake caused by the high blood concentration of phenylalanine in these animals. When amino acids which are transported on a carrier distinct from that for phenylalanine are used, there is no difference between the rate of incorporation into brain protein of intraventricularly or systemically administered radioactive amino acid.

Synthesis of the catecholamines and serotonin appears to be regulated at the first step, which is the hydroxylation of the dietary amino acid to the immediate precursor of the active amine. For serotonin synthesis, it is now fairly well established that not only is tryptophan hydroxylase the rate-limiting step of the pathway, but it is controlled by the availability of tryptophan in the central nervous system. The K_m of tryptophan hydroxylase is approximately equal to the normal intracerebral concentration of tryptophan, so that any increase in brain tryptophan will lead to enhanced hydroxylation. Since it is also known that there is a considerable excess of 5-hydroxytryptophan decarboxylase activity compared with the hydroxylase, this means that an increase in the brain tryptophan concentration will lead directly to an increase in brain serotonin formation. It has been shown that a great many drugs which are known to increase the brain serotonin concentration do so by increasing the concentration of tryptophan in the central nervous system. The only exception that has been noted to date is the class of drugs that inhibit monoamine oxidase. These drugs increase the brain concentration of serotonin and other amines by reducing oxidative catabolism, not by enhancing synthesis. Thus, the rate of brain synthesis of serotonin is regulated by the access of tryptophan into the brain.

Tryptophan is unique among amino acids in that it is transported in the blood bound to serum albumin. Under normal circumstances, about 90% of the 9–16 mg/l of tryptophan in blood is bound to albumin, and only about 10% is freely diffusible. Any factor that disturbs the equilibrium of tryptophan binding would be expected to affect its uptake into the brain (and other tissues), by increasing the amount of tryptophan that is freely diffusible. Two factors which have been shown to compete with tryptophan for albumin binding are salicylates and non-esterified fatty acids. Following either salicylate (for example aspirin) ingestion, or elevation of serum non-esterified fatty acid, the brain concentrations of tryptophan and serotonin are increased considerably, although the total serum tryptophan concentration is not increased, and indeed may even be less than normal.

There is some evidence in the literature that the region in the ventro-medial hypothalamus that regulates appetite (the so-called satiety centre) may well be serotoninergic. On refeeding a fasted animal, there is an increase in total serum tryptophan, which occurs at the same time as the serum non-esterified fatty acid is elevated from fasting. Therefore, the diffusible serum tryptophan concentration is considerably higher than normal. Much of this tryptophan comes from the pancreas, where it accumulates during overnight fasting. The tryptophan appears to be mainly in the β-cells of the Islets of Langerhans, and may be associated with insulin. Drug-induced diabetes, caused by β-cell destruction by alloxan or strepto-zotocin, leads to abolition of this tryptophan accumulation on fasting; moreover, the release after refeeding occurs at the same time as insulin release. It is possible that tryptophan release from the pancreas acts as a signal to the hypothalamic satiety centre, where it acts as the immediate precursor of the neurotransmitter, serotonin.

The concentration of tyrosine in the brain is considerably higher than the K_m of tyrosine hydroxylase, so it appears unlikely that catecholamine synthesis is regulated in the same way as is serotonin synthesis, i.e. by availability of the precursor amino acid. Brain phenylalanine and tyrosine hydroxylases are inhibited in vitro by catecholamine accumulation, so it is prob-able that this pathway is regulated by a conventional feed-back mechanism.

The function of the biogenic amines in the brain

The term 'biogenic amines' is generally used to cover dopamine, noradrenaline and serotonin, which, as was shown in Chapter 6, are synthesized and catabolized by parallel pathways. Although dopamine is the immediate precursor of noradrenaline, it has a neurotransmitter function in its own right, and there is good evidence in the literature that there are two separate pools of brain dopamine, one associated with the formation of noradrenaline, and the other concerned with dopaminergic transmission.

Work by Jouvet and coworkers (summarized in a review by Jouvet, 1969) has indicated that the sleep-inducing system of the mammalian brain is located in the serotoninergic neurons of the midline raphe system of the brain stem. Selective destruction of the raphe system of cats, by electrical coagulation, leads to severe and permanent insomnia. The degree of insomnia, loss of brain serotonin and the degree of destruction of the raphe system (assessed histologically *post mortem*) are all significantly correlated. Administration of chloromethamphetamine, which is a central serotonin depletor, or *p*-chlorophenylalanine, which inhibits serotonin synthesis by inhibition of tryptophan hydroxylase, leads to insomnia in experimental animals. The duration of such drug-induced insomnia is proportional to the dose of the drug given, and *p*-chlorophenylalanine-induced insomnia can be specifically reversed by administration of 5-hydroxytryptophan, the immediate precursor of serotonin.

Monoamine oxidase inhibiting drugs suppress specifically that phase of sleep known as paradoxical or rapid eye movement sleep, during which dreaming is believed to occur. It has therefore been suggested that the transition from slow-wave sleep (characterized by a slow wave pattern on electro-encephalogram) to paradoxical sleep requires the oxidative degradation of monoamines. Electrical coagulation of parts of the *locus coeruleus*, the major monoamine oxidase containing region of the brain, has resulted in experimental animals which are capable of slow-wave sleep, but not of paradoxical sleep.

Arousal reactions have been shown to be mediated by the noradrenergic neurons of the reticular formation of the mid-brain. Electrical coagulation of this very diffuse neuronal network has not been successful, but chemical destruction has shown that animals in which the reticular formation has been largely destroyed are incapable of normal arousal.

In Parkinson's disease there is a massive cellular necrosis in the *substantia nigra* of the brain, the region that contains most of the brain dopamine not associated with noradrenaline formation. Parkinsonism is characterized by rigidity of the limbs, tremor, and an inability to initiate voluntary movement. As well as the idiopathic form of the disease (for which no aetiological factor can be identified), there are two forms that are clinically indistinguishable, one arising from chronic manganese poisoning, which was first identified among manganese miners in South America; and the other, a post-encephalitic form, associated with patients now in late middle age, who suffered from encephalitis in their youth.

Electrical coagulation of the *substantia nigra* of experimental animals gives rise to a loss of ability to initiate voluntary movement of the type seen in Parkinsonism in human beings. The other two signs, the rigidity of the limbs, and the tremor, are believed to be 'negative signs', due to over-activity of neuronal tracts because of a failure of normal regulatory mechanisms. If this is so, it suggests that dopamine, as well as being a stimulatory neurotransmitter in the *substantia nigra*, may also function as an inhibitory transmitter, preventing or modulating the firing of neurons under other chemical stimuli.

Together with neuronal degeneration in Parkinsonism, there is a considerable loss of brain dopamine, as would be expected; the loss of dopamine appears to occur before the neuronal degeneration. In a series of patients who died with hemiplegic Parkinsonism (disability of one side of the body only) *post mortem* examination showed that the level of dopamine on one side of the brain was considerably below normal, while the level on the other side, corresponding to the unaffected side of the body, was almost normal. This can be taken as further evidence for the involvement of dopamine in the disease.

Because of this, attempts have been made to raise the brain dopamine level in Parkinsonian patients by administration of DOPA (3,4-dihydroxyphenylalanine, the immediate precursor of the transmitter amine). Dopamine itself cannot be administered peripherally to raise the brain level, since it does not cross the blood–brain barrier. The use of DOPA in this way has been dramatically successful in many patients, leading to rapid remission of symptoms, and the clinical improvement has been shown to persist for a considerable time. However, the dose of DOPA necessary is very high, as much as 10–12 g/day in some cases. This is because there is a considerable amount of DOPA decarboxylase in many peripheral tissues, including the liver, kidneys and lungs. Many patients are unable to tolerate such high doses because of serious side effects including nausea, involuntary movements, and in some cases serious psychiatric disturbances. A more recent development in treatment has been the use of specific inhibitors of DOPA decarboxylase which do not penetrate the blood–brain barrier, and therefore act only on the peripheral enzyme. Using such inhibitors, it is possible to reduce the dose of DOPA very considerably, since very much more is available for uptake into the brain, with a much lower incidence of side effects.

The role of amines in the sleep system, and in neurological disorders has been clearly established partly using animal models, and partly because the clinical state of Parkinsonism is well defined. Attempts to implicate amines in psychiatric disturbances suffer from the problems of psychiatry, and the necessarily subjective nature of psychiatric diagnosis and classification of diseases. A further problem is that there are few animal models of psychiatric disturbances. Most investigations have therefore relied on measurement of amines and their metabolites in blood and urine, a procedure that is obviously not very satisfactory, since the brain metabolism of amines is only a very small part of their whole body metabolism. There have been a few studies on amines in cerebro-spinal fluid, which is a closer reflection of brain metabolism, but even this is not ideal, and it is not easy to obtain samples of cerebro-spinal fluid by lumbar puncture from any patient, and even less from one who is psychiatrically disturbed.

There is a considerable amount of evidence, mainly circumstantial, that abnormalities of central amine metabolism may be involved in the aetiology of some psychiatric disorders. Drugs such as reserpine, which deplete the brain biogenic amines, lead to sedation and the development of a depressive state. A similar effect is noted with many drugs which inhibit amine synthesis. The two most widely used classes of anti-depressant drugs are the tricyclic compounds such as imipramine, and the monoamine oxidase inhibitors. Both classes of compound increase the availability of amines in presynaptic neurons. The tricyclic compounds, as noted above, act by enhancing the activity of the membrane amine uptake mechanisms, so conserving more of the amine after its release for transmission. The monoamine oxidase inhibitors act by reducing the post-synaptic oxidative catabolism of the amines, so leaving more for the presynaptic re-uptake mechanism.

In general, because of the dangers of monoamine oxidase inhibitors, tricyclic compounds are tried first, although there is no way, as yet, of telling which class of compound will be effective for any one patient. As well as its role in the central nervous system in the catabolism of neurotransmitters, monoamine oxidase is present in liver and other mitochondria, where it acts to oxidize not only endogenously-formed monoamines, but also those taken in the diet. Therefore, any patient taking monoamine oxidase inhibitors must avoid foods known to be rich in the pharmacologically active monoamines, especially tyramine and tryptamine. Such foods include cheese, many fermented and pickled products, and yeast extract.

There have been a number of attempts to decide whether the primary amine deficiency in psychological depression is one of serotonin or catecholamines. *Post mortem* studies of patients who committed suicide while depressed have shown, in some cases, that the brain level of 5-hydroxy-indole-acetic acid was considerably lower than in control subjects (for example, road accident victims). This was interpreted as indicating a reduced level or turnover of serotonin. It has also been shown that some depressed patients have a reduced ability to decarboxylate 5-hydroxytryptophan while depressed, and this returns to normal on recovery. Premenstrual depression, and depression in women taking oral contraceptive steroids, have been attributed to increased tryptophan catabolism by the kynurenine pathway in the liver, thus reducing the amount of tryptophan available for serotonin synthesis in the brain, and also reducing the availability of pyridoxal-*P* because of the increased need for this cofactor in the kynurenine pathway (see page 174).

A number of reports have suggested that in some depressed patients, administration of relatively large amounts of tryptophan, together with monoamine oxidase inhibitors, has a considerably faster and greater effect than the monoamine oxidase inhibitors alone. However, other workers have shown similar effects of DOPA therapy, thus implicating catecholamine deficiency rather than serotonin deficiency.

It is possible that catecholamine and serotonin deficiency represent two different classes of psychological depression, but there is little evidence of this, and classification of depression is by no means uniform from one psychiatric team to another. An alternative hypothesis has been proposed, which suggests that either amine in reduced amount can lead to a similar clinical picture. The basis of this hypothesis is that an imbalance between the dopaminergic and serotoninergic systems is the determinant factor, and hyperactivity of one system would be as harmful as underactivity of the other.

Some evidence for this viewpoint was obtained by a series of experiments by Wada and coworkers (1963). They used alteration in the response of trained animals to an unpleasant stimulus as an index of behavioural modification. They showed that drugs which either increased brain serotonin or reduced catecholamines led to a similar state, in which the response was considerably impaired. Conversely, treatments which either decreased brain serotonin or increased the level of catecholamines led to an improvement in the conditioned behaviour, and generally made the animals more alert.

It has been shown that administration of DOPA, as a precursor of the catecholamines, not only leads to the expected increase in catecholamine levels, but also to a reduction in cerebral serotonin. This has been attributed to competition for decarboxylation by the adventitious hydroxyamino acid, which is normally only formed in catecholaminergic neurons, and therefore cannot compete with hydroxytryptophan. Administration of hydroxytryptophan as a serotonin precursor similarly decreases brain catecholamines, but administration of tryptophan, which must be hydroxylated by a specific hydroxylase, does not, although it does lead to an increase in serotonin.

There have been many attempts to identify a biochemical abnormality in the schizophrenic diseases. None to date has stood the test of time, possibly at least partly because of the diffuse nature of the schizophrenias, and the extreme difficulty of reaching any agreement on diagnosis. A number of hallucinogenic drugs induce a schizophreniform state, and many of these bear a structural resemblance to biogenic amines. It was therefore considered that schizophrenia may be the result of endogenous production of a hallucinogen. However, the psychoses induced by mescaline, lysergic acid derivatives, dimethyltryptamine and other hallucinogens are all clinically distinguishable from schizophrenia, and these drugs are no longer regarded as providing a useful model of the clinical disease.

Pollin and coworkers (1961) showed that administration of methionine or tryptophan to some schizophrenics, together with monoamine oxidase inhibitors, led to a considerable worsening of their clinical state, followed by a rebound period, during which they were somewhat improved. It was suggested that the action of methionine was to enhance an abnormal methylation of one of the brain amines, thus leading to synthesis of a hallucinogenic compound. However, neither glycine nor serine, both important donors to the one-carbon pool for methyl transfer, had any effect on these patients. Furthermore, there is little evidence of the occurrence of any abnormally methylated compound in schizophrenics.

Friedhoff and van Winkel (1962) believed that they had isolated such a compound from schizophrenic urine when they discovered a substance which showed up as a pink spot after multiple staining on paper chromatography. 'Pink spot' was subsequently identified by one group of workers as dimethoxyphenylethylamine, although others have claimed that it is p-tyramine, the decarboxylation product of tyrosine. Subsequently, it was shown that 'pink spot' is also present in the urine of normal subjects, although in lesser amount than in chronically hospitalized schizophrenics. Few workers in the field now believe that it has any connection with schizophrenia; it is probably the result of intestinal bacterial action. The greater amounts in hospitalized patients have been attributed to chronic constipation, which is frequently encountered in psychiatric hospitals.

The exacerbation of schizophrenic symptoms on administration of tryptophan is of interest in view of a report by Bender and Bamji (1974) that serum tryptophan in a small group of hospitalized schizophrenics was abnormally low. This was accompanied by a reduction in the albumin binding of the amino acid, so that any administered tryptophan would presumably be more readily and immediately available for uptake into the brain.

Coppen and coworkers (1973) have shown that in a small group of depressed patients, although the total serum tryptophan concentration was normal, the percentage bound to albumin was increased, thus presumably reducing the tryptophan readily available for uptake into the brain. In recovered depressive patients the albumin binding of tryptophan was normal.

It is therefore possible that control of synthesis of serotonin by variation in the binding of tryptophan to serum albumin may be important in the aetiology of some psychiatric disorders.

γ-Aminobutyric acid (GABA)

The formation of GABA by decarboxylation of glutamate was discussed on page 91, where it was noted that all the available evidence suggests that in brain the pathway of GABA formation is not a minor shunt pathway alternative to α-oxo-glutarate decarboxylation, but the major route of citrate metabolism. There does not appear as yet to have been any investigation of the possibility of GABA formation from arginine (by the γ-guanidobutyramide pathway) in the mammalian central nervous system. GABA was first identified as a neurotransmitter in the peripheral nervous system of invertebrates. In mammals, it is not found in the peripheral system at all, but is present in relatively large amounts in the diencephalon and corpora quadrigemina of the brain.

GABA is generally an inhibitory transmitter; that is, release of GABA inhibits the firing of a neuron under the influence of another transmitter. It is generally assumed that there are two afferent neurons into a synapse at which GABA is involved, one producing the stimulatory transmitter, and the other producing GABA to modulate the response. The importance of this inhibitory transmission is shown in avitaminosis B_6, or in the presence of specific antimetabolites, when animals convulse spontaneously because of the absence of GABA.

Glutamate decarboxylase, the enzyme responsible for the production of GABA from glutamate, has a low affinity for pyridoxal-P, and it has been observed that in avitaminosis B_6 there is a considerable increase in the production of the apoenzyme in the brain, presumably as a mechanism to chelate as much as possible of the available cofactor. This contrasts with DOPA decarboxylase, which is almost unaffected by avitaminosis B_6; this enzyme has a very high affinity for pyridoxal-*P*, and therefore would be expected to be fully saturated with cofactor even under conditions of severe deficiency.

Other compounds

The evidence that dopamine, noradrenaline and serotonin have roles in chemical transmission in the central nervous system is extremely strong, as is that implicating acetylcholine. GABA is also almost certainly a neural transmitter, although the evidence for this is not as good as that for the others. A great many other amino acids and derivatives have also been proposed as neurotransmitters, including glutamate, aspartate, glycine and taurine [formed from cysteine by *S*-oxidation and decarboxylation (see page 131)]. However, there is relatively little evidence as yet for the participation of these compounds in brain function, and their role must be considered unproven.

A number of amines, including tyramine, tryptamine and phenylethylamine, have been identified in the central nervous system, and have been considered to have some function. The origin of these compounds is obscure, since there is a considerable amount of evidence that the parent amino acids, tyrosine, tryptophan and phenylalanine, are not substrates for mammalian decarboxylases. In the absence of any proven mechanism for their synthesis, any claims as to their function in the brain must be regarded as highly tentative.

Further reading

Chase, T. N. and Murphy, D. L. (1973). Serotonin and central nervous system function. *Ann. Rev. Pharmacol.*, **13**, 181–197.
Cooper, J. R., Bloom, F. E. and Roth, R. H. (1970). *Biochemical basis of neuropharmacology*. Oxford University Press.
Cotzias, G. C., Papavasiliou, P. S. and Gellene, R. (1969). Modification of Parkinsonism—chronic treatment with L-DOPA. *New Engl. J. Med.*, **280**, 337–345.
Glassman, A. (1969). Indoleamines and affective disorders. *Psychosomat. Med.*, **31**, 107–114.
Hornykiewicz, O. (1966). Dopamine and brain function. *Pharmacol. Rev.*, **18**, 925–964.
Levin, E. and Scicli, G. (1969). Brain barrier phenomena. *Brain Res.*, **13**, 1–12.
de Robertis, E. (1971). Molecular biology of synaptic receptors. *Science*, **171**, 963–971.
Schildkraut, J. J. (1965). The catecholamine hypothesis of affective disorders: a review of supporting evidence. *Amer. J. Psychiatr.*, **122**, 509–522.
Snyder, S. S. (Ed.) (1972). *Perspectives in neuropharmacology: a tribute to Julius Axelrod*. Oxford University Press.
Symposium proceedings. (1973.) Dynamic aspects of the synapse. *Brain Res.*, **62**, 299–597.

References cited in the text are listed in the bibliography

CHAPTER 8

NUTRITIONAL ASPECTS OF AMINO ACIDS

Arnold E. Bender

Professor of Nutrition, Queen Elizabeth College, University of London

Protein must be consumed by man and other animals since their tissues, enzyme systems, transport mechanisms and many hormones are protein in composition. An infant born at 3·5 kg becomes an adult of 60 kg and the difference includes about 11 kg of protein—obvious evidence that the diet must contain protein.

However, the mature adult whose weight remains constant still requires a regular supply of dietary protein to replace the continuing losses involved in the dynamic equilibrium of the tissues as described earlier.

The total protein turnover in the average adult is about 300 g per day of which about 40 g is lost from the body and must be replaced from the diet. Nitrogen is used as an index both of protein consumed and urea lost simply because of the ease of analysis. Not all dietary nitrogen is protein, some foods are relatively rich in purines, free amino acids (which are as useful as whole proteins) and other forms of nitrogen. The term 'crude protein', which is total N multiplied by 6·25 is a useful approximation of dietary protein although it is more accurate to determine true protein N and multiply by the correct factor, namely 5·7 for cereals, 6·38 for milk and 6·25 for most other foods.

Essential amino acids

Since most tissues are composed of all the 20 amino acids, all are needed for growth and repair. Some, however, can be synthesized in the body so long as nitrogen, usually in the form of other amino acids, is available from the diet. Hence the distinction between those amino acids that cannot be synthesized and must therefore be provided in the diet ready-made, the so-called essential amino acids, and those that can be synthesized, so-called non-essential amino acids. However, enough protein or nitrogen must be consumed to take care of the needs for the synthesis of non-essentials as well as providing ready-made essential amino acids.

The evidence for the segregation of the amino acids into these two categories came from a series of classical experiments of Rose, first on rats and eventually on human subjects.

Under special circumstances non-essentials can become essential. For example when benzoic acid is fed in large enough doses the detoxication compound, hippuric acid, requires the synthesis of such large amounts of glycine that this amino acid becomes growth-limiting and could, under these circumstances, be classed as essential.

The experimental evidence for so classifying the amino acids in man is based not on growth, but on the maintenance of nitrogen balance in adults. Arginine and histidine are not essential by this criterion but it is accepted, from indirect evidence, that they are essential for infants. In Rose's experiments the dietary level of all amino acids except one was fixed and the one under investigation was varied in quantity until the subject was neither gaining nor losing nitrogen, i.e. he was in N equilibrium. This amount was taken as the dietary need. An illustration of the large degree of individual variation of dietary requirements of human beings was the observation that in a group of only 30 subjects the need for lysine covered a two-fold range.

Since dietary protein must supply the amino acids needed for tissue synthesis some foods will contain mixtures of amino acids in proportions approximating more closely to the composition of human protein tissues than other foods. This is the principle of protein quality—quality from the dietary point of view—discussed below.

Dietary needs

It was stated above that the losses from the body average about 40 g per day but this is only an approximation. It is not only subject to a considerable degree of biological variation, but may vary from day to day with changes in conditions and environment.

Determination of the requirements of protein are therefore imprecise. Estimations of vitamin requirements, for example, are assisted by the appearance of specific symptoms when a deficiency state is reached, so that clinical observation of population groups correlated with dietary intake can be used to establish limits of adequacy and inadequacy. With protein, however, there are no specific signs of deficiency in adults—the problem of infants is a separate one.

Over the years of nutritional research the recommended amounts of protein have varied considerably from 100 g per day to 30 g, from 1 g per kg body weight to 0·5 g. Some of these figures were based on observation of healthy people or on experimentation, others were based on the method of totalling the body's 'obligatory nitrogen losses' and adding a varying safety factor.

The currently-accepted recommendations are those of the Expert Committee of the World Health Organization (Energy and Protein Requirements 1973) which do not differ in the basis of calculations from those of the UK Department of Health and Social Security (1969) although the final recommended intakes (as distinct from calculated requirements) do differ.

The obligatory nitrogen losses include: (i) urine (from continuing tissue degradation) as urea, uric acid, allantoin and creatinine together with ammonium salts formed in the kidney; (ii) faeces (from undigested foods approximating to 5 % of dietary protein, shed lining of intestine, bacteria and residues of digestive juices); (iii) sweat, which will vary with conditions, and (iv) small amounts in hair, nails, skin cells and menstrual loss. Losses from the four sources are measured directly on human volunteers but errors are inevitably introduced when taking average values from small numbers of volunteers (possibly about 100 subjects can be collected together from the literature for such calculations) and applying the results to the population as a whole.

The calculation, shown in detail in Table 8.1 involves the following principles. The total average nitrogen loss is calculated and an allowance made for individual

Table 8.1. Calculation of protein requirement

	Obligatory N losses on protein-free diet	
	mg N/kg body wt	mg N per unit basal energy (kJ)
Urine	37	0·33
Faeces	12	0·10
Skin	3	0·03
Miscellaneous	2	0·02
Total	54	0·48

	per kg body wt
Requirement to replace obligatory losses	54 mg
Additional amount to maintain N balance +30%	66·2 mg
Additional amount to cover individual variation +30%	86 mg
Expressed as protein (× 6·25)	0·54 g
Allow for protein quality at 75%	0·72 g
Recommended intake for 65 kg man	47 g/day

Joint FAO/WHO Expert Committee: Energy and Protein requirements, WHO Tech. Rpt. Series, No. 522, Geneva 1973.

variation. Until the 1973 WHO Report it was assumed from the limited evidence available that the shape of the distribution curve meant that about 97% of the individual values fell within 2 standard deviations of the mean, i.e. 20%. The 1973 Report suggests that this should be 30%.

If this amount of 'perfect' protein is supplied then all (or at least 97%) of the subjects will obtain their minimum protein needs. In other words, if one replaces exactly the obligatory nitrogen losses then this should satisfy the protein requirements. However, it has been shown that when this is done the individual is still in slight negative nitrogen balance and additional protein is needed to maintain balance. The WHO 1973 Report suggests that 30% extra dietary protein is needed for this purpose. Hence obligatory losses plus 30% for individual variation and 30% for N balance = recommended intake.

Finally, this figure is based on the assumption that the dietary protein is composed of amino acids in exactly the proportions required by the tissues, i.e. 'perfect' protein, so a factor has to be included to allow for deviations from 'perfection'.

The difference between *requirement* and *recommended intake* is that the latter is set high enough to take care of individuals with above-average needs. For proteins, the WHO *recommended intakes* are 30% higher than average *require-*

ments (for vitamins the figure is 20%). This assumes that the requirements of energy and other nutrients are adequately supplied.

The UK Recommended Intakes Committee adopts a more practical attitude towards eating. The Report (1969) lists firstly, minimum requirements which

Table 8.2. U.K. recommendations and requirement for protein

		Body wt (kg)	Minimum requirement protein as per cent energy	Recommended* (g/day)
Infant	0–3 months	4·6	9·5	
	3–6 months	6·6	7·4	20
	6–12 months	8·3–9·5	6·6–6·4	
Children	1–2 years	11·4	6·3	30
	3–5 years	16·5	6·1	40
	7–9 years	25·1	5·7	53
Boys	9–12 years	31·9	5·8	63
	12–15 years	45·5	6·6	70
	15–18 years	61·0	6·7	75
Girls	9–12 years	33·0	6·1	58
	12–15 years	48·6	7·6	58
	15–18 years	56·1	7·0	58
Men		65	5·0–6·7	65–90
Women		55	6·9–7·0	51–63
Pregnancy			7·3	60
Lactation			8·1	68

* It is recommended that 10% of diet should come from protein.

Recommended Intakes of Nutrients for UK Dept. of Health & Social Security. Rept. no. 120, HMSO, 1969.

approximate to those calculated above (Table 8.1). This would provide a most unattractive diet of 5–6% protein. It *recommends* that people should continue to eat the type of diet that is commonly eaten in this country, namely one containing about 10% protein. Certainly extra work does not require extra protein, the figure is the same for adults of the same body size whether they are at rest, engaged in sedentary work or extremely active, but if the active worker eats more food of the same kind (as he is most likely to do) then he will consume more protein the more energy he uses (and consumes). So the UK figures for *recommended* protein (not required protein) intakes increase with activity while those of WHO, and also USA, remain constant (Table 8.2).

Extras

Estimates of protein needs, and indeed needs of all nutrients, apply in the first instance to young, healthy subjects who have been under investigation. It must be emphasized that the recommended intakes assume that all other nutrients are being ingested in adequate amounts, and they do not take account of any extra needs incurred through ill-health other than 'the daily stresses of coughs and

196

colds'. Needs for nutrients in disease are not only greater but vary enormously so no figure can possibly be established.

Extra protein is required for conditions such as growth in children, pregnancy and lactation, as shown in Table 8.2. Such figures are arrived at, respectively, from weight increments of children or the foetus, and for milk secretion during lactation.

Figures for RDI's sometimes differ between different authorities for a variety of reasons: (i) there are sometimes differences of scientific opinion between conclusions drawn from inadequate evidence; (ii) further information leads to modifications of figures introduced in subsequent reports; (iii) the increments added to take account of individual variations are often a matter of opinion rather than being firmly based on scientific evidence; (iv) there may be national policy reasons for setting a figure at higher or lower levels.

Quality

As stated above, all figures for RDI are, in the first instance, based on the assumption that the dietary protein is composed of amino acids in exactly the proportions needed for tissue synthesis, i.e. they are 'perfect' proteins.

As might be expected some proteins resemble the body requirements of amino acids more closely than others and so are of higher 'quality'. The quality of proteins depends on their amino acid composition, and can be expressed in a number of ways.

Firstly, the amounts and proportions of the amino acids for maintenance for men and women have been established, Table 8.3, so it is possible to compare

Table 8.3. Composition of amino acid reference pattern, expressed as g amino acid per 100 g protein

	Reference pattern	Cow's milk	Egg
Lysine	4·2	7·8	6·3
Leucine	4·8	9·9	9·0
Isoleucine	4·2	6·4	6·8
Phenylalanine	2·8	4·9	6·0
tyrosine	2·8	5·1	4·4
Methionine	2·2	2·4	3·1
cystine	2·0	0·9	2·3
Threonine	2·8	4·6	5·0
Tryptophan	1·4	1·4	1·7
Valine	4·2	6·9	7·4

the chemical composition of the food protein with these target values. The value of the protein for tissue synthesis is limited by that amino acid present in least relative amount, the so-called 'limiting amino acid'. This can be expressed as 'protein score'. This is the limiting amino acid expressed as a percentage of the target figure for this amino acid. For example wheat contains 2·1 g lysine per 100 g protein compared with the target value of 4·2 so that protein score for wheat is 50. If lysine is added then this amino acid is no longer limiting and, in fact, threonine becomes the limiting factor. The bread plus lysine now has a protein score of 75.

The drawback to this method of assessing protein quality, although it is often used, is that not all the amino acid present is biologically available; some part may be present in a linkage that is not hydrolysed during digestion. All chemical analyses of protein composition are preceded by acid hydrolysis which releases all the amino acid. This is particularly true of lysine, which has been the most thoroughly investigated of the non-available amino acids, but other amino acids can also be rendered non-available. Lysine can be linked through its ε-amino group with a reducing sugar or carbonyl group and it is this linkage that is stable to enzymic hydrolysis. The non-available linkages of other amino acids have not been established.

This type of linkage takes place when proteins are heated, especially in the presence of reducing sugars and moisture, and depends on time and temperature reached. It is not a practical problem in most food processing and domestic cooking procedures but only in rather special circumstances such as roasting of meat or the explosive puffing of certain types of breakfast cereals. In some proteins, cross-links are formed between the ε-amino groups of lysyl residues and the β-carboxyl groups of aspartyl or the γ-carboxyl groups of glutamyl residues. These links are resistant to digestion by mammalian proteases, and the lysine involved is therefore unavailable.

Before the human needs for each amino acid were established, amino acid composition of food proteins was compared with that of egg, which is completely utilizable, and the ratio of limiting amino acid in the food to that in egg was termed chemical score. In practice that figure differs little from protein score.

Before it was evident that protein quality depended on the amino acid composition, quality was assessed by biological assay on experimental animals, the method is still commonly used to avoid the problem of non-availability of amino acids.

The protein food is fed to experimental animals under conditions where all the nutrients are freely available so that protein is the limiting factor, i.e. it is fed at relatively low protein levels, conventionally 10% to a young rat. The usefulness of the protein for growth and metabolic function is a measure of its quality. The proportion of food protein (in practice, food nitrogen) that is retained in the body is the measure of quality and is termed net protein utilization. This may be determined either by the difference between intake and output (urine plus faeces) or the amount retained in the body estimated through carcase analysis.

A parallel measure ignores losses in digestion and expresses the result as the proportion of the absorbed nitrogen that is retained, rather than the dietary nitrogen that is retained. This is termed Biological Value (Table 8.4). It is equal to NPU only when digestibility is 100%, otherwise BV is always greater than NPU.

BV of human milk and egg protein (as measured on rat) are 1 (expressed as a ratio); for meat, cow's milk, fish, the value is 0·75; rice 0·6; wheat 0·5; many peas and beans 0·35–0·50; and for any protein that is completely lacking in one of the essential amino acids, such as gelatin, the value is zero.

Table 8.4. Measures of protein quality

$$\text{Biological value (BV)} = \frac{\text{Retained nitrogen}}{\text{Absorbed nitrogen}}$$

$$\text{Net protein utilization (NPU)} = \frac{\text{Retained nitrogen}}{\text{Dietary nitrogen}}$$

$$= \text{BV} \times \text{Digestibility}$$

Protein efficiency ratio (PER) = Gain in wt (g)/g protein eaten

$$\text{Net protein retention (NPR)} = \frac{\text{Gain in wt} + \text{loss of wt of non-protein group of animals}}{\text{protein eaten}}$$

These figures, of course, apply to the single protein under investigation, which is a somewhat academic laboratory exercise carried out to establish the properties of the protein. In practice, no one ever eats single proteins and we need then to know the NPU of the diet as a whole. When a mixture of protein foods is consumed they complement one another, that is a relative lack of an amino acid in one protein is compensated by a relative surplus in another so that the mixture can have an NPU greater than the mean. For example maize has a BV of 0·36 and is limited by lysine; pea flour has a BV of 0·40 and is limited by methionine. A mixture of equal parts of the proteins from these two sources has a BV of 0·70—nearly as good as that of meat at 0·75. In general, cereals are limited by lysine and pulses by methionine, so that many of the traditional mixtures of foods eaten in many parts of the world automatically complement one another.

In practice it is found that even in the worst-fed countries of the world the NPU of the diet is 0·5–0·6, compared with 0·7–0·8 in the best-fed countries, such as UK where the proteins are largely drawn from meat, wheat and milk. So protein quality is not a matter of vital importance in diets as a whole. Where protein quality becomes a matter of importance is where the quantity is marginal. Since quantity can compensate for quality any short-comings in quality are tantamount to a shortage of quantity. Such conditions exist in areas where the main foods are the starchy roots such as cassava or arrowroot or fruits such as plantains where protein content is as little as 2-4% and also of low quality. Protein quality becomes a matter of importance when one is seeking sources of additional protein with which to supplement a diet.

These two methods of measuring protein quality, Biological Value and net protein utilization, depend upon nitrogen balance; another commonly used method is termed 'protein efficiency ratio' which depends upon growth (although this, in turn, must depend on N accretion in the body). Protein efficiency ratio, PER, is the weight gain per gram of protein eaten, and is usually determined at

10% dietary protein level. The best proteins have a PER of about 4·4, proteins with an NPU of 0·4 cannot support growth, i.e. PER is zero.

In comparisons of protein quality, for example in seeking protein sources for the preparation of baby foods, or to supplement staple foods such as bread, casein is often taken as a standard of comparison. This is only because it is readily available in relatively purified form by precipitation from milk; it has PER about 2·3 and NPU of 0·70.

As stated earlier, quantity compensates for quality and if the recommended daily intake of 'perfect' protein is 45 g per day, this need could be fulfilled by 90 g of protein of NPU 50. These variations in quality are taken care of in the RDI laid down by the World Health Organization (see Table 8.3).

The non-availability of amino acids, i.e. their linkage in forms that are not hydrolysed during digestion, are little understood except for lysine. The linkage between the ε-amino group of lysine and reducing sugars is termed the Maillard or browning reaction and is shown in the brown outer part of roast meat or the brown colour of meat extract. It adds flavour to prepared foods and the loss in nutritive value is rather small and unimportant.

Protein as a source of energy

The mature adult who is turning over 300 g of protein a day is losing 40 g of this from the body. Such losses take place by deamination and excretion of the nitrogen as urea, and oxidation of the carbon skeleton to carbon dioxide and water with the liberation of 17 kJ (4 kcal) per g.

The same path is followed by dietary protein in excess of requirements for tissue replacement. Amounts beyond the (approximately) 40 g per day are converted into urea, carbon dioxide and water with the liberation of 17 kJ per g.

In the mature adult, the total dietary protein is included in the food available for energy. Although a subject consuming exactly the 40 g of protein that is being excreted is using this entirely for tissue replacement, he is making use of the energy from the 40 g of tissue protein being degraded, i.e. 160 kJ. If his intake is higher, say 100 g per day, 40 g is used to replace tissue losses and the remaining 60 g is oxidized for energy—160 kJ plus 240 kJ. So even although part of the dietary protein is used for tissue synthesis the whole of the intake is available as a source of energy (so long as the subject is in N equilibrium) and the energy content of a diet includes the protein as well as the fat and carbohydrate.

In growth, pregnancy and convalescence, where protein tissues are being increased, some part of the dietary protein, beyond the 40 g needed for every-day replacement, stays in the body and is not oxidized. However, this amounts to only a few grams per day and is usually ignored when calculating the energy content of the diet. For example a schoolchild may grow by 2·5 kg per year which is only 7 g of tissue per day, equivalent to about 1·5 g of protein.

The body appears to have first call on the energy of the diet, meaning that when fats and carbohydrates are inadequate to supply the energy needs, some part of the dietary protein is oxidized to supply energy. This becomes of great importance in poorly-fed areas and in elderly persons where food intake is restricted for a variety of reasons. A diet that is deficient in energy (i.e. inadequate in quantity) is likely also to be deficient in protein. When the diet is deficient in both energy and protein it is of limited use only adding extra protein, since much of this will be oxidized, therefore additional energy foods are needed in the first instance.

When the energy content of foods is measured by combustion in a bomb calorimeter, the protein is completely oxidized to carbon dioxide, water and nitrogen dioxide; in the body the nitrogen is excreted as urea which still contains 6·9 kJ per g. Allowances must therefore be made for the incomplete combustion that takes place in the body—protein provides 23.9 kJ per g in the calorimeter and 17 kJ per g in the body.

Nitrogen balance

During growth, pregnancy, athletic training and convalescence the body is laying down extra protein—the intake is greater than the losses and the subject is consequently in positive protein (nitrogen) balance. During starvation, or under conditions leading to muscle wastage, the subject is in negative nitrogen balance.

Table 8.5. Representative protein losses

1. Before surgery	
Bleeding peptic ulcer	90 g (over 5 days)
Burn	30 g (in one day)
Fracture of long bone	140–190 g (over 10 weeks)
2. During operation (due to blood loss)	
Gastric surgery	9–18 g
Pneumonectomy	20–60 g
Thyroidectomy	3–12 g
3. Catabolic response after surgery	
Herniotomy	18 g over 10 days
Gastric resection	50–175 g over 5–10 days
Appendicitis	50 g over 10 days

Large scale destruction of tissue occurs in conditions such as trauma, surgical shock, burns and toxaemia. The losses vary with the severity of damage, the state of protein 'reserves' and other conditions, but the size of the losses, judged against a background of a daily requirement in health of 40 g per day, indicates the problem involved in restoration during convalescence. The surgical trauma associated with removal of the appendix can cause the loss of 160–230 g of protein; fracture of the femur can result in an 800 g loss; a limb burn, which includes loss of damaged tissue, exudation of tissue fluid and the mobilization and loss of protein reserves, can amount to 1000–1250 g. Even 7 days bed-rest, i.e. inactivity of the muscles, results in the loss of about 300 g of protein (see Table 8.5).

The losses are largely the result of a general increase in catabolism, thought to be under hormonal influence, whereby the tissue proteins are mobilized, hydrolysed to amino acids—it is thought in preparation for tissue repair—and then deaminated, oxidized and the nitrogenous portion excreted in large quantities in the urine. Losses are less in subjects already suffering from depletion of their protein reserves but cannot be prevented by feeding large quantities of protein before the damage occurs.

Protein stores

The losses referred to above imply some form of reserve or store of protein in the well-fed subject, and this has been the subject of much controversy over many years. There is no specific site of storage nor any indication that there is any chemical difference between stored protein and tissue structure. Certainly, within a few days of protein deprivation there are considerable losses from the liver, which might therefore be regarded as a store. Prolonged shortages lead to losses from less essential tissues, such as muscle, in order to maintain the integrity of more essential tissues, such as liver, heart etc. Subjects can withstand prolonged periods of either protein deficiency or total starvation with consequent atrophy of muscles but, if re-fed, complete, or apparently complete, recovery takes place.

An inadequate intake of protein leads to a form of adaptation whereby the turnover of amino acids is reduced with a consequently greater economy of nitrogen utilization.

The result of this adaptation is that there is no sharp line of demarcation between adequate and inadequate intake of protein. In fact it is not possible to diagnose whether or not a subject is receiving adequate intake of protein foods unless the shortage is both severe and prolonged. In infants there is certainly a slowing and eventually a cessation of growth with appearance of the protein-energy deficiency disease called kwashiorkor but no such indication is apparent in adults. The minimum requirements of adult man are small, that is, as shown in Table 8.2 only 5–6% of the energy needs come from protein. It is difficult to compile a diet, or at least a palatable diet, lower than this in protein. Even peoples subsisting on starchy roots such as cassava containing only 2–4% protein invariably add small amounts of protein-rich foods. Even if they did consume inadequate amounts of protein there is no clear evidence of any sign of ill-health; only after lengthy periods of months or years is there a fall in serum proteins.

The converse of the discussion of protein losses from stores is the building up of such stores when the subject consumes excessive amounts of protein. He will, under such conditions, go into positive nitrogen balance, i.e. store extra protein in the body, but there is no particular site of storage, merely an overall increase in many different tissues. This has defeated attempts to assess protein needs from N balance. It might be thought that one could increase or decrease the dietary protein intake until the subjects passed in and out of N balance and so arrive at a figure for the amount required. This does not happen since it is possible, as indeed it is with some other nutrients, such as calcium, to attain balance on many different levels of intake. If a well-fed subject reduces his protein intake he goes in negative N balance only temporarily, then strikes a balance at the lower level of intake — presumably with lower reserves than previously. Similarly, if he changes from a low to a higher protein intake he goes into positive balance, temporarily, and then attains nitrogen equilibrium at the new, higher, level of intake, presumably with a higher state of protein reserves. There is no evidence to indicate which level of reserves is most beneficial.

Food problems

No problem of protein shortage exists in the western world since almost all foods contain enough to satisfy at least minimum needs. An overall shortage of food will certainly result in a protein deficiency, both from inadequate intake and from oxidation of such protein as is fed for the purpose of providing energy. Many protein-rich foods are available, especially for infant feeding, but they are usually not necessary.

In the underfed countries of the world there is little problem so far as adults are concerned, although it is not clear whether they would benefit from extra protein. The main problem is that of babies who are growing rapidly; they require proportionately more protein than do adults. The disease termed kwashiorkor is based on a protein deficiency when the energy intake is possibly near adequate, compared with marasmus where the total diet is in short supply; both are termed protein-energy malnutrition.

The infant problem arises from weaning babies on to inadequate foods, and much effort has been devoted to producing baby foods rich in protein based on foodstuffs such as oilseed residues, fish meal and milk powder.

As regards future developments, it has always been more expensive in terms of land and effort to produce protein-rich foods rather than starchy foods, so new sources of protein and new methods of improving protein quality have been sought. Protein quality can be increased as has been indicated earlier, by supplementing with the limiting amino acids. These are lysine in many cereal foods and methionine in many animal and other vegetable foods. Lysine is manufactured on a commercial scale and is used for this purpose; methionine is also manufactured on a commercial scale but its strong flavour has limited its supplemental value to animal feeds. Other approaches have been to produce protein-rich foods by novel procedures such as factory-scale growth of yeasts, algae, fungi and bacteria, either for human food or animal feed, as well as breeding varieties of common plants richer in protein and higher in protein quality.

Further reading

Bender, A. E. (1973). *Nutrition and dietetic foods.* Leonard Hill Books, Aylesbury, Bucks.

Davidson, S., Passmore, R. and Brock, J. F. (1972). *Human Nutrition and dietetics.* 5th edition. Churchill–Livingstone, Edinburgh.

APPENDIX I

THE AMINO ACIDS

In the table below, the structures and some chemical properties of the amino acids are listed. For those which are incorporated into proteins, the conventional three-letter and single-letter codes are also listed, as are the codons found in mRNA corresponding to the amino acids. Where either adenine or guanine can be found in the third place of a codon, the symbol *Pu* is used. Similarly, *Py* is used to indicate either of the pyrimidines, cytidine or uracil, and *Nu* to indicate any nucleotide. Amino acids marked with an asterisk are those which are dietary essentials for man.

Amino acid	Structure	Mol. wt	pK_a	Codon
Alanine Ala (A)	CH_3—CH—COOH | NH_2	89·1	2·35 9·87	GC*Nu*
β-Alanine	CH_2—CH_2—COOH | NH_2	89·1	3·55 10·24	n/a
Allysine (α-Amino-caproic-δ- semialdehyde)	HC=O | $(CH_2)_3$ | CH—COOH | NH_2	145·2	Not determined	n/a
α-Amino adipic acid	CH_2—COOH | CH_2 | CH_2—CH—COOH | NH_2	161·2	2·14 (α) 4·21 (ε) 9·77	n/a
γ-Aminobutyric acid (GABA)	CH_2—COOH | CH_2—CH_2—NH_2	103·1	4·03 10·56	n/a
Arginine Arg (R)	NH_2 | C=NH | NH | $(CH_2)_3$ | CH—COOH | NH_2	174·2	1·83 8·99 12·48 (guanido)	CG*Nu*⎫ AG*Pu*⎭

Amino acid	Structure	Mol. wt	pK_a	Codon
Argininosuccinic acid	NH$_2$ · · · · CH$_2$—COOH | · · · · · · · · | CH$_2$—NH—C=NH—CH—COOH | CH$_2$ | CH$_2$—CH—COOH · · · · · · · | · · · · · · · NH$_2$	290·3	1·62 ⎤ 2·70 ⎬ COOH 4·26 ⎦ 9·58 (α-NH$_2$) >12 (guanido)	n/a
Asparagine AsN or Asp-NH$_2$	CO—NH$_2$ | CH$_2$—CH—COOH · · · · · | · · · · · NH$_2$	132·1	2·1 8·84	AA*Py*
Aspartic acid Asp (D)	COOH | CH$_2$—CH—COOH · · · · · | · · · · · NH$_2$	133·1	1·99 (α) 3·90 (γ) 9·90	GA*Py*
Citrulline	· · · · · · O · · · · · · ‖ CH$_2$—NH—C—NH$_2$ | CH$_2$ | CH$_2$—CH—COOH · · · · · | · · · · · NH$_2$	175·2	Not determined	n/a
Cystathionine	· · · · · · · · · NH$_2$ · · · · · · · · · | CH$_2$—CH$_2$—CH—COOH | S | CH$_2$—CH—COOH · · · · · | · · · · · NH$_2$	222·3	Not determined	n/a
Cysteine Cys (C)	CH$_2$—SH | CH—COOH | NH$_2$	121·2	1·92 8·35 10·46 (—SH)	UG*Py*
Cystine (Cys)$_2$	· · · · · · NH$_2$ · · · · · · | S—CH$_2$—CH—COOH | S—CH$_2$—CH—COOH · · · · · · · · | · · · · · · · · NH$_2$	240·2	<1·0 2·1 8·02 8·71	n/a
Diaminopimelic acid	NH$_2$ | CH$_2$—CH—COOH | CH$_2$ | CH$_2$—CH—COOH · · · · · | · · · · · NH$_2$	190·2	1·8 2·2 8·8 9·9	n/a

Amino acid	Structure	Mol. wt	pK_a	Codon
Dihydroxy-phenylalanine (DOPA)	HO—[ring]—CH_2—CH—COOH, OH, NH_2	197·2	2·32 8·72 9·96 11·79 (OH)	n/a
Di-iodotyrosine	HO—[ring with I, I]—CH_2—CH—COOH, NH_2	433·0	2·12 6·48 (OH) 7·82	n/a
Ethionine	CH_2—S—CH_2—CH_3 CH—COOH NH_2	163·2	Not determined	n/a
Glutamic acid Glu (E)	COOH CH_2 CH_2—CH—COOH NH_2	147·1	2·10 (α) 4·07 (δ) 9·47	GA*Pu*
Glutamine GlN *or* Glu-NH_2 (Q)	CO—NH_2 CH_2 CH_2—CH—COOH NH_2	146·1	2·17 9·13	CA*Pu*
Glycine Gly (G)	CH_2—COOH NH_2	75·1	2·35 9·78	CG*Nu*
Histidine His (H)	N⟋⟍N [imidazole]—CH_2—CH—COOH NH_2	155·2	1·80 6·04 (imidazole) 9·76	CA*Py*
Homocysteine	CH_2—SH CH_2—CH—COOH NH_2	117·2	2·22 8·87 10·86	n/a
Homoserine	CH_2—OH CH_2—CH—COOH NH_2	119·1	2·71 9·62	n/a
Hydroxylysine	CH_2—NH_2 CH—OH CH_2 CH_2—CH—COOH NH_2	162·2	2·13 8·62 9·67	n/a

Amino acid	Structure	Mol. wt	pK_a	Codon
3-Hydroxyproline Hyp	(pyrrolidine ring with —OH, —COOH, N—H)	131·1	1·82 9·66	n/a
4-Hydroxyproline Hyp	HO— (pyrrolidine ring) —COOH, N—H	131·1	1·82 9·66	n/a
5-Hydroxytryptophan (5-HTP)	HO—(indole ring, N—H)—CH_2—CH—COOH, NH_2	220·2	Not determined	n/a
* Isoleucine (Ile) (I)	CH_3—CH_2—CH(CH_3)—CH(NH_2)—COOH	131·2	2·32 9·76	AUA AUPu
Kynurenine	(benzene ring)—C(=O)—CH_2—CH(NH_2)—COOH, ring—NH_2	208·2	Not determined	n/a
* Leucine Leu (L)	CH_3—CH(CH_3)—CH_2—CH(NH_2)—COOH	131·2	2·33 9·74	UUPu CUNu
* Lysine Lys (K)	CH_2—NH_2 | CH_2 | CH_2 | CH_2—CH(NH_2)—COOH	146·2	2·16 9·18 (α) 10·79 (ε)	AAPu
β-lysine	CH_2—NH_2 | CH_2 | CH_2 | CH(NH_2)—CH_2—COOH	146·2	Not determined	n/a
* Methionine Met (M)	CH_2—S—CH_3 | CH—COOH | NH_2	149·2	2·13 9·28	AUG
Ornithine	CH_2—NH_2 | CH_2 | CH_2—CH(NH_2)—COOH	132·2	1·71 8·69 (α) 10·76 (δ)	n/a

Amino acid	Structure	Mol. wt	pK_a	Codon
5-Oxo-proline (pyroglutamic acid)		129·1	3·32	n/a
* Phenylalanine Phe (F)		165·2	2·16 9·18	UU*Py*
Proline Pro (P)		115·1	1·95 10·64	CC*Nu*
Saccharopine	CH₂—NH—CH—COOH | | CH₂ CH₂ | | CH₂ CH₂ | | CH₂ COOH | CH—COOH | NH₂	275·3	Not determined	n/a
Serine Ser (S)	CH₂—OH | CH—COOH | NH₂	105·1	2·19 9·21	UC*Nu* AG*Py*
* Threonine Thr (T)	CH₃ | CH₂—OH | CH—COOH | NH₂	119·1	2·09 9·10	AC*Nu*
Thyroxine (T₄)		776·9	2·2 6·45 (OH) 10·1	n/a

Amino acid	Structure	Mol. wt	pK_a	Codon
Tri-iodothyronine (T$_3$)	OH group with I substituents, O linkage, I, I, CH$_2$—CH—COOH, NH$_2$	651·0	2·2 8·40 (OH) 10·1	n/a
* Tryptophan Trp (W)	indole ring, CH$_2$—CH—COOH, NH$_2$	204·2	2·43 9·44	UGG
Tyrosine Tyr (Y)	HO—ring—CH$_2$—CH—COOH, NH$_2$	181·2	2·20 9·11 10·13 (OH)	UAPy
* Valine Val (V)	CH$_3$, CH$_3$—CH—COOH, NH$_2$	117·1	2·29 9·74	GUNu

APPENDIX II

INBORN ERRORS OF AMINO ACID METABOLISM

Throughout the text, defects of amino acid metabolism have been noted where they are of clinical importance, or where the elucidation of the metabolic defect has led to greater understanding of normal pathways. Most of the diseases listed on the following pages are extremely rare, and indeed, for some there are only one or two reports in the literature. The frequencies per million live births for the N. American and European populations of some of the more common diseases are as follows: phenylketonuria, 80; cystinuria, 70; Hartnup's disease, 40; histidinaemia, 40; hyperprolinaemia, 20; argininosuccinic aciduria, 4; maple syrup urine disease, 3.

Disease	Signs	Blood	Urine	Intelligence	Enzyme defect
Alkaptonuria	Urine darkens on standing, cartilage pigmented, arthritis	—	Homogentisic acid	Normal	Homogentisic acid oxidase
Cystathioninuria	—	—	Cystathionine	Retarded or normal	Cystathionase (may be vitamin B_6 dependency)
Cystinuria	Urinary calculi of cysteine	—	Cys, Lys, Arg and Orn	Normal	Renal transport mechanism for Cys and basic amino acids
Familial goitre	Hypothyroid goitre		—	(a) Normal	Failure of thyroid I^- uptake
				(b) Cretinous	Failure of tyrosine iodination
				(c) Cretinous	Iodotyrosine coupling enzyme
				(d) Cretinous	Iodotyrosine deiodinase
				(e) Normal	Low thyroglobulin synthesis
		High thyrotropin	—	(f) Cretinous	Impaired thyroid response to thyrotropin
Hartnup disease	Photosensitive pellagrous rash	Total amino acids low	High neutral amino acids, abnormal Trp metabolites	Normal	Failure of intestinal and renal neutral amino acid transport
Histidinuria	Speech defect	—	His, imidazole lactate, pyruvate and acetate	Retarded in some cases	Histidase
Homocystinuria	Dislocation of lens of eye, fine sparse hair	Homocysteine and Met high	Homocysteine	Retarded in 60% of cases	Cystathionine synthetase

Disease	Signs	Blood	Urine	Intelligence	Enzyme defect
Hydroxy-kynureninuria	Growth retardation, bone abnormalities, pellagrous rash	—	Hydroxykynurenine, kynurenine	Retarded	?Kynureninase
Hydroxyprolinaemia	—	Hydroxyproline	Hydroxyproline	Severely retarded	Hydroxyproline oxidase
Hyperammonaemia	Periodic ammonia intoxication, vomiting, protein intolerance	High NH_4^+	—	Normal	Carbamyl phosphate synthetase
(a) Argininaemia		High NH_4^+ and Arg	Arg, Lys, Orn	Normal	Arginase
(b) Argininosuccinic aciduria		High NH_4^+ and argininosuccinate	Argininosuccinate	Normal	Argininosuccinase
(c) Citrullinaemia		High NH_4^+ and citrulline	Citrulline	Retarded	Argininosuccinate synthetase
(d) Hyperornithin-aemia		High NH_4^+ and Orn	Orn	Normal	Ornithine carbamyl transferase
Hyperglycinaemia (a) Ketotic	Grown retardation, ketosis, fits; fatal in 1st year of life	Acetone and other neutral ketones	Ketones	Retarded	Unclear
(b) Non-ketotic	Fits, failure to thrive	Gly high	Gly	Retarded	glycine oxidase or glycine cleavage system
Hyperlysinaemia	Growth retardation, muscle weakness, abnormal EEG	Lys high	Lys (and saccharopine)	Retarded	Saccharopine dehydrogenase
Hypermethioninaemia	Irritability, somnolence	Met high	General amino aciduria, esp Met	Normal	?Methionine S-adenosyl transferase
Hyperprolinaemia	Congenital renal defects, haematuria	Pro high	Pro, Gly and Hyp	Retarded	Proline oxidase

Disease	Signs	Blood	Urine	Intelligence	Enzyme defect
Hypervalinaemia	Failure to thrive, inability to suckle, nystagmus, vomiting	Val high	Val	Normal	?Valine aminotransferase
Isovalericacidaemia	Vomiting, acidosis, lethargy, coma, characteristic odour	Isovaleric acid high	Short chain fatty acids	Retarded	Isovaleryl CoA dehydrogenase
Kynureninuria	—	—	Kynurenine	Normal	Partial defect of kynurenine hydroxylase
Maple syrup urine disease	Vomiting, feeding difficulties, poor muscle tone, maple syrup odour in urine	Val, Leu and Ile, high	Val, Leu and Ile, and branched chain ketones	Retarded	Branched chain oxoacid decarboxylase
Oxoprolinuria	—	Oxoproline high	Oxoproline, low urea	Slightly retarded	Oxoprolinase
Pendred's syndrome	Euthyroid goitre, nerve deafness	—	—	Normal	Partial defect of tyrosine iodination
Phenylketonuria	—	High Phe, low Tyr	Phenylpyruvate, lactate and acetate	Very severely retarded	Phenylalanine hydroxylase
Tyrosinaemia	Failure to thrive, vomiting, diarrhoea	High Tyr, low phosphate	p-Hydroxyphenyl-pyruvate, lactate and acetate	Normal	p-Hydroxyphenyl-pyruvate oxidase

Further reading

Stanbury, J. B., Wyngaarden, J. B. and Fredrickson, D. S. (Eds). *The metabolic basis of inherited disease*. Third Edition. McGraw-Hill Inc, New York. (1972.)

Scriver, C. R. and Rosenberg, L. E. *Amino acid metabolism and its disorders*. W. B. Saunders, Philadelphia. (1973.)

SYSTEMATIC ENZYME NOMENCLATURE

Throughout the text, only trivial names have been used for enzymes to aid clarity and simplicity. The systematic Enzyme Commission numbers for these enzymes are listed here, in alphabetical order of the trivial names in the text, according to: *Enzyme Nomenclature: Recommendations (1972) of IUPAC-IUB*, Elsevier, Amsterdam, 1973.

Three classes of enzymes have not been included in this list: aminotransferases, EC 2.6.1.X; amino acid decarboxylases, EC 4.1.1.X; amino acid racemases, EC 5.1.1.X. Other enzymes not listed below have not yet been ascribed systematic names and EC numbers.

N-Acetyl glutamate synthetase   2.3.1.35
N-Acetyl glutamic-γ-semialdehyde dehydrogenase   1.2.1.38
N-Acetyl-γ-glutamokinase   2.7.2.8
Acetyl ornithinase   3.5.1.16
O-Acetyl serine sulphur transferase   4.2.99.8
Acyl-SCoA dehydrogenase   1.3.99.3
Adenase   3.5.4.2
Adenylosuccinase   4.3.2.2
Adenylosuccinate synthetase   6.3.4.4
Agmatine ureohydrolase   3.5.3.11
Alanine dehydrogenase   1.4.1.1
Aldehyde oxidase   1.2.3.1
Allantoicase   3.5.3.4
Allantoinase   3.5.2.5
ω-Amidase   3.5.1.3
D-Amino acid oxidase   1.4.3.3
L-Amino acid oxidase   1.4.3.2
α-Amino adipic acid dehydrogenase   1.2.1.31
α-Amino adipic semialdehyde–glutamate reductase   1.5.1.10
δ-Amino laevulinate dehydrase   4.2.1.24
δ-Amino laevulinate synthetase   2.3.1.37
Aminomuconic semialdehyde dehydrogenase   1.2.1.32
Angiotensinase   3.4.99.3
Anthranilate phosphoribosyl transferase   2.4.2.18
Anthranilate synthetase   4.1.3.27
Arginase   3.5.3.1
Arginine glycine amidinotransferase   2.1.4.1
Arginine oxidase   1.13.12.1
Argininosuccinase   4.3.2.1
Argininosuccinate synthetase   6.3.4.5
Asparaginase   3.5.1.1
Asparagine synthetase   6.3.1.1

Aspartase   4.3.1.1
Aspartate carbamyl transferase   2.1.3.2
Aspartic-β-semialdehyde dehydrogenase   1.2.1.11
Aspartokinase   2.7.2.4
ATP-phosphoribosyl transferase   2.4.2.17
Betaine aldehyde dehydrogenase   1.2.1.8
Bromelain   3.4.22.5
γ-Butyrobetaine hydroxylase   1.4.11.1
Carbamyl phosphate synthetase—using ammonia   2.7.2.5
Carbamyl phosphate synthetase—using glutamine   2.7.2.9
Carboxypeptidase A   3.4.12.3
Carboxypeptidase B   3.4.12.2
Carboxypeptidase C   3.4.12.1
Catechol-O-methyl transferase   2.1.1.6
Choline dehydrogenase   1.1.99.1
Chorismate mutase   5.4.99.5
Chymotrypsin   3.4.21.1
Collagenase   3.4.24.3
Creatine phosphokinase   2.7.3.2
Crotonase   4.2.1.17
β-Cyano-alanine synthetase   4.4.1.9
β-Cystathionase   4.4.1.8
γ-Cystathionase   4.4.1.1
Cystathionine β-synthetase   4.2.1.22
Cystathionine γ-synthetase   4.2.99.9
Cysteamine oxygenase   1.13.11.19
Cysteine oxidase   1.13.11.20
Dehydroquinate dehydratase   4.2.1.10
Desamido NAD amidotransferase   6.3.5.1 and 6.3.5.5
Diamine oxidase   1.4.3.6
Diaminopimelic acid epimerase   5.1.1.7
Dihydrofolate reductase   1.5.1.3
Dihydroxyacid dehydratase   4.2.1.9
Dopamine-β-hydroxylase   1.14.17.1
Elastase   3.4.21.11
Ficin   3.4.22.3
Formamidase   3.5.1.9
Formiminoglutamate formimino transferase   2.1.2.5
Fumaryl acetoacetate hydrolase   3.7.1.2
Glutamate dehydrogenase   1.4.1.2
Glutamate synthetase   2.6.1.53
Glutaminase   3.5.1.2
Glutaminase II   2.6.1.15
Glutamine fructose-6-P amidotransferase   5.3.1.19
Glutamine synthetase   6.3.1.2
γ-Glutamyl cyclotransferase   2.3.2.4
γ-Glutamyl cysteine synthetase   6.3.2.2
γ-Glutamyl transpeptidase   2.3.2.2
Glutaric semialdehyde dehydrogenase   1.2.1.20
Glutathione reductase   1.6.4.2
Glutathione-S-transferase   2.5.1.12, 2.5.1.13 and 2.5.1.14
Glutathione synthetase   6.3.2.3
Glycerate dehydrogenase   1.1.1.29
Glycerate kinase   2.7.1.31

Glycerate-2-phosphohydrolase   3.1.3.20
Glycerate phosphomutase   2.7.5.3 and 2.7.5.4
Glycinamide ribonucleotide synthetase   6.3.4.13
Glycine amidinotransferase   2.1.4.1
Glycine oxidase 1.4.1.10
Glycyl dipeptidase   3.4.13.1 and 3.4.13.2
Glyoxylate carboxyligase   4.1.1.47
Glyoxylate oxidase   1.2.3.5
Guanase   3.5.4.3
γ-Guanidobutyrate amidinohydrolase   3.5.3.7
Histaminase   1.4.3.6
Histamine methyl transferase   2.1.1.8
Histidase   4.3.1.3
Histidinol dehydrogenase   1.1.1.23
Histidinol-P phosphatase   3.1.3.15
Homo-aconitase   4.2.1.36
Homocitrate synthetase   4.1.3.21
Homocysteine methyl transferase   2.1.1.10
Homogentisic acid oxidase   1.13.11.5
Homoserine dehydratase   4.4.1.1
Homoserine dehydrogenase   1.1.1.3
Homoserine kinase   2.7.1.39
3-Hydroxyanthranilic acid oxygenase   1.10.3.5
γ-Hydroxyglutamate dehydrogenase   1.1.99.2
β-Hydroxy-isobutyric acid dehydrogenase   1.1.1.31
β-Hydroxy-isobutyryl-SCoA hydrolase   3.1.2.4
Hydroxymethyl glutaryl-SCoA lyase   4.2.1.18
γ-Hydroxy-α-oxo-glutarate aldolase   4.1.3.16
p-Hydroxyphenylpyruvate hydroxylase   1.13.11.27
Hydroxyproline oxidase   1.1.1.104
Hypotaurine oxidase   1.8.1.3
Imidazole glycerol-P dehydratase   4.2.1.19
Imidazolone propionate hydrolase   3.5.2.7
Indole glycerol phosphate synthetase   4.1.1.48
Iodinase   1.11.1.8
Isopropylmalate synthetase   4.1.3.12
Kynureninase   3.7.1.3
Kynurenine hydroxylase   1.14.13.9
D-Lactate dehydrogenase   1.1.1.28
L-Lactate dehydrogenase   1.1.1.27
Lactate racemase   5.1.2.1
Lysine acetyl transferase   2.3.1.32
Lysine-2-3-amino-mutase   5.4.3.2
D-α-Lysine mutase   5.4.3.4
L-β-Lysine mutase   5.4.3.3
Lysine-oxoglutarate oxidoreductase   1.5.1.7
Lysine oxygenase   1.13.12.12
Lysyl hydroxylase   1.14.11.4
Maleyl-acetoacetate isomerase   5.2.1.2
Meso-diaminopimelic acid decarboxylase   4.1.1.20
Methionine-S-adenosyl transferase   2.5.1.6
β-Methylcrotonyl-SCoA carboxylase   6.4.1.4
Methylmalonic semialdehyde dehydrogenase   1.2.1.27
Methylmalonyl-SCoA mutase   5.4.99.2

Monoamine oxidase   1.4.3.4
Nitrate reductase   1.7.99.4
Nitrilase   3.5.5.1
Nitrite reductase   1.7.99.3
Nitrogenase   1.7.99.2
5′-Nucleotidase   3.1.3.5
Nucleotide pyrophosphatase   3.6.1.9
Ornithine carbamyl transferase   2.1.3.3
Ornithine mutase   5.4.3.1
α-Oxo-acid decarboxylase   4.1.1.1
Papain   3.4.22.2
Pepsin   3.4.23.1
Phenylalanine hydroxylase   1.14.16.1
Phenylethanolamine-N-methyl transferase   2.1.1.28
Phenylserine aldolase   4.1.2.26
Phosphoglycerate dehydrogenase   1.1.1.95
Phosphoribosyl-AMP cyclohydrolase   3.5.4.19
Phosphoribosyl-formimino AIC-RP isomerase   5.3.1.16
Phosphoribosyl pyrophosphate amidotransferase   2.4.2.14
Phosphoserine phosphatase   3.1.3.3
Porphobilinogen deaminase   4.3.1.8
Prephenate dehydratase   4.2.1.51
Prephenate dehydrogenase   1.3.1.12
D-Proline reductase   1.4.1.6
Prolyl hydroxylase   1.14.11.2
Putrescine propylamine transferase   2.5.1.16
Pyridoxal oxidase   1.1.1.107
Pyridoxal phosphokinase   2.7.1.35
Pyridoxine oxidase   1.1.1.65
Δ^1-Pyrroline-2-carboxylate reductase   1.5.1.1
Δ^1-Pyrroline-5-carboxylate reductase   1.5.1.2
Pyruvate oxidase   1.2.3.3
Saccharopine dehydrogenase—glutamate forming   1.5.1.9
Saccharopine dehydrogenase—lysine forming   1.5.1.7
Serine-O-acetyl transferase   2.3.1.30
Serine deaminase   4.2.1.13 and 4.2.1.16
Serine hydroxymethyl transferase   2.1.2.1
Shikimate dehydrogenase   1.1.1.25
Shikimate kinase   2.7.1.71
Subtilisin   3.4.21.14
Succinic semialdehyde dehydrogenase   1.2.1.16 and 1.2.1.24
N-Succinyl-diaminopimelic acid deacylase   3.5.1.18
Thioredoxin dehydrogenase   1.6.4.5
Threonine aldolase   2.1.2.1
Threonine deaminase   4.2.1.16
Threonine dehydrogenase   1.1.1.103
Threonine synthetase   4.2.99.2
Thrombin   3.4.21.5
Trypsin   3.4.21.4
Tryptophanase   4.1.99.1
Tryptophan hydroxylase   1.14.16.4
Tryptophan pyrrolase   1.13.11.11
Tryptophan synthetase   4.2.1.20
Tyrosinase   1.14.18.1

BIBLIOGRAPHY

Afting, E-G., Katsunuma, T. and Holzer, H. (1972). Comparative studies on the inactivating enzymes for pyridoxal enzymes from yeast and the rat. *Biochem. Biophys. Res. Commun.*, **47**, 103–110.

Alivisatos, S. G. A. (1965). Enzymatic interactions of histamine with pyridine coenzymes. *Fed. Proc.*, **24**, 769–773.

Ames, B. N. and Dubin, D. T. (1960). The role of polyamines in the function of bacteriophage DNA. *J. Biol. Chem.*, **235**, 769–775.

Baldwin, E. (1966). *An introduction to comparative biochemistry*. 4th Edition. Cambridge Univ. Press.

Barnes, M. J. and Kodicek, E. (1972). Biological hydroxylations and ascorbic acid, with special reference to collagen metabolism. *Vit. and Horm.*, **30**, 1–43.

Bayoumi, R. A., Kirwan, J. R. and Smith, W. R. D. (1972). Some effects of dietary vitamin B_6 deficiency and 4-deoxy-pyridoxine on GABA metabolism in rat brain. *J. Neurochem.*, **19**, 569–576.

Bender, D. A. and Bamji, A. N. (1974). Serum tryptophan binding in chlorpromazine-treated chronic schizophrenics. *J. Neurochem.*, **22**, 805–809.

Bentley, J. P. and Hanson, A. N. (1969). The hydroxyproline of elastin. *Biochim. Biophys. Acta*, **175**, 339–344.

Bergerson, F. J., Turner, G. L. and Appleby, C. A. (1973). Studies on the physiological role of leghaemoglobin in soybean root nodules. *Biochim. Biophys. Acta*, **292**, 271–282.

Berl, S., Takagaki, G., Clarke, D. D. and Waelsch, H. (1962). Metabolic compartments *in vivo*: ammonia and glutamic acid metabolism in brain and liver. *J. Biol. Chem.*, **237**, 2562–2569.

Buchanan, B. B. and Arnon, D. I. (1970). Ferredoxins: chemistry and function in photosynthetic, nitrogen-fixing and fermentative metabolism. *Adv. Enzymol.*, **33**, 119–176.

Cardinale, G. C., Rhoads. R. E. and Udenfriend, S. (1971). Simultaneous incorporation of $^{18}O_2$ into succinate and hydroxyproline by collagen proline hydroxylase. *Biochem. Biophys. Res. Commun.*, **43**, 537–543.

Carnahan, J. E., Mortenson, L. E., Mower, H. F. and Castle, J. E. (1960). Nitrogen fixation in cell-free extracts of *C. pasteurianum. Biochim. Biophys. Acta*, **44**, 520–535.

Chalupa, W. (1972). Metabolic aspects of non-protein nitrogen utilisation in ruminant animals. *Fed. Proc.*, **31**, 1152–1164.

Colombini, C. E. and McCoy, E. E. (1970). Vitamin B_6 metabolism: the utilisation of ^{14}C-pyridoxine by the normal mouse. *Biochem.*, **9**, 533–538.

Colombo, J. P., Richterich, R., Donath, A., Spake, A. and Rossi, E. (1964). Congenital lysine intolerance with periodic ammonia intoxication. *Lancet*, **i**, 1014–1015.

Cook, G. C. (1973). Independent jejunal mechanisms for glycine and glycyl-glycine transfer in man *in vivo. Brit. J. Nutr.*, **30**, 13–19.

Cooper, A. J. L. and Meister, A. (1972). Isolation and properties of highly purified glutamine transaminase. *Biochem.*, **11**, 661–671.

Coppen, A., Eccleston, E. G. and Peet, M. (1973). Total and free tryptophan concentrations in the plasma of depressive patients. *Lancet*, **ii**, 60–63.

Dancis, J., Hutzler, J., Cox, R. P. and Woody, N. C. (1969). Familial hyperlysinaemia with lysine–oxo-glutarate reductase insufficiency. *J. Clin. Invest.*, **48**, 1447–1452.

Dixon, R. A. and Postgate, J. R. (1972). Genetic transfer of nitrogen fixation from *K. pneumoniae* to *E. coli. Nature*, **237**, 102–103.

Efron, M. L. (1965). Familial hyperprolinaemia. *New Engl. J. Med.*, **272**, 1243–1254.

Efron, M. L., Bixby, E. M. and Pryles, C. V. (1965). Hydroxyprolinaemia. *New Engl. J. Med.*, **272**, 1299–1309.

Efron, M. L., Bixby, E. M., Hockaday, T. D. R., Smith, L. H. and Meshorer, E. (1968). Hydroxyprolinaemia: (ii) the origin of free hydroxyproline, collagen turnover, the evidence for a biosynthetic pathway in man. *Biochim. Biophys. Acta*, 165, 238–250.

Fellows, F. C. I. (1973). Biosynthesis and degradation of saccharopine, an intermediate of lysine metabolism. *Biochem. J.*, 136, 321–327.

Friedhoff, A. J. and van Winkel, E. (1962). Isolation and characterisation of a compound from the urine of schizophrenics. *Nature*, 194, 897–898.

Frimpter, G. W., Andelman, R. J. and George, W. F. (1969). Vitamin B_6 dependency syndromes. *Amer. J. Clin. Nutr.*, 22, 794–805.

Goldberg, B., Epstein, E. H. and Shor, C. J. (1972). Precursors of collagen secreted by cultured human fibroblasts. *Proc. Nat. Acad. Sci. U.S.A.*, 69, 3655–3659.

Grove, J. A., Gilbertson, T. J., Hammerstedt, R. H. and Henderson, L. M. (1969). The metabolism of D- and L-lysine specifically labelled with ^{15}N. *Biochim. Biophys. Acta*, 184, 329–337.

Henderson, G. B. and Snell, E. E. (1971). Vitamin B_6 responsive histidine deficiency in mutants of *S. typhimurium*. *Proc. Nat. Acad. Sci. U.S.A.*, 68, 2903–2907.

Hendrickson, H. R. and Conn, E. E. (1969). Cyanide metabolism of higher plants: (iv) purification and properties of β-cyano-alanine synthetase of the blue lupin. *J. Biol. Chem.*, 244, 2632–2640.

Hill, B. E., Rowell, F. J., Gupta, R. N. and Spenser, I. D. (1972). Biosynthesis of vitamin B_6. *J. Biol. Chem.*, 247, 1869–1882.

Houslay, M. D. and Tipton, K. F. (1973). The nature of the electrophoretically-separable forms of rat liver monoamine oxidase. *Biochem. J.*, 135, 173–186.

Ivanov, V. I. and Karpeisky, M. Y. (1969). Dynamic three-dimensional model for enzymic transamination. *Adv. Enzymol.*, 32, 21–53.

Johansson, S., Lindstedt, S. and Tiselius, H-G. (1968). Metabolism of $^3H_8$-pyridoxine in mice. *Biochem.*, 7, 2327–2332.

Jouvet, M. (1969). Biogenic amines and the states of sleep. *Science*, 163, 32–41.

Kapeller-Adler, R. (1965). Histamine catabolism *in vitro* and *in vivo*. *Fed. Proc.*, 24, 757–765.

Katunuma, N., Tomino, I. and Nishino, H. (1966). Glutamine isoenzymes in rat kidney. *Biochem. Biophys. Res. Commun.*, 22, 321–328.

Katunuma, N., Matsuda, Y. and Kuroda, Y. (1970). Phylogenic aspects of different regulatory mechanisms of glutamine metabolism. *Adv. Enz. Reg.*, 8, 73–81.

Katunuma, N., Kominami, E. and Kominami, S. (1971a). A new enzyme that specifically inactivates the apo-protein of pyridoxal enzymes. *Biochem. Biophys. Res. Commun.*, 45, 70–75.

Katunuma, N., Kito, K. and Kominami, E. (1971b). A new enzyme that specifically inactivates the apo-protein of NAD-dependent dehydrogenases. *Biochem. Biophys. Res. Commun.*, 45, 76–81.

Krebs, E. G. and Fischer, E. H. (1964). Phosphorylase and related enzymes of glycogen metabolism. *Vit. and Horm.*, 22, 399–410.

Krebs, H. A. (1973). The discovery of the ornithine cycle of urea synthesis. *Biochem. Educ.*, 1, 19–23.

Lefauconnier, J-M., Portemer, C., de Billy, G., Ipatchi, M. and Chatagner, F. (1973). Redistribution of pyridoxal-*P* in the male rat as a result of repeated injections of hydrocortisone. *Biochim. Biophys. Acta*, 297, 135–141.

Magendie, F. (1829). *An elementary compendium of physiology for the use of students*. 3rd edition (transl. E. Milligan). Carfree, Edinburgh; Longmans, Green, London. Quoted in Munro, H. N. and Allison, J. B. (1964). *Mammalian Protein metabolism*. Vol. I, Academic Press, New York and London.

Martinez-Carrion, M., Turano, C., Riva, F. and Fasella, P. (1967). Evidence of a critical histidine residue in soluble aspartate aminotransferase. *J. Biol. Chem.*, 242, 1426–1430.

220

Maurer, R. and Crawford, I. P. (1971). Tryptophan synthetase β_2 subunit: the primary structure of the pyridoxyl peptide from the *Pseudomonas putida* enzyme. *J. Biol. Chem.*, **246**, 6625–6630.

Meister, A. (1968). The synthesis and utilisation of glutamine. *Harvey Lect.*, **68**, 139–178.

Meister, A. (1973). On the enzymology of amino acid transport. *Science*, **180**, 33–39.

Miller, R. L. (1971). Chromatographic separation of the enzymes required for hydroxylation of lysine and proline residues of protocollagen. *Archs. Biochem. Biophys.*, **147**, 339–342.

Morris, D. R. and Pardee, A. B. (1965). A biosynthetic ornithine decarboxylase in *E. coli. Biochem. Biophys. Res. Commun.*, **20**, 697–702.

Morris, D. R. and Pardee, A. B. (1966). Multiple pathways of putrescine biosynthesis in *E. coli. J. Biol. Chem.*, **241**, 3129–3135.

Mudd, S. H. (1971). Pyridoxine-responsive genetic disease. *Fed. Proc.*, **30**, 970–976.

Mycek, M. J., Clarke, D. D., Neidle, A. and Waelsch, H. (1959). Amine incorporation into insulin as catalysed by transglutaminase. *Archs. Biochem. Biophys.*, **84**, 528–540.

McCoy, E. E., Henn, S. W. and Colombini, C. E. (1972). The effect of neuropharmacological agents on the metabolism of vitamin B_6 in the brain. In Ebadi, M. and Costa, E. (Eds) *Advances in biochemical psychopharmacology.* Vol. 4. *The role of vitamin B_6 in neurobiology.* Raven Press, New York and North Holland, Amsterdam.

McDermot, C. E., Casciano, D. A. and Gaertner, F. H. (1973). Isolation and characterisation of a hydroxykynureninase from homogenates of adult mouse liver. *Biochem. Biophys. Res. Commun.*, **51**, 813–818.

Nicholls, A., Snaith, M. L. and Scott, J. T. (1973). The effect of oestrogen therapy on plasma and urinary levels of uric acid. *Brit. Med. J.*, (i), 449–451.

Pabst, M. J., Kuhn, J. C. and Somerville, R. L. (1973). Feed-back regulation in the anthranilate aggregate from wild-type and mutant strains of *E. coli. J. Biol. Chem.*, **248**, 901–914.

Patterson, M. K. and Orr, G. R. (1968). Asparagine biosynthesis by Novikoff hepatoma. *J. Biol. Chem.*, **243**, 376–380.

Pearce, L. A. and Schanberg, S. M. (1969). Histamine and spermine content in brain during development. *Science*, **166**, 1301–1303.

Perry, J. and Chanarin, I. (1973). Formylation of formate as a step in physiological folate absorption. *Brit. Med. J.*, (ii), 588–589.

Pestaña, A., Sandoval, I. V. and Sols, A. (1971). Inhibition by homocysteine of serine dehydratase and other pyridoxal-5-*P* enzymes of the rat through cofactor blockage. *Archs. Biochem. Biophys.*, **146**, 373–379.

Pinell, S. R., Krane, S. M., Kenzora, J. E. and Glimcher, M. J. (1972). A heritable disorder of connective tissue: hydroxylysine deficient collagen disease. *New Eng. J. Med.*, **286**, 1013–1020.

Pisano, J. J., Finlayson, J. S. and Peyton, M. P. (1969). Chemical and enzymic detection of protein cross-links. *Biochem.*, **8**, 871–876.

Pollin, W., Cardon, P. V. and Kety, S. S. (1961). Effects of amino acid feedings on schizophrenic patients treated with iproniazid. *Science*, **133**, 104–105.

Recsei, P. A. and Snell, E. E. (1970). Histidine decarboxylase of *Lactobacillus* 30a: (vi) mechanism of action and kinetic properties. *Biochem.*, **9**, 1493–1497.

Regoeczi, E., Irons, L., Koj, A. and McFarlane, A. S. (1965). Isotopic studies of urea metabolism in rabbits. *Biochem. J.*, **95**, 521–532.

Rhoads, R. E. and Udenfriend, S. (1968). Purification and properties of collagen proline hydroxylase from new-born rat skin. *Archs. Biochem. Biophys.*, **139**, 329–339.

van't Riet, J., Knook, D. L. and Planter, R. J. (1972). The role of cytochrome b_1 in nitrate assimilation and nitrate respiration in *K. aerogenes. FEBS Lett.*, **23**, 44–46.

Riley, W. D. and Snell, E. E. (1970). Histidine decarboxylase of *Lactobacillus* 30a: (v) origin of the enzyme-bound pyruvate and separation of non-identical sub-units. *Biochem.*, **9**, 1485–1491.

Schoenheimer, R. (1942). *The dynamic state of body constituents*. Harvard Univ. Press, Cambridge, Mass.

Shapiro, B. M. and Stadtman, E. R. (1970). The regulation of glutamine synthesis in micro-organisms. *Ann. Rev. Microbiol.*, **24**, 501–524.

Shimizu, H., Kakimoto, Y. and Sano, I. (1964). The determination and distribution of polyamines in the mammalian central nervous system. *J. Pharm. Exp. Ther.*, **143**, 199–204.

Simell, O., Visakorpi, J. K. and Donner, M. (1972). Saccharopinuria. *Archs. Dis. Child.*, **47**, 52–55.

Singh, V. K. and Sung, S. C. (1972). The effect of spermidine on DNA-dependent RNA polymerase from brain cell nuclei. *J. Neurochem.*, **19**, 2885–2888.

Snell, E. E. (1972). Relation of chemical structure to metabolic activity of vitamin B_6. In Ebadi, M. S. and Costa, E. (Eds) *Advances in biochemical psychopharmacology*. Vol. 4. *The role of vitamin B_6 in neurobiology*. Raven Press, New York and North Holland, Amsterdam.

Stadtman, E. R., Shapiro, B. M., Kingdon, H. S., Woolfolk, C. A. and Hubbard, J. S. (1968). Cellular regulation of glutamine synthetase activity in *E. coli*. *Adv. Enz. Reg.*, **6**, 257–289.

Stadtman, T. C. (1963). Anaerobic degradation of lysine (ii) cofactor requirements and properties of soluble enzyme system. *J. biol. Chem.*, **238**, 2766–2773.

Starcher, B. C., Partridge, S. M. and Elsden, D. F. (1967). Isolation and partial purification of a new amino acid from reduced elastin. *Biochem.*, **6**, 2425–2432.

Tabor, C. W. and Tabor, H. (1966). Transport system for 1,4-diaminobutane, spermidine and spermine in *E. coli*. *J. Biol. Chem.*, **241**, 3714–3723.

Tucci, A. F. and Ceci, L. N. (1972). Control of lysine biosynthesis in yeast. *Archs. Biochem. Biophys.*, **153**, 751–754.

Vender, J., Jayarman, K. and Richenberg, H. V. (1965). Metabolism of glutamate in a mutant of *E. coli*. *J. Bacteriol.*, **90**, 1304–1308.

Visek, W. J. (1972). Effects of urea hydrolysis on cell life-span and metabolism. *Fed. Proc.*, **31**, 1178–1193.

Wada, J. A., Wrinck, J., Hill, D., McGeer, P. L. and McGeer, E. G. (1963). Central aromatic amine levels and behaviour. *Archs. Neurol.*, **9**, 69–80.

Walser, M., Lund, P., Ruderman, N. B. and Coulter, C. W. (1973). Synthesis of essential amino acids from their α-oxo analogues by perfused rat liver and muscle. *J. Clin. Invest.*, **52**, 2865–2877.

Winter, H. C. and Arnon, D. I. (1970). The nitrogen fixing system of photosynthetic bacteria: (i) preparation of a cell-free system from *Chromatium*. *Biochim. Biophys. Acta*, **197**, 170–179.

Yamaguchi, K., Sakakibara, S., Asamizu. J. and Ueda, I. (1973). Induction and activation of cysteine oxidase of rat liver. *Biochim. Biophys. Acta*, **297**, 48–59.

Yoshida, T. and Kikuchi, G. (1969). Physiological significance of the glycine cleavage system in human liver as revealed by the study of a case of hyperglycinaemia. *Biochem. Biophys. Res. Commun.*, **35**, 577–583.

Yoshida, T. and Kikuchi, G. (1970). Major pathways of glycine and serine catabolism in rat liver. *Archs. Biochem. Biophys.*, **139**, 380–392.

Youdim, M. B. H., Collins, G. G. S. and Sandler, M. (1969). Multiple forms of rat brain monoamine oxidase. *Nature*, **223**, 626–628.

Zeller, E. A. (1965). Identity of histaminase and diamine oxidase. *Fed. Proc.*, **24**, 766–768.

INDEX